The Radiology
of the
Postoperative Hip

The Radiology of the Postoperative Hip

MATTHEW FREEDMAN, M.D.

Associate Professor of Radiology
Director of Orthopedic Radiology
University of Maryland
School of Medicine
Assistant Professor of Radiology
The Johns Hopkins Medical Institutions

Incorporating many cases from the collection of
JACK W. BOWERMAN, M.D.
Director of Orthopedic Radiology
The Russell H. Morgan Department of Radiology
The Johns Hopkins Medical Institutions

A WILEY MEDICAL PUBLICATION
JOHN WILEY & SONS
New York • Chichester • Brisbane • Toronto

Library of Congress Cataloging in Publication Data:

Freedman, Matthew.
   The radiology of the postoperative hip.

   1. Hip joint—Radiography. 2. Hip joint—Surgery.
I. Title. [DNLM: 1. Hip—Radiography. 2. Hip—
Surgery. WE855 F853r]
RD772.F73   617′.58   79-12411
ISBN 0-471-04416-4

Printed in the United States of America

10 9 8 7 6 5 4 3 2 1

This book is dedicated to my mother,
Florence Bernstein Freedman,
whose many books served as
an inspiration for this one.

Preface

Because disease of the hip is common, because of the importance of the hip to the individual, and because of the marked biomechanical stress placed upon it, many of the best minds and many of the most innovative procedures in orthopedic surgery have been devoted to the treatment of hip disease. By surveying in detail the radiologic changes of orthopedic surgery of the hip, one can gain an appreciation of the fundamental principles of orthopedic radiology; these principles are applicable in other parts of the body as well.

The orthopedist, in dealing with a patient with a hip problem, has many techniques available for his consideration. Although the orthopedist's aim is to restore the hip to normal function, unfortunately restoration of normal function is often unachievable. Thus the orthopedist must choose a procedure that restores those aspects of hip functioning most important to the patient. A sedentary person places different values on the functioning of his or her hip than a laborer or an athlete. A construction worker must know that his hip will not give way. The amateur athlete needs mobility, the patient with muscle weakness (from a stroke or meningomyelocele) needs stability. Thus the procedure must be tailored to the individual.

Because each procedure carries a risk of failure, and because each procedure has its own expected duration of success, it is important not to think of each technique as final.

The orthopedist, in choosing a procedure, must always have in mind an alternative strategy should the procedure fail. The radiologist must always consider each picture as a way station in the progress of the patient's hip disability and always be alert for the early detection of a complication; a constant awareness of the often transient nature of the orthopedist's success is imperative.

The introduction gives an overview of the basic techniques and appliances available for the treatment of hip disease and of the common types of radiographic changes seen following surgery. The subsequent chapters are concerned with the methods available for the treatment of specific diseases in child and adult. Each of the later chapters contains a discussion of the principles behind the treatment of a disease; the available procedures and their normal radiographic appearance are also discussed. This is followed by a discussion of complications and how they may be detected.

In many chapters, examples are given so that the reader can test himself, so to speak, on the material just covered by reviewing the radiographs and then reading the related text. The final chapter is a discussion of the applications of computed tomography and tracer imaging techniques in the evaluation of the hip and the results of surgery.

Matthew Freedman

Acknowledgments

This book is the result of the influence of the many fine orthopedists and radiologists with whom I have had the privilege of working and from whom I have learned so much. I should especially like to thank Dr. H. Todd Stradford, who convinced me that there really was a role for a radiologist interested in orthopedics. Special thanks also belong to Dr. Robert Robinson, chairman of the Department of Orthopedics at the Johns Hopkins Medical Institutions, for his many helpful criticisms of the manuscript. I should also like to thank Drs. Richard Maurer, Lynn Staheli, and Mac Madenwald, past directors of orthopedics at the United States Public Health Service Hospital in Seattle; Dr. Louis A. Goldstein, chairman emeritus of the Department of Orthopedics at the University of Rochester and Dr. Jack Devanny, of his staff; Drs. John Adams and Henry Feffer, chairman and associate chairman at the George Washington University Medical Center; Lee Riley and Steven Kopits at the Johns Hopkins Medical Institutions, as well as the many other staff members and residents of these departments whose patient care efforts contributed so greatly to the contents of this book.

I should also like to thank Dr. Stanley Rogoff, director of Diagnostic Radiology at the University of Rochester, who encouraged my initial pursuit of this topic for presentation at a resident seminar; John Dorst, for his many helpful criticisms of this manuscript; and Drs. Stanley Siegelman and Martin Donner, who provided me with the time and facilities for preparing this manuscript. I should also like to thank the many fine residents and staff members in diagnostic radiology who helped me find cases and who helped review the manuscript.

My consistently excellent handwriting decipherer and typist, Mrs. Kristy McDonald, deserves special thanks, as do the excellent photographers, Henri Hessels and Willie Ragsdale, and our librarian, Michael Houck.

And special thanks to my family, John, Jenny, Miriam, and Gladys, who accepted the disarray of papers and time so that this book might finally be finished.

Contents

INTRODUCTION

1. Basic Techniques   3
2. Principles of the Radiologic Evaluation of Appliances   29
3. A Radiologic Approach to the Complications of Hip Surgery   46

Part 1. THE CHILD'S HIP

4. Congenital Displacement of the Hip   59
5. Surgery in Neurogenic Dysfunction of the Hip   79
6. Legg-Calve-Perthes Disease   89
7. Slipped Capital Femoral Epiphysis   110
   Conclusion   119

Part 2. THE ADULT'S HIP

Section A: Fractures of the Proximal Femur   121

8. Fractures of the Femoral Neck   123
9. Femoral Head Replacements   145

10. Intertrochanteric Fractures   172
11. Fracture Through Metastases: A Brief Note   201

Section B: Arthritis of the Hip   207

12. Intertrochanteric Osteotomies for Degenerative Joint Disease   209
13. The Cup Mold Arthroplasty   218
14. The Total Hip Replacement   227
15. Salvage Procedures—The Girdlestone Arthroplasty   289
16. Hip Fusion   293
17. Tracer Imaging and Computed Tomography in Disease of the Hip   299

POSTSCRIPT   304

Index   305

The Radiology
of the
Postoperative Hip

INTRODUCTION

1
Basic Techniques

Orthopedic procedures of the hip are classified into four types. These are fracture treatment, osteotomies, arthroplasties, and arthrodeses. In the child, hip disease may also make necessary procedures to lengthen or shorten the femur or the tibia or to control the growth of the greater trochanter.

Fracture Treatment

The orthopedist treating a patient with a fracture has several specific goals. In the acute period he or she is concerned with relief of pain, the prevention of additional injury (especially to nerves and vessels), the treatment of any systemic effect of the fracture (blood loss, fat emboli), associated injuries, the reduction of the deformity, and stabilization of the fracture. In dealing with the acute problems, his goal is to prevent or minimize any long-term disability that could result from the fracture. He is concerned with the eventual function of the injured part of the body. Age and metabolic status are important factors in the response of bone to activity, disease, trauma, and surgery. Coexistent diseases may limit the extent of possible correction. A person viewing only the radiograph has a limited knowledge of the patient's associated problems and of the compromise necessary to balance the treatment of the acute problems with the long-term result. Because of this, it is essential that the radiologist's interpretation not be judgmental.

Two major methods of hip-fracture treatment are available: fracture reduction with stabilization and prosthetic replacement of the fractured bone or of the total joint. Restoration of normal anatomy, while theoretically desirable, is often not practical or necessary. The aim of fracture reduction is to achieve maximum function with sufficient stability to permit the bone fragments to unite without displacement or functionally significant angulation. The prime method of achieving stability is by correct alignment of the bone fragments. Once this alignment is achieved, it must be held in position until union has occurred. Several different kinds of external supports may be used, such as traction, splints, or casts; however, greater stability results from internal fixation with pins, nails, or various appliances. These devices are not substitutes for an adequate and stable reduction; they simply help to maintain it. If the reduction is not stable, the pin, nail, or appliance will usually fail and the reduction will be lost. For this reason, the appearance of the appliance used is of less importance than the adequacy of the reduction. If malreduction is recognized, reoperation or the addition of external fracture-support methods (traction, cast, etc.) can help to prevent long-term disability.

Osteotomies

The term osteotomy has two different meanings: one broad and one narrow. In its broad sense, osteotomy is a procedure in which bone is cut. Since most open orthopedic operative procedures on the hip involve cutting bone, most procedures involve osteotomies. In its narrow sense osteotomy is a procedure in which the bone is cut in order to change its alignment. This change in alignment will usually have an effect on the alignment of the joint as well. Less commonly, an osteotomy does not involve realignment of the bone—the bone is cut and allowed to heal in the same position. Specific uses of this type of osteotomy in patients with degenerative arthritis of the hip and in patients undergoing hip-fusion operations will be discussed in the appropriate sections.

Osteotomies are named by the change in the alignment resulting from the osteotomy. Thus there are internal and external rotational osteotomies (Figure 1-1), varus and valgus osteotomies (Figure 1-2a,b and 1-3a,b), medial displacement osteotomies (Figure 1-4), flexion and extension osteotomies, and combinations of all of these. Angulation of the bone can be achieved in two ways: by adding a wedge of bone (the opening wedge osteotomy, Figure 1-5a,b), or by removing a wedge of bone (the closing-wedge osteotomy, Figures 1-2 and 1-3). In young children, angulation can be achieved without adding or removing a wedge of bone, transverse osteotomy with repositioning and fixation is usually sufficient.

It is necessary to maintain the position of the bone fragments following the osteotomy and, as with fractures, this can be done by external support with traction, splints or casts or by internal fixation devices.

Arthroplasty

An arthroplasty is a surgical procedure in which the joint is reshaped, or part or all of the joint is replaced by a prosthesis. Arthroplasties include procedures in which portions of bone or cartilage are removed from the articular surfaces of the joint, procedures in which some material is interposed between the two sides of the joint (the interposition arthroplasty with fascia and the cup mold arthroplasty [Figure 1-6], in which a metallic cup is interposed), prosthetic replacement of the femoral head (Figure 1-7) or acetabulum, and total joint replacements (Figure 1–8). These procedures are discussed in detail in subsequent chapters.

Arthrodesis

An arthrodesis is a fusion across a joint preventing motion. There are two basic types: the intra-articular fusion (Figure 1-9) and the extra-articular fusion (Figure 1-10). Combinations of the two procedures are common. Arthrodeses can be combined with proximal femoral osteotomies to minimize stress at the surgical site. Bone graft and/or metallic appliances can be used to help hold the arthrodesis site immobile until it fuses. Arthrodeses are discussed in Chapter 16.

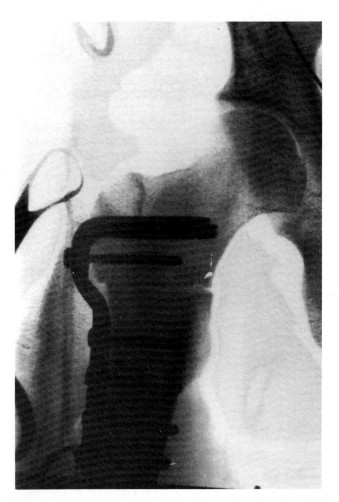

Figure 1-1. An intraoperative view of a rotational osteotomy of the proximal femur performed for treatment of degenerative arthrosis of the hip. Note the lack of alignment of the femoral cortices.

ORTHOPEDIC APPLIANCES

When the orthopedist chooses an appliance to use for a particular patient, he is guided by his past experience. There are many different types of orthopedic appliances

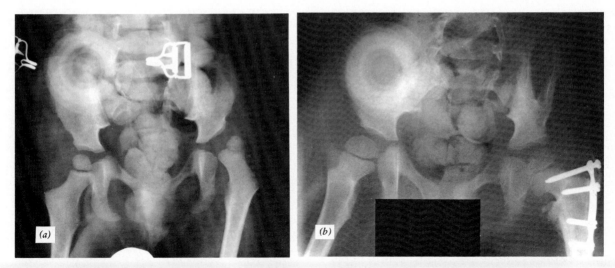

Figure 1-2. Preoperative and postoperative views of varus intertrochanteric osteotomy performed for paralytic subluxation of the hip secondary to a meningomelocoele. (*b*) The hole in the left ilium is secondary to a Sharrard muscle transfer operation.

and several manufacturers of each kind, and thus the selection process can be quite complex. From the viewpoint of the radiologist, however, it is acceptable to deal with these appliances by dividing them into several small groups. Within each group there are many minor differences that will affect the structural strength, ease of insertion, and durability of the appliance. These differences may affect the frequency with which we might see appliance failure, but they do not affect the ways in which the appliances may fail. In this book, the groups will be named generically whenever possible; however, occasionally eponyms will be used to discuss related designs of commonly used varieties. This does not mean that the named appliance is necessarily better than the others in its group. In the same manner, the use of a particular manufacturer's design does not imply that it is better, but only that it is acceptable and examples of its use were available to the author.

The generic types of appliances are:

Pins (Figure 1-11*a,b*)
Pins are long, thin devices designed to be pushed or drilled into place. They can be smooth or serrated (Figure 1-12) but do not have a spiral (screw) thread. They usually lack a broadened end, but there are pins with a broad end for ease of removal (Figure 1-13). Pins usually are thin enough so that excess length can be cut off easily.

Screws (Figures 1-14, 1-15)
Screws are analogous to those used in carpentry or metal work. Each has a spiral screw thread and may have a straight, cross, or hexagonal slit in its top to help in turning the screw, which is usually inserted with a screwdriver.

Bolts (Figure 1-16*a,b*)
Bolts usually pass through the bone to allow the placement of a nut or cap on the far end. They are analogous to carpentry bolts. Because of the nut or cap, bolts usually do not pull out; but, because of the separate nut, they are more difficult to insert. Bolts are usually turned with a wrench.

Lag Bolts or Lag Screws (Figure 1-17)
These devices are different from bolts in that they are tapered and do not have nuts or caps. They thus resemble screws but can be turned by a wrench or a screwdriver. They have an exaggerated, broad screw thread.

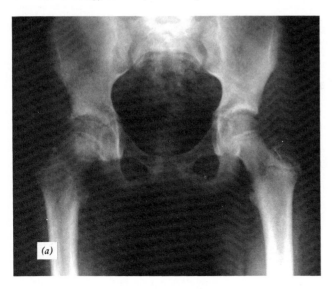

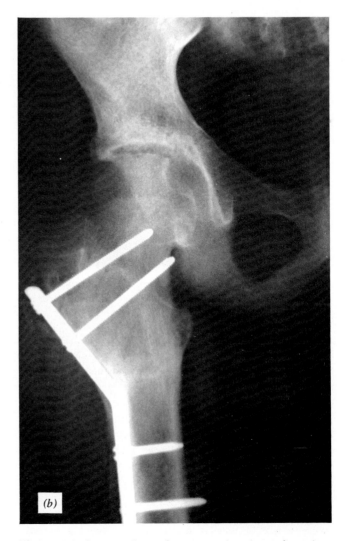

Staples
Staples can be used to bridge the two sides of an osteotomy to help stabilize the alignment.

Nails (Figures 1-18, 1-19*a,b*)
Nails are designed to be driven (hammered) into place. Often the tract is partially drilled first to prevent the bone from cracking. These nails usually are much broader than carpentry nails and often have fins on them to prevent rotation.

Side Plates (Figure 1-18)
Side plates are metallic plates placed on the side of the bone for support. In hip surgery, these plates are often adapted to permit a hip nail to be bolted to them (Figure 1-20). Conversely, certain hip nails are one-piece nail and side-plate assemblies (Figuer 1-21*a,b*).

Blade Plates (Figures 1-22, 1-23)
A blade plate is a combination of a side plate with a wide flat, U or V shaped blade that can be inserted into the bone. The angle of the blade to the plate varies from 90 to 180°. Blade plates are often used to hold osteotomies in proper position during healing. Straight blade plates (180°) are also called splines (Figure 1-23).

Figure 1-3. Preoperative and postoperative views of a valgus subtrochanteric osteotomy performed as treatment for slipped capital femoral epiphysis.

Femoral Head Replacements
These are metallic devices that replace the femoral head; usually a substantial portion of the neck is included. There are two types of replacement heads; the stem prosthesis (Figure 1-24), in which a stem of metal passes from the femoral neck through the lateral femoral cortex (this device is no longer used but is still occasionally seen), and

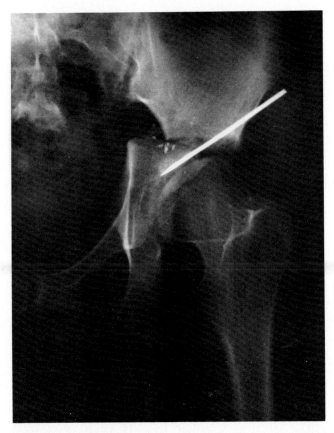

Figure 1-4. Medial displacement osteotomy of the acetabulum (the Chiari operation) for residua of congenital displacement of the hip in a young adult. A pin is used to hold the fragments in the new position.

the intramedullary form (Figure 1-25), in which the replacement head is attached to an anchoring stem placed in the medulla of the bone. This stem or anchor may be fenestrated to permit the ingrowth of bone to anchor it, or it may be smooth to permit easy removal and replacement if necessary.

Cups (Figure 1-26)

These are cup-shaped (without the handle) devices made to fit between the femoral head, or, less often the shaft (Figure 1-27), and the acetabulum. They are used in an interposition arthroplasty and serve to mold the damaged

joint into a new and hopefully better and more congruous joint.

Acetabular Replacments (Figure 1-28)

Such devices (cups, for example), are now rarely used but are available for specific purposes.

Joint Replacements

There are several generic types of joint replacements. The joints can have metal-on-metal articulations (Figure 1-29a,b), metal-on-plastic articulations (Figure 1-30a,b), or plastic-on-plastic articulations. The femoral-head component can sit centrally (Figure 1-30) or eccentrically (Figure 1-31) within the acetabular component. The components can be press fitted (i.e., tightly fitted) into the bone or placed in a plastic, polymethylmethacrylate, a space filler that fills in any gaps between the prosthesis and the bone. The femoral head can be held in the acetabulum by the patient's muscle power (and thus can sublux or dislocate) or it can be fitted through a cap on the acetabular component which is intended to prevent dislocation.

Polymethylmethacrylate

Polymethylmethacrylate is a plastic polymer commonly used in orthopedic surgery, especially in hip surgery. Its name is often shortened to methylmethacrylate or methacrylate. Methylmethacrylate is radiolucent on a radiograph and appears as a lytic area within bone (Figure 1-32). It is common for the manufacturers of orthopedic devices to add sterile barium to methylmethacrylate to make it radiopaque (Figure 1-33b). The degree of radiopacity varies with the amount of barium added. Methylmethacrylate is used to achieve three objectives. The first is as a space filler to replace bone that has been removed from the body, either by a surgeon or by disease (osteoporosis or lytic neoplasms in bone). Large quantities of the plastic are occasionally used in this manner (Figure 1-33a,b). The second objective is to bind the prosthesis tightly to bone. By filling every micro- and macro-outpouching of the surgical cavity in the bone, a very firm interdigitation fit (called an interference fit) may be achieved. The third objective is to spread and diffuse the

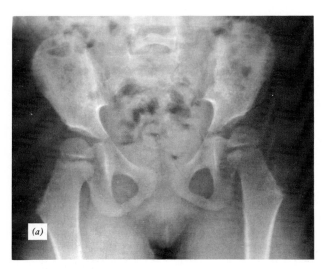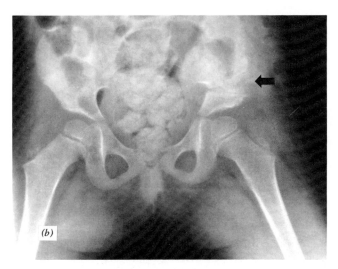

Figure 1-5. Preoperative and postoperative views of an opening wedge osteotomy of the ilium (the Salter innominate bone osteotomy) performed as treatment for congenital subluxation of the hip. (*a*) The preoperative film demonstrates an increased left acetabular angle. (*b*) The postoperative film demonstrates an iliac bone osteotomy with a wedge of bone placed in the osteotomy to hold the fragments apart in their new position.

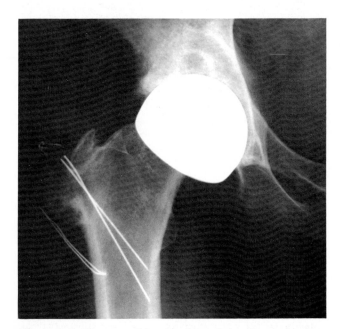

Figure 1-6. The cup mold arthroplasty. A metallic cup has been placed between the femoral head and the acetabulum.

force transmitted from the appliance to the bone. A force applied to a small area of the prosthesis-methacrylate interface is spread outward through the methacrylate to a larger surface of medullary bone. Diffusion of the force permits the bone to absorb the applied stress without fracturing. Diffusion of the force also prevents or limits osetoclastic resorption, which is the normal response of medullary bone to excessive pressure with its probable resultant microfractures. This force diffusion helps prevent loosening of the prosthesis. Because of this last property of methacrylate, it is important that the plastic be placed in sites of expected stress. With the femoral component, the stress of weight bearing tends to shift the prosthesis in the bone into varus deformity and to telescope it further into the medullary cavity (Figure 1-34). Thus it is said to be important that methacrylate be placed medial to the proximal portion of the prosthesis, adjacent to the calcar of the femur, lateral to the distal portion of the prosthesis, and distal to the tip of the prosthesis. When methylmethacrylate is not used (and is thus not available to diffuse the force), the prosthesis must be designed to

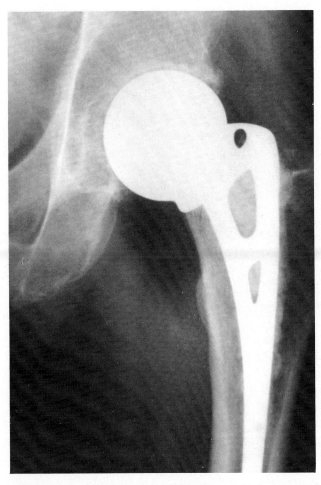

Figure 1-7. A femoral head replacement arthroplasty: the Austin-Moore prosthesis. This prosthesis has been placed in polymethylmethacrylate.

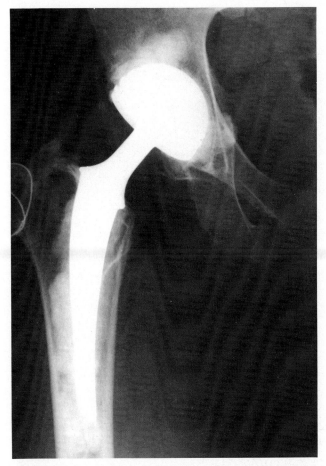

Figure 1-8. A total hip replacement: The Harris prosthesis. Both acetabulum and femoral head and neck have been replaced by this prosthesis. The prosthesis is held in place by polymethylmethacrylate.

transfer a substantial portion of the weight to the cortex of the bone, expecially to the medial cortex of the femoral neck, the calcar femoris, which is the strongest portion of the bone of the femoral neck (Figure 1-35).

PRINCIPLES OF THE USE OF APPLIANCES

In the treatment of fractures, appliances help to hold the reduction but cannot stabilize a poor reduction. When used to try to support an unstable reduction, an appliance will frequently bend or break. If it is strong enough to resist the stress placed on it, then the appliance will cut through the bone, and, even though the appliance has not changed its position, the bone fragments will.

The tendency for the femoral head or prosthesis to sublux or dislocate is often dependent on the presence of ante- or retroversion, both of which are poorly evaluated on the frontal radiograph of the hip. The lateral radiograph should be of adequate quality and carefully in-

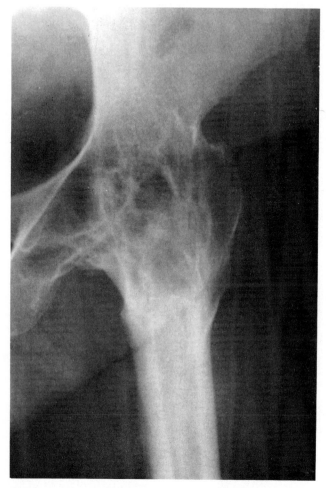

Figure 1-9. An intra-articular fusion. The joint space has been crossed by trabecular bone.

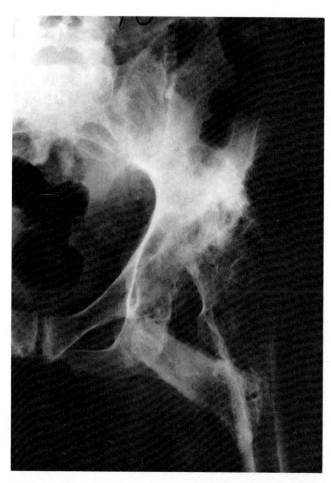

Figure 1-10. A combined intra- and extra-articular fusion. A supporting buttress of bone has been placed from the ischium to the femoral shaft. In addition, the joint space has been obliterated by trabecular bone crossing from the femoral neck to a pseudo (or displaced) acetabulum.

terpreted. The cross-table lateral is the best for this assessment.

In the treatment of fractures of the proximal femur, the major early stress on the reduction is external rotation resulting from the patient's position in bed. The lateral view best demonstrates the extent of bony support of the posterior portion of the femur and is the best predictor of stability or loss of reduction.

There is no single position of an appliance or a prosthesis. The position will vary with the needs of the patient for mobility or stability. This will be discussed in appropriate areas later.

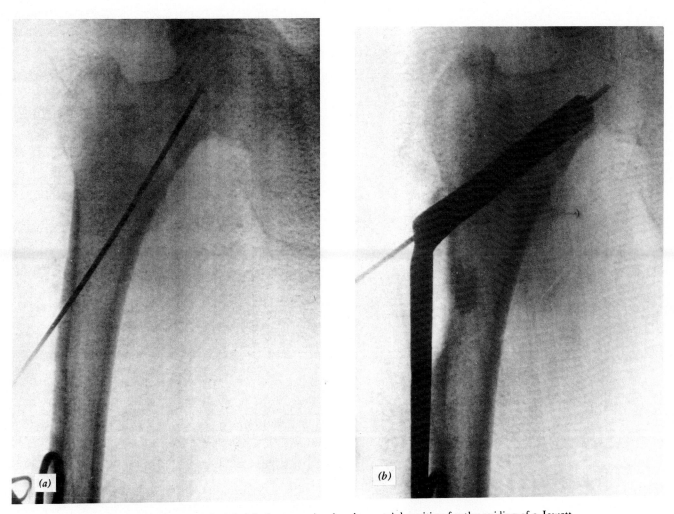

Figure 1-11. A nonthreaded Steinmann pin placed as a trial position for the guiding of a Jewett hip nail. (*a*) The pin shown in an unwanted position. (*b*) The pin has been replaced and the Jewett nail has been guided over the new pin to achieve proper position for the nail.

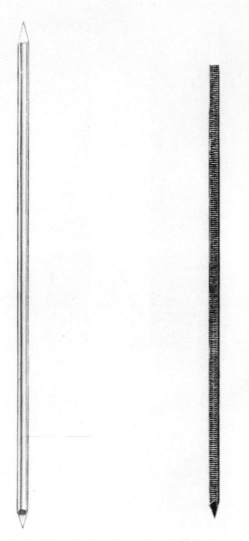

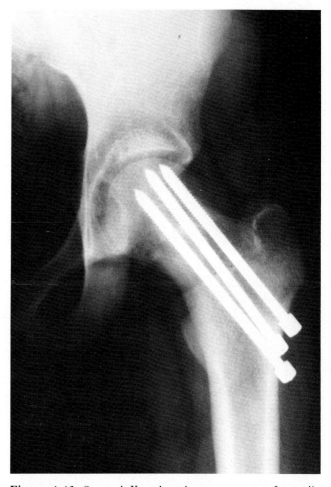

Figure 1-13. Serrated Knowles pins as treatment for undisplaced femoral neck fracture. The serrations are not a spiral thread for ease of insertion, but serve to increase the holding power in the cancellous bone. The enlarged end is to aid in removal should this prove necessary.

Figure 1-12. Threaded and nonthreaded Steinmann pins. (Courtesy DePuy).

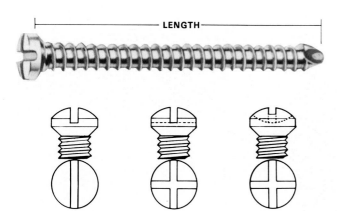

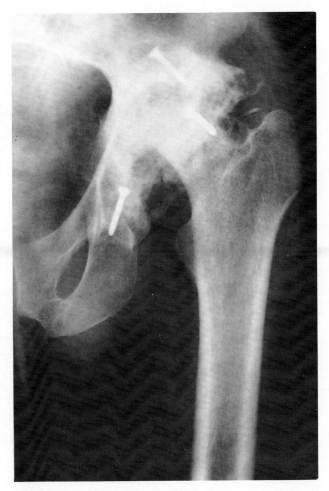

Figure 1-14. Drawing of screws with different types of head. (Courtesy DePuy.)

Figure 1-15. Screws used to help stabilize fragments of a comminuted acetabular fracture.

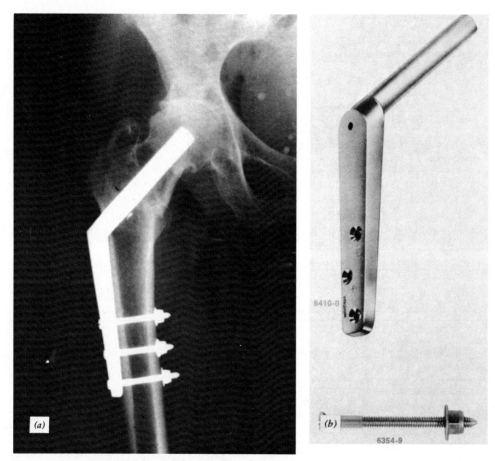

Figure 1-16. (*a*)Three bolts with nuts holding the side-plate portion of a Holt nail in treatment of an intertrochanteric fracture of the femur. (*b*) Drawing of Holt nail and a Barr bolt. (Courtesy Howmedica®.)

14

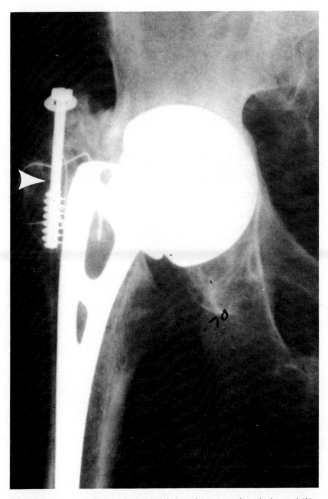

Figure 1-17. A lag bolt (arrow) has been used to help stabilize the greater trochanter. The patient also has a femoral head replacement prosthesis (Austin-Moore) placed into the cup of a cup mold arthroplasty. (The combination is an early form of the total hip replacement.)

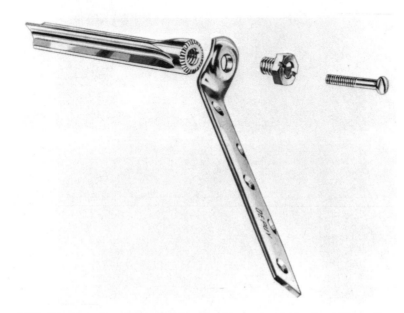

Figure 1-18. Drawing of a tri-flanged hip nail with separate side plate. The nail can be used with or without the side plate. (Courtesy DePuy).

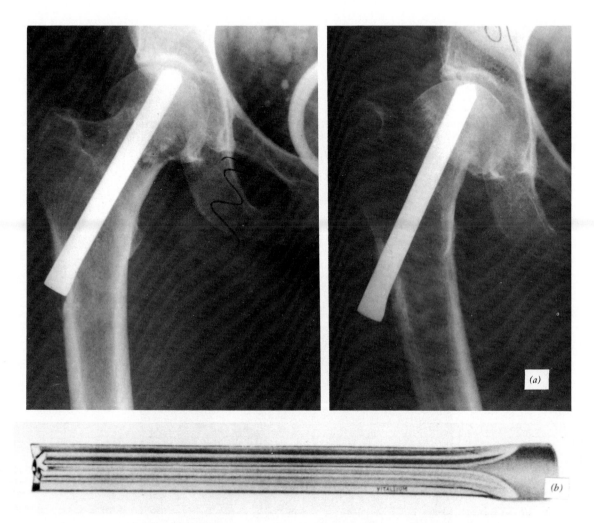

Figure 1-19. (*a*) Flanged hip nail of Smith-Petersen type, used in treatment of a femoral neck fracture. (*b*) Drawing, Smith-Petersen nail. (Courtesy Howmedica®.)

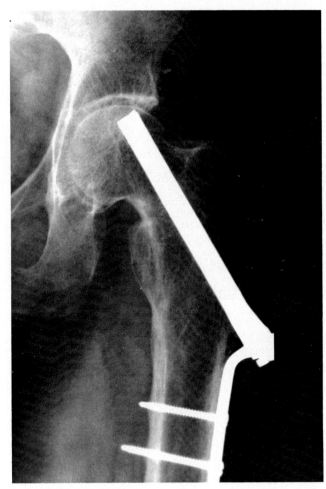

Figure 1-20. Triflanged hip nail bolted to a separate side plate in treatment of a femoral neck fracture.

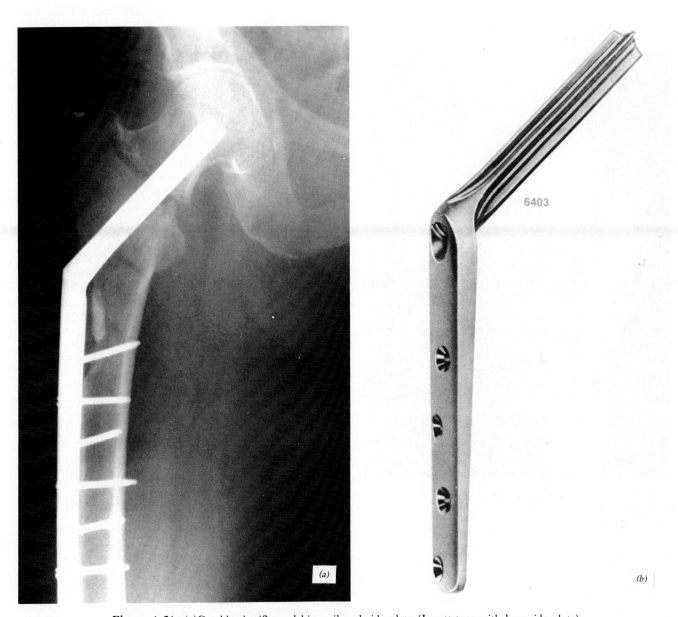

Figure 1-21. (*a*)Combined triflanged hip nail and side plate (Jewett type with long side plate) for stabilization of intertrochanteric fracture with iatrogenic subtrochanteric cortical disruption. (*b*) Drawing, Jewett appliance (Courtesy Howmedica®.)

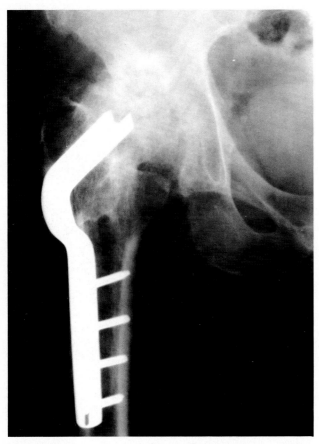

Figure 1-22. A blade plate combination that stabilizes a medial displacement osteotomy used as treatment of degenerative arthrosis of the hip.

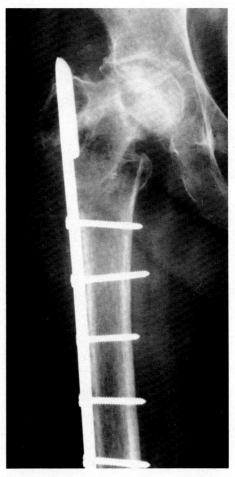

Figure 1-23. A 180°-angled blade plate or spline. This was used to permit vertical impaction without medial or lateral displacement of an intertrochanteric medial displacement osteotomy. This osteotomy was performed as treatment of avascular necrosis and degenerative arthrosis of the hip.

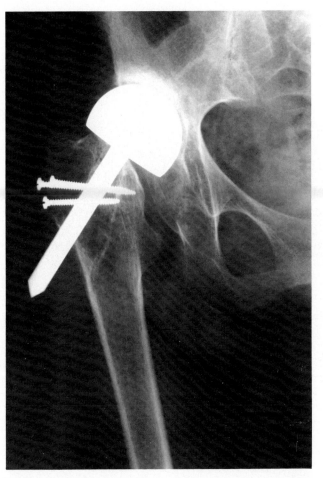

Figure 1-24. A stem femoral head prosthesis (a variant of the Judet prosthesis).

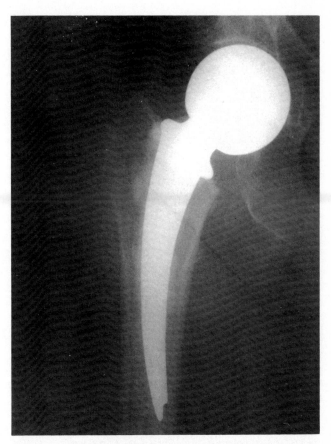

Figure 1-25. An intramedullary femoral head prosthesis. Muller type, stabilized with radiopaque methylmethacrylate.

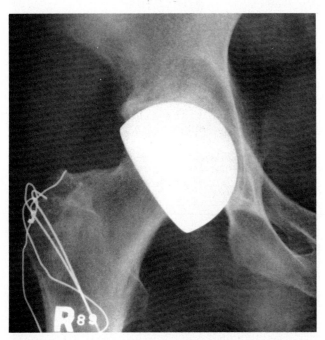

Figure 1-26. A cup mold arthroplasty, with the metal cup placed on the reshaped femoral head. (The broken wires in the greater trochanter are of no consequence, since the greater trochanter osteotomy had healed before wire breakage.)

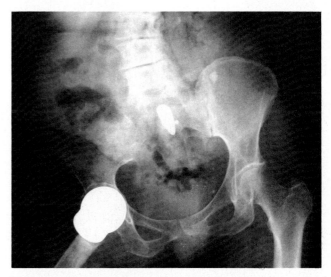

Figure 1-27. A cup mold arthroplasty in which the cup has been placed on the femoral shaft.

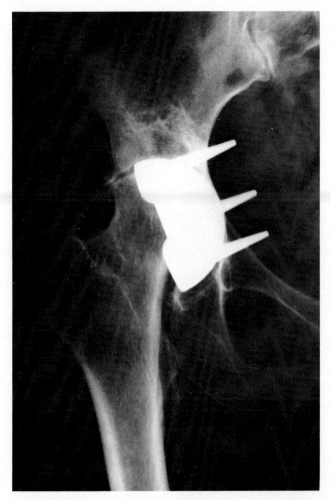

Figure 1-28. A Urist cup used as an acetabular replacement.

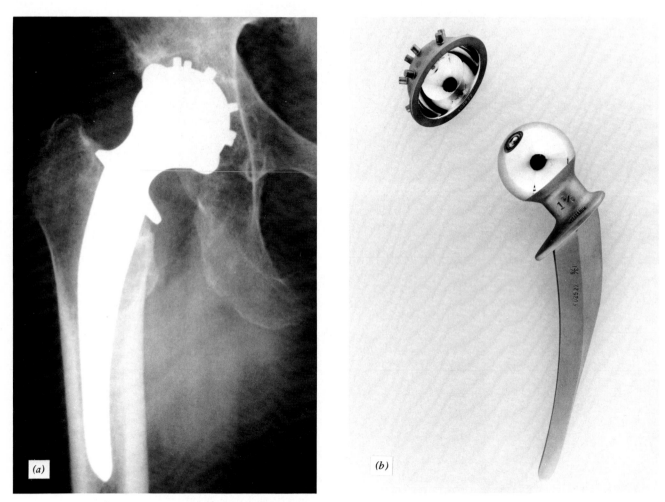

Figure 1-29. (*a*) A metal-on-metal total hip replacement. (Mckee-Farrar prosthesis.) (*b*) The McKee-Farrar prosthesis.

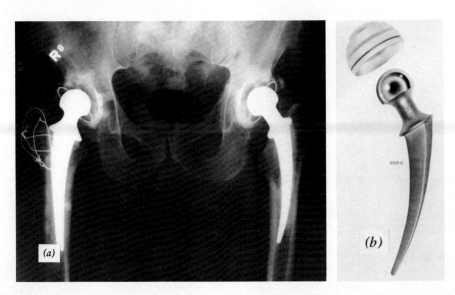

Figure 1-30. (*a*)Two variants of a metal-on-plastic total hip replacement (both variants of the Charnley-Muller prosthesis). (*b*) Drawing of the Charnley-Muller prosthesis. (Courtesy Howmedica®.)

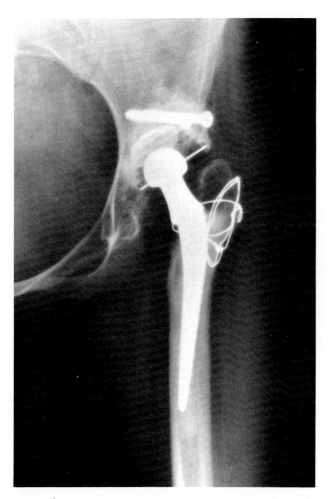

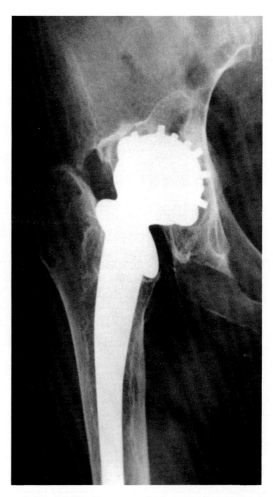

Figure 1-31. Total hip replacement with an eccentric seating of the femoral head in the plastic acetabulum component (Turner-Aufranc prosthesis).

Figure 1-32. McKee-Farrar total hip replacement prostheses in radiolucent methylmethacrylate. The lucent methacrylate can be identified by the thin rim of sclerotic bone surrounding it, in both the acetabulum and the femur.

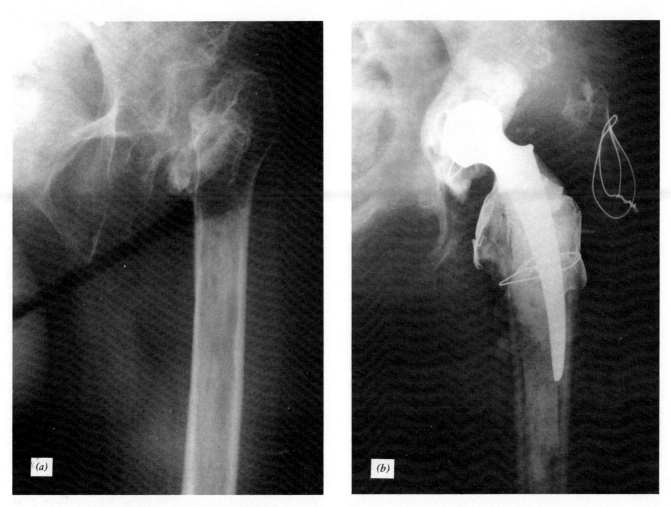

Figure 1-33. Radiopaque methylmethacrylate used in large quantity to stabilize a Charnley-Muller prosthesis in markedly osteoporotic femoral bone. (*a*) Preoperative view. (*b*) Postoperative view.

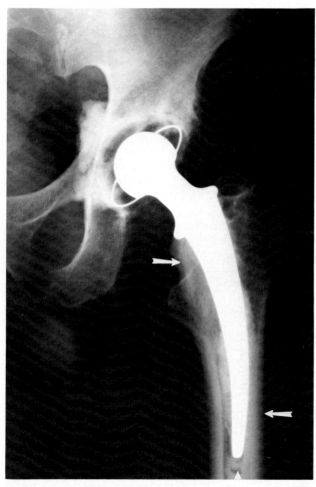

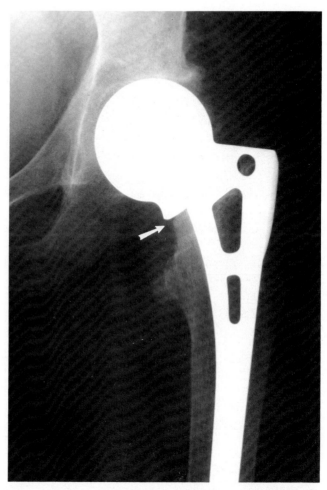

Figure 1-34. Charnley-Muller total hip replacement prosthesis in radiopaque methylmethacrylate. Arrows indicate major sites of stress.

Figure 1-35. Femoral head replacement prosthesis (Austin-Moore). No methacrylate. The flange at the base of the prosthetic femoral neck sits on the true femoral neck (arrow), transmitting much of the force of weight bearing from the prosthesis to the femoral cortex.

2
Principles of the Radiologic Evaluation of Appliances

THE RESPONSE OF BONE TO A METAL APPLIANCE

The Child

In growing bone, periosteal new bone may partially encase a metallic side plate. If it does, there will usually be no separation between the metal and the periosteal new bone. At the site where the nail penetrates through the cortex into the medullary portion of bone of a child, one will occasionally see a failure or partial failure of bone growth of both cortical and medullary bone on the epiphyseal side of the metal plate, usually with firm apposition of bone to the metal on the diaphyseal side of the plate (Figure 2-1). Occasionally, large cortical defects also occur on the epiphyseal side of the metal plate (Figure 2-2). These defects occcur only in growing bone and presumably represent an uneven remodeling of bone or inhibition of the growth of bone.

The Adult or Child

In the child or adult, the bone next to the appliance may have three different appearances: trabecular bone adjacent to the appliance (Figure 2-3); a thin rim of sclerotic bone along the surface of the appliance (Figure 2-4a,b); or a thin (less than 1 mm) zone of lucency separating the sclerotic bone from the metal—histologically this is fibrous tissue and does not indicate loosening (Figure 2-4a,b).

The tip of the stem of an intramedullary appliance may be surrounded by an increase in the amount of in-tramedullary bone (Figure 2-5a,b). This may be seen as an area of increased density near the tip and distal to the tip of the prosthesis or as a definite buttress of bone extending inward from the medial or lateral cortex of the femur to the tip of the prosthesis. This sclerosis also occurs with loose prostheses, where it is accentuated (Figure 2-6).

Many, but not all, hip appliances result in some redistribution of the pathways by which stress is transferred from the trunk to the leg. When this occurs, there is often hypertrophy of the bone that receives additional stress and atrophy of the bone that receives less stress. Thus, if a hip nail and side plate are carrying additional stress, there may be a thickening of the lateral cortex of the femur near the prosthesis. If an intramedullary prosthesis is transferring stress to the shaft distal to the femoral neck, the medial portion of the femoral neck may atrophy (Figure 2-7). This atrophy of the femoral neck does not indicate loosening or infection but is an expected consequence of the lack of stress applied to the bone. This transference of compressive force distally may account for the denser bone seen near the tip of an intramedullary prosthesis.

Zone of Radiolucency Around Blade Due to Slight Motion

Bone Resorption Between Appliance and Flexible Portion of Bone

It is quite common to see a thin zone of bone resorption (demarcated by a thin band of sclerotic bone) surrounding

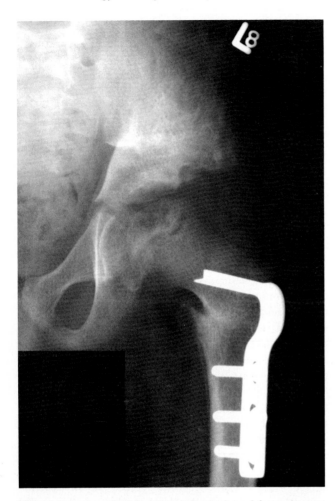

Figure 2-1. A small defect is seen in the lateral femoral cortex proximal to the metal plate. This is a normal finding in children. The patient had a varus osteotomy and a supra-acetabular osteotomy (Salter type) for treatment of Legg-Perthes disease.

pliance in the femoral neck. This bone resorption is minimal near the side plate and maximal near the proximal (or free) end of the appliance, and it is this pattern that permits the observer to differentiate it from the resorption occurring because of loosening or infection. With loosening, resorption will occur both along the nail and near the side plate. Infection often causes asymmetric or uneven resorption that may be contained near the side plate and not near the free end of the appliance (Figure 2-9); such resorption may also surround the nail with uneven radiolucency unexplainable as the result of motion or differences in flexibility of bone and metal (Figures 2-10, 2-11).

Radiolucency around the metal appliance can also be caused by a shift in bone fragments occurring after internal fixation. The radiolucency resulting from these shifts is

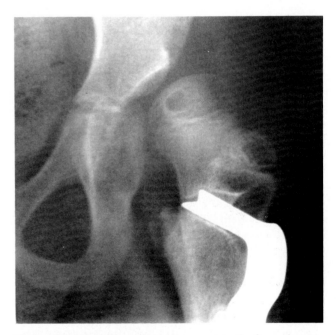

Figure 2-2. Marked resorption is present in the femoral cortex proximal to the side plate. This is an unusual exaggeration of the normal response; it suggests possible infection, though none was present in this case. This is a patient 16 months post varus osteotomy performed as treatment of valgus deformity of the femur with hip subluxation due to spastic diplegia. The valgus deformity has recurred.

the nail portion of a nail and side-plate appliance or around the blade of a blade-plate appliance; this resorption is caused by minimal motion between the bone and the appliance (Figure 2-8a,b). This motion occurs because bone and metal differ in flexibility. As a person walks, there is minimal give in the bone, which pivots on the femoral shaft and then springs back to normal position. Because metal is less flexible than bone, there is often minimal bone resorption around the portion of the ap-

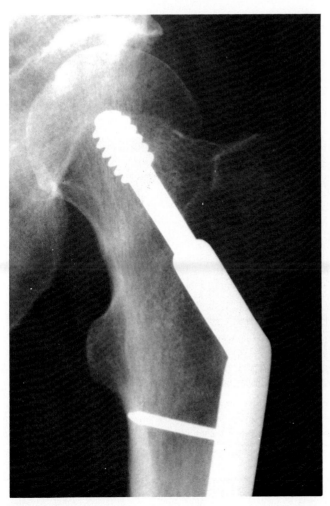

Figure 2-3. Four months following internal fixation of a mid-femoral neck fracture, the trabecular bone appears to be touching the metal appliance. (Richard-type compression screw.)

usually predictable and is related to the alignment of the fragments and their relative stabilities (Figure 2-12,*a,b,c,d*; Figure 2-13*a,b*).

The Response of Bone to Methylmethacrylate

With Radiolucent Methylmethacrylate
When barium is not added to methylmethacrylate, the methylmethacrylate is radiolucent. Thus, on radio-graphs, there is an absence of bone in areas where methylmethacrylate is present. Because most of the radiographic density of bone is due to cortical bone and only a small portion is due to trabecular bone, a large amount of trabecular bone must be displaced by the methacrylate before its disappearance becomes detectable. (This is analogous to the difficulties encountered in the detection of lytic medullary metastases.) Thus, when radiolucent methacrylate is used, a viewer of the radiograph may have no clue to its presence or location. This is the usual situation in the early postoperative period in almost all patients (Figure 2-14) and persists in a minority over many years.

Most patients, however, develop a thin rim of sclerotic bone (less than 1 mm thick) partially or circumferentially around the radiolucent methacrylate, so that its presence may be inferred (Figure 2-15). This sclerotic rim usually takes 6 to 12 months to develop.

With Radiopaque Methylmethacrylate
The amount of barium added to methylmethacrylate varies and therefore the density of the methacrylate also varies. In the acute period, the radiopaque methacrylate can be seen sitting within the medullary portion of bone. Because of the difficulty of identifying trabecular bone, it is not possible to tell whether the entire surgical cavity within the bone has been filled with methacrylate except where the methacrylate approaches the cortex. The amount of methacrylate used varies with the surgeon's preference and with the patient's degree of osteoporosis. After 6 to 12 months, many of the patients develop a thin band of sclerotic bone (less than 1 mm thick), which lies less than 1 mm away from the radiopaque methacrylate. The intervening gap is radiolucent and histologically is filled with immature or mature fibrous tissue. Evaluation of this radiolucent zone is of great importance.

The Radiolucent Line Around Radiopaque Methylmethacrylate

Most patients develop a thin zone of radiolucency around their radiopaque methylmethacrylate (Figure 2-16). A zone of 1 mm or less is expected, but in some patients, the zone is wider than 1 mm. In these cases there are several possible etiologies. The zone of radiolucency can be thicker

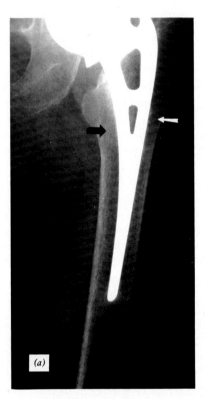

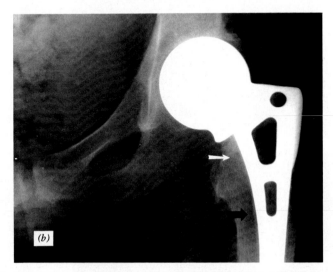

Figure 2-4. Two patients with Austin-Moore prostheses used for treatment of femoral neck fractures. In each, portions of the stem are directly surrounded by sclerotic bone (white arrows) and portions where a thin zone of radiolucency separates the metal from the zone of sclerosis (black arrow). The gap between the flange of the prosthesis and the femoral neck in Figure 2-4a is a normal finding; see also Figure 2-7.

than 1 mm in some patients without problems, but the thicker it is the greater the chance of a complication. In asymptomatic patients the gap may exceed 1 mm because the methacrylate was never tightly apposed to the bone at the time of surgical placement. This situation commonly occurs in the acetabulum; it seems to be more common in the inferomedial and superolateral aspect of the acetabulum and probably occurs in the anterior portion of the acetabulum as well (Figure 2-17a,c). Because of the potential occurrence of gaps between the bone and the methacrylate, any apparent increase in the thickness of the gap, especially in the acetabulum, may be due to slight changes in the position of the patient or to a different cen-

tering or angulation of the beam. The author has seen several asymptomatic patients whose perimethacrylate zone of radiolucency widened and narrowed from film to film depending on the centering of the radiograph. One must be very careful not to overcall loosening of the acetabular prosthesis because of minimal changes in the size of the zone of radiolucency. This same problem theoretically could occur in the femur, but the author has never seen it.

A wide zone of radiolucency may also be caused by loosening of the prosthesis. Periprosthetic infection may cause diffuse or focal widening of the zone of radiolucency. These complications are discussed in Chapter 3.

Radiolucent Line Between Prosthesis and Methacrylate

Radiolucency between the prosthesis and the methacrylate has a different meaning from that of the zone of radiolucency between the methacrylate and the bone. Since bone is a living tissue, it can react to stress placed upon it; metal and methacrylate do not resorb in response to stress. Separation between the prosthesis and the methacrylate usually is not due to a change in either structure. Most commonly, the radiolucency results from jiggling or slight movement of the prosthesis within its methacrylate bed during the time that the methacrylate is hardening (Figure 2-17a,b,c). If this is the case, the radiolucency should be present on the first postoperative film and should not change as long as the radiographic positioning and the position of the leg do not change. When a zone of radiolucency develops between the prosthesis and the

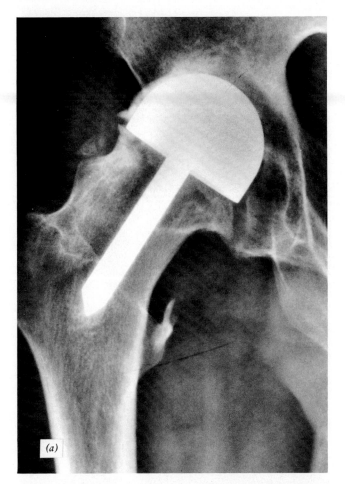

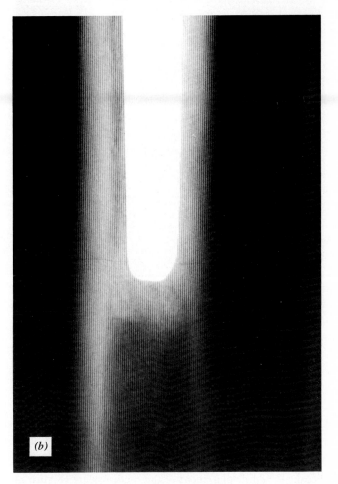

Figure 2-5. Two patients with different forms of femoral head replacement prostheses. In each there is an increase in the density of trabecular bone at the tip of the prosthesis. This is due to a normal transfer of stress distally. (a) A variant of the Judet stem prosthesis. (b) An Austin-Moore prosthesis.

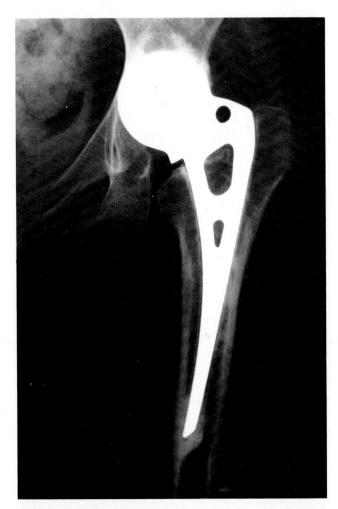

Figure 2-6. Marked buttressing of the tip of this loose Austin-Moore prosthesis is present. As seen 10 years after Austin-Moore prosthetic replacement of the femoral head and neck for an un-united femoral neck fracture.

methacrylate after the methacrylate has hardened, and if the radiographic views are truly comparable, this change indicates a loosening of the prosthesis associated with breakage and displacement of the methacrylate (Figure 2-18a,b). Since it is uncommon for all of the methacrylate surrounding the prosthesis to fragment equally, added stress may be placed on the prosthesis, causing it to break. Fracture of the stem of the prosthesis may be very difficult

to identify and should be searched for diligently in patients in whom the methacrylate is broken.

Methacrylate and the Change in the Elasticity of Bone

The metal prosthesis has a flexibility different from normal bone, and thus a thin zone of radiolucency can develop at the bone-metal junction. This is usually filled in

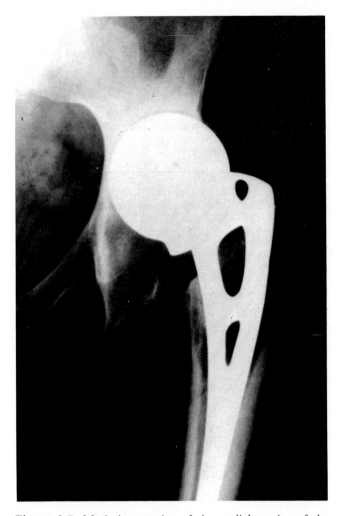

Figure 2-7. Marked resorption of the medial portion of the femoral neck is present. At surgery, this Austin-Moore prosthesis was tightly seated in the femoral canal.

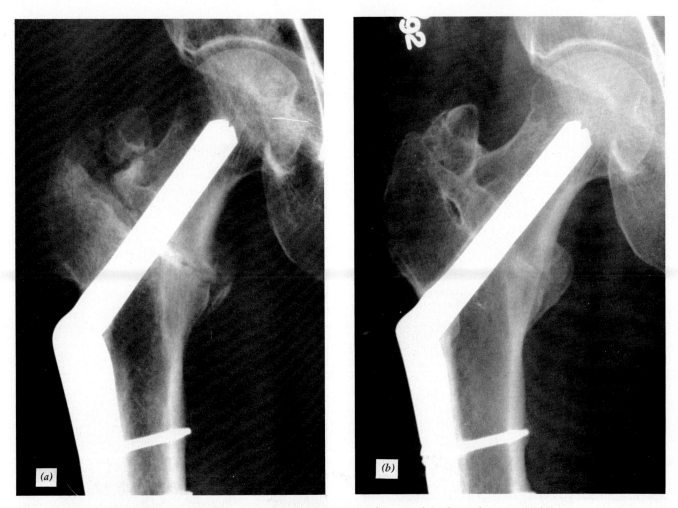

Figure 2.8. (*a*) Partially united high intertrochanteric fracture of the femur four months following fracture and internal fixation with a Jewett nail side-plate appliance. (*b*) Three years following fracture and internal fixation, a radiolucent stripe can be seen adjacent to the superior margin of the nail, bordered by a thin zone of sclerosis. The radiolucent zone is wider near the free proximal end of the nail and narrower near its base. This is the type of resorption seen when the bone is less rigid than the metal and gives a little with each step.

with fibrous tissue to compensate partially for the difference in elasticity. Methacrylate is also stiffer than bone, but since it may fill so much of the medullary area of the bone, the stresses may be transmitted to the cortex of the bone rather than to medullary bone. Because of this it is possible to see, on some patients, a thickening of the cortex

just distal to the tip of the femoral prosthesis and its methacrylate (Figure 2-17*a,c*). Occasionally periosteal lamellae may be present there and should not be interpreted as having pathologic significance. Care must be taken, however, not to miss a stress fracture in this location.

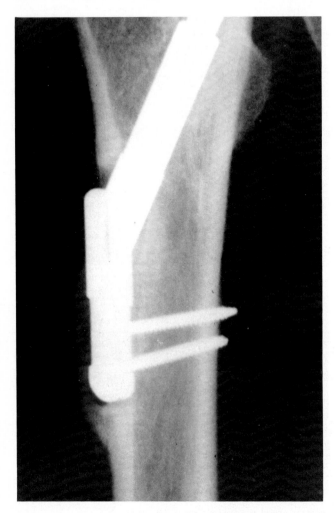

Figure 2-9. An infected Massie nail demonstrates bone resorption around the side plate with the screws still properly seated and with only minimal resorption around the intramedullary portion of the appliance.

The Effect That Prior Hip Surgery Has on the Appearance Following a Second Operation

Throughout the book many examples will be seen in which patients have had a second procedure performed on a previously operated hip. Often the residua of the previous operation can be inferred from the final film (Figure

2-19a,b). In addition to the specific changes or realignment of these operations, there is a frequently seen marked wavy or irregular periosteal reaction around the proximal femur weeks to months following the second operation (Figure 2-20a,b); this common and somewhat worrisome periosteal reaction is a normal, nonpathologic response.

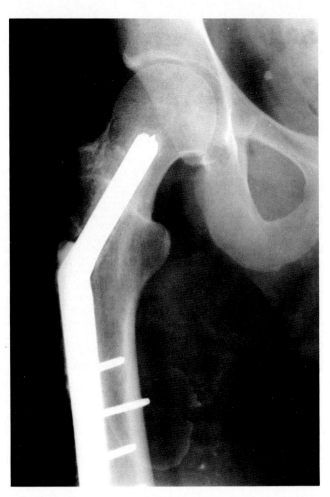

Figure 2-10. An infected Jewett appliance. There is resorption around the intramedullary portion of the nail, with no loosening of the screws or side plate. The zone of resorption encircles the intramedullary portion of the nail, a pattern not explainable as the result of different degrees of flexibility of bone and metal. Thus, the changes should represent infection. (Film made during a sinus tract contrast injection.)

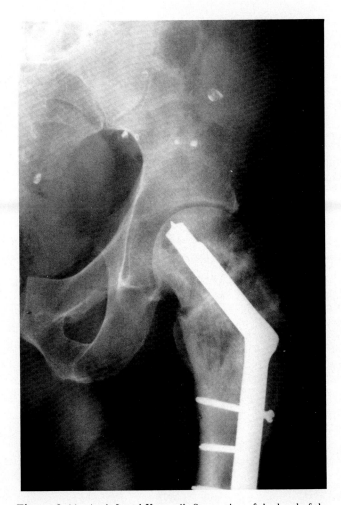

Figure 2-11. An infected Ken nail. Separation of the head of the proximal screw from the side plate indicates loosening of the side plate. The resorption around the portion of the nail in the femoral head and neck is uneven in its margins. This implies infection.

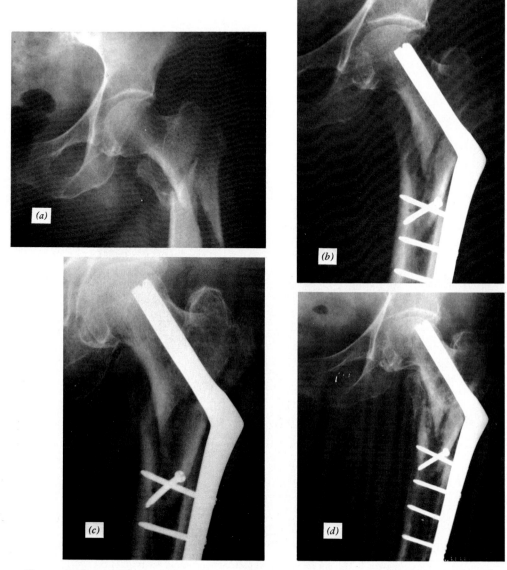

Figure 2-12. (*a*) This unstable intertrochanteric and subtrochanteric fracture occurred in a 77-year-old woman who bent over to pick up a child's play ball in the street. (*b*) Eight days following reduction and internal fixation with a Jewett nail, the alignment is much improved, but the fragments are still unstable. Reduction and fixation were performed to decrease pain and simplify nursing care. (*c*) Five days later, a gap has appeared between the distal portion of the nail and the greater trochanter fragment, due to a shift in the fragment. The patient was kept nonweight bearing for five months following fracture. (*d*) Eight months following fracture, the bone has shifted slightly in relation to the nail. The gap between the distal portion of the nail and the bone is now more symmetrical due to slight shift in the position of the fragments. the nail has also slightly shifted its position within the femoral head.

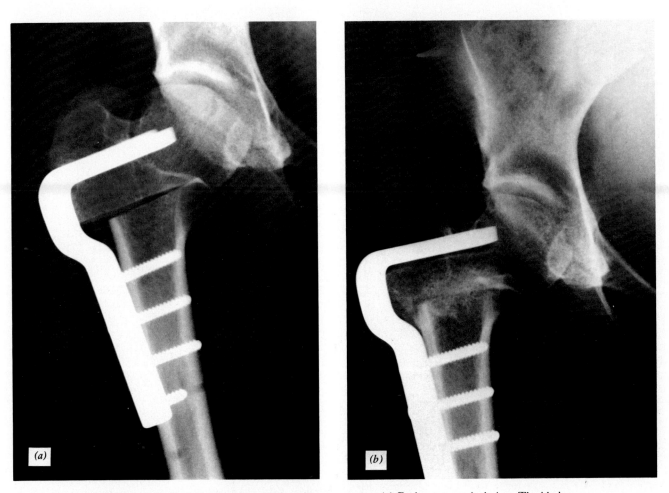

Figure 2-13. Varus and medial displacement osteotomy. (*a*) Early post surgical view. The blade holds the bone fragments slightly distracted. (*b*) Four months later, the fragments have shifted into contact. A bony gap is present inferior to the blade of the blade plate, a consequence of the shift.

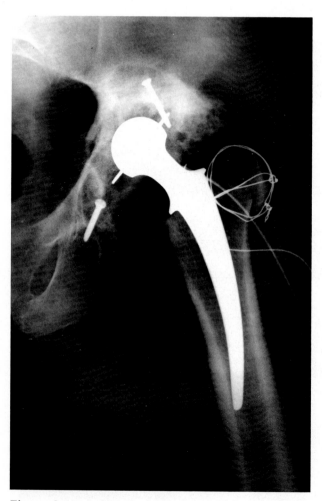

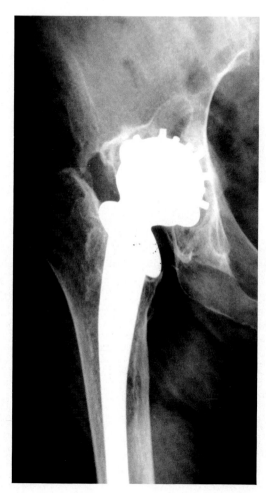

Figure 2-14. A Charnley-Muller total hip replacement implanted in radiolucent methylmethacrylate shortly following surgery. The location of the methacrylate is not visible. Total hip replacement used as treatment for degenerative arthritis following acetabular fracture.

Figure 2-15. A McKee-farrar total hip prosthesis placed in radiolucent methylmethacrylate. There is a thin band of sclerotic bone surrounding the methacrylate both within the acetabulum and within the femoral shaft.

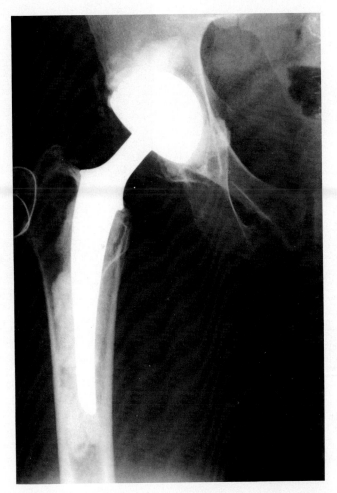

Figure 2-16. A Harris total hip replacement implanted in radiopaque methylmethacrylate. Surrounding the acetabular methacrylate is a thin zone of radiolucency, which in turn is surrounded by a thin rim of sclerotic bone. The methacrylate surrounding the femoral prosthesis deomonstrates both the lack of interface with trabecular bone (near the greater trochanter) and the approximation of the cortex bone (indicative of complete filling of the surgical cavity). These are all normal features of the methacrylate bone interface.

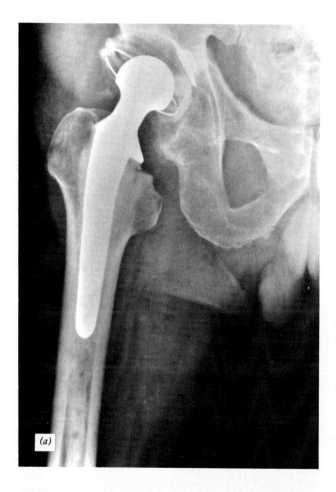

(a)

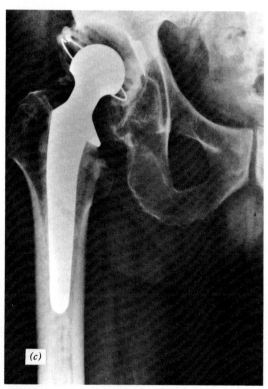

(c)

Figure 2-17. Variant of Turner-Aufranc total hip replacement prosthesis, showing gap between acetabular methacrylate and inferomedial portion of the acetabulum and minimal gap between the femoral prosthesis and the methacrylate—early films. (*a*) Early postoperative view. (*b*) Close-up showing a small gap between the prosthesis and the methacrylate. (*c*) One-year follow-up demonstrating no change in the acetabular methacrylate-bone gap or in the femoral prosthesis-methacrylate gap. Thickening of the femoral cortex near the distal lateral portion of the prosthesis has developed, a response to the redistribution of stress.

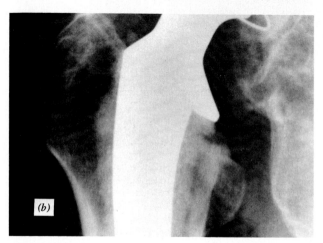

(b)

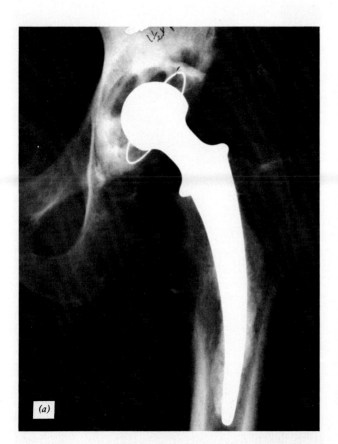 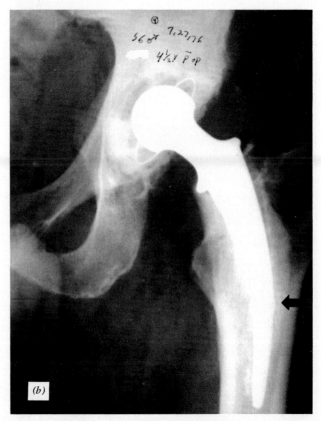

Figure 2-18. Charnley-Muller total hip prosthesis. A gap between the methacrylate and the prosthesis has developed between the two studies, indicating loosening. The slight irregularity near the lower third of the femoral component (arrow) represents a fracture of the prosthesis. (*a*) 1½ years following surgery. 4½ years following surgery.

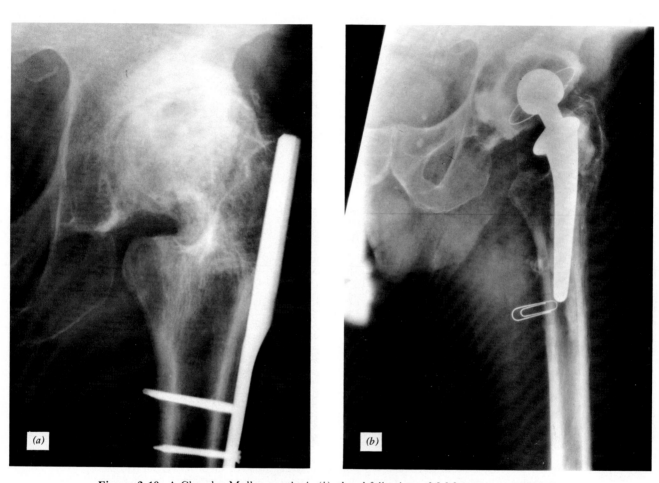

Figure 2-19. A Charnley-Muller prosthesis (*b*) placed following a McMurray-type medial displacement osteotomy (*a*). The abnormal relationship of the greater trochanter to the femoral neck remnant and the holes of the screws can be seen. Abundant periosteal reaction is a normal finding following a second operation on the proximal femur and does not indicate infection. (*a*) McMurray osteotomy. (*b*) Charnley-Muller prosthesis.

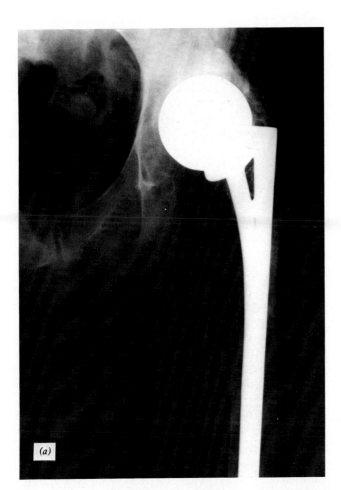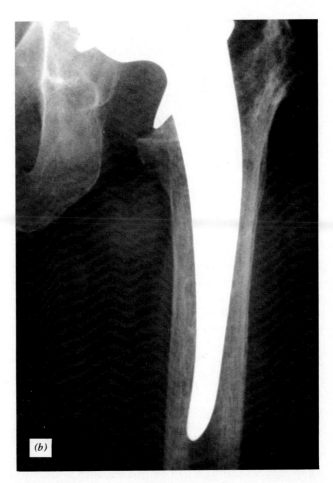

Figure 2-20. A McKee-Farrar prosthesis placed following removal of a painful Austin-Moore prosthesis. (*a*) A long-stem Moore prosthesis replaced a painful Thompson prosthesis used for a femoral neck fracture. Moderate heterotopic bone developed following surgery, limiting motion. Both the limitation of motion and the pain led the patient to seek additional surgery. (*b*) A McKee-Farrar prosthesis was used, placed in lucent methacrylate. Wavy periosteal reaction is seen along the lateral aspect of the femur, due to reoperation. There is no clinical evidence of loosening or infection. Slight thickening of the femoral cortex near the tip of the femoral component is also present [compare to the cortical thickness in (*a*)] and has developed following the removal of the Moore prosthesis.

3

A Radiologic Approach to the Complications of Hip Surgery

Complications of hip surgery are of three types: (1) complications of the original disease which would occur with or without therapy, such as the loss of femoral-head cartilage following slippage of the capital femoral epiphysis; (2) complications representing an expected recurrence of deformity or wearing out of the appliance, such as the frequent recurrence of deformity following surgery for neurogenic hip disease; and (3) the complications occurring on a scattered individual basis, which may reflect either failures of the surgical technique or failures of the patient's body to respond to therapy adequately, such as infection, loosening, dislocation, and the development of heterotopic bone. This chapter gives an overview of these complications, each of which will be discussed in more detail in subsequent chapters.

SUBLUXATION AND DISLOCATION

Stability of the hip joint depends on the balance between the shape and alignment of the proximal femur and acetabulum and the strength and direction of muscle pull across the joint. Fascial strength is also of importance. Changes in the shape of the acetabulum, changes in the angulation and rotation of the femur, damage to fascial planes during surgery, and change in the effective active length of muscles may all contribute to instability. Preexisting muscle weakness may affect the final stability and may influence the selection of the type and positioning of an appliance.

Although it is of prime importance to place the nail or prosthesis in a position stable enough to prevent its displacement within the bone, the position selected must also reflect the desired balance between joint stability and mobility. In general, the more stable the position chosen for the femoral-acetabular alignment, the less mobile the hip. In the patient with strong muscles, a position that provides maximum mobility will be chosen, while in the patient with weak muscles (due to age or neurologic disease) a position of greater stability is sought. While generalization is difficult, a first approximation of proper positioning can be given. The details of specific procedures for specific diseases are discussed in subsequent chapters.

JOINT ALIGNMENT

In the normal person, the major movements of the hip are rotation, flexion, and abduction, with less motion necessary for adduction and extension. The orientation of the normal acetabular opening, laterally and anteriorly, provides for the major movements. The normal antever-

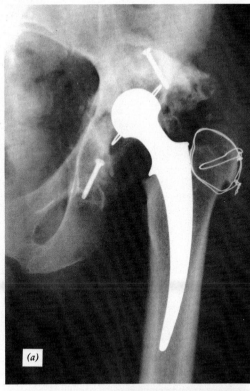

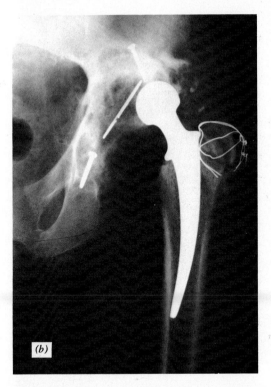

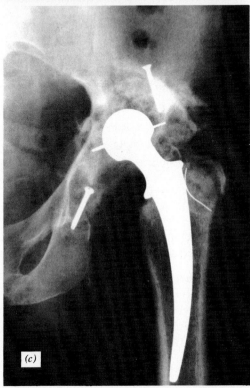

Figure 3-1. A Charnley-Muller total hip replacement prosthesis with the acetabular cup (marked by the wire) approximately 50° off horizontal. (*a*) Located, one day after surgery. (*b*) Dislocated later the same day (the femoral head is no longer centered within the wire ring acetabular marker). (*c*) Located following surgical replacement of the acetabular component, now at approximately 25°.

sion of the femoral neck also permits increased flexion by limiting impingement of the thigh against the abdomen. In general, the hip becomes unstable if the opening of the acetabulum or an acetabular prosthesis is directed more than 50° laterally (Figure 3-1). The degree of anterior opening is less well defined and more difficult to measure, but with most acetabular prostheses, 10 to 15° is preferred. Decreasing the lateral opening of the acetabulum or its prosthesis will usually increase stability but limit abduction. The acceptable degree of anterior opening of the acetabulum or its prosthesis is directly related to the degree of femoral anteversion present. While a 0° anterior opening would be stable with the leg in extension, impingement of the femur against it (with subluxation) would occur in flexion, unless moderate femoral antever-

47

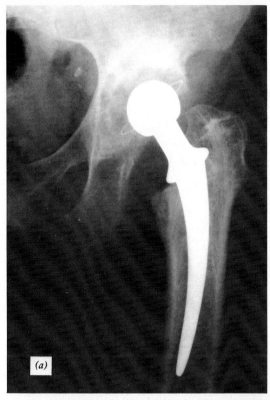

(a)

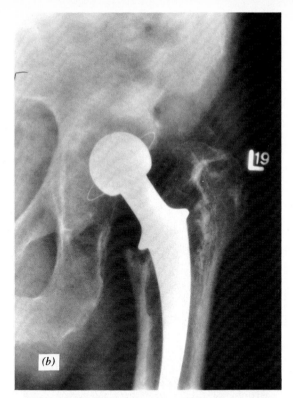

(b)

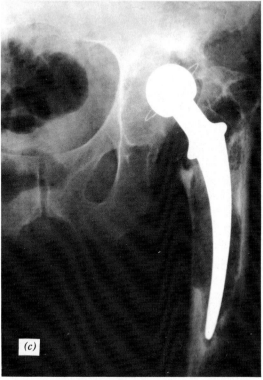

(c)

Figure 3-2. Progressive evidence of loosening of a Charnley-Muller total hip replacement. (*a*) One month following surgery, the area of medullary bone removed and replaced by radiolucent methacrylate is not visible. (*b*) Eighteen months later, resorption of the medial femoral cortex is present, indicative of loosening or infection. (*c*) Thirty months later, the amount of cortical resorption has increased, as has the pain. Arthrography and surgery confirmed the loosening of the femoral prosthesis. Resorption of cortex is an unusual, but very helpful, sign of loosening.

sion were also present. Retroversion of the proximal femur will also result in impingement against the acetabular prosthesis, resulting in instability. Posterior opening of the acetabulum can result in posterior subluxation with the hip flexed. The ideal position is a balance between acetabulum and femur and between stability and mobility.

EVALUATION OF MUSCLE LENGTH AND DIRECTION OF PULL

From a radiologic vantage, only two hip muscle groups need to be evaluated; the glutei, particularly the gluteus medius, which inserts on the greater trochanter, and the iliopsoas (inserting on the lesser trochanter). Both play important roles in the functioning and stability of the hip.

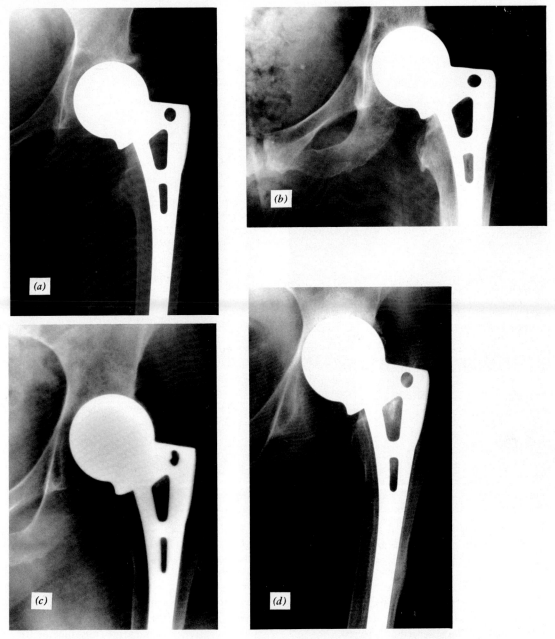

Figure 3-3. Austin-Moore prosthesis, with initial normal response of medullary bone, followed by loosening with outward shift of the sclerotic margin of the bone. (*a*) Three months following surgery, there is no evidence of delineation of the medullary bone from the Austin-Moore prosthesis. (*b*) Ten months following surgery, a thin band of sclerotic bone is present approximately 1 mm away from the metal prosthesis. This is a normal finding. (*c*) Twenty-three months following surgery, the appearance is unchanged. (*d*) Five and one-half years following surgery, the zone of radiolucency has increased as the sclerotic band of bone has been displaced outward This

(*Continued on next page*)

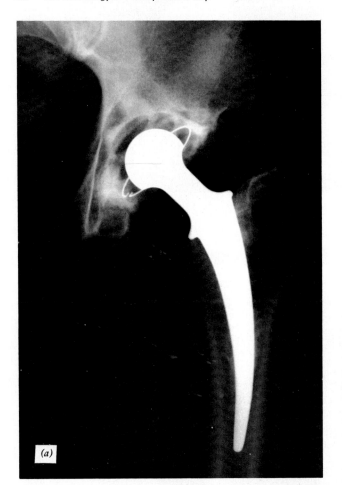
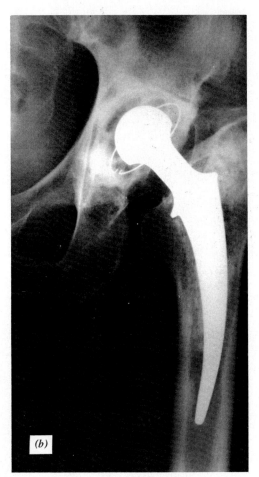

Figure 3-4. A Charnley-Muller total hip prosthesis with loosening of the femoral component. (*a*) Properly seated prosthesis in minimally radiopaque methacrylate. (*b*) Thirty-two months later, the prosthesis has sunk into the femoral canal, indicating loosening.

Together they hold the hip joint reduced. While many abnormalities of the muscles cannot be detected radiographically, a few can be observed or inferred.

Maintenance of muscle length is an important factor in preserving the strength and stability of the hip. Muscles are strongest at specific effective lengths. The tolerance for

variance of this length is somewhat variable but is relatively limited for the glutei. Side-to-side or preoperative-to-postoperative comparative measurements of both the vertical height from the greater trochanter to the level of the acetabulum and the effective length of the femoral neck should be made. When surgery is expected to result in

increase in the band of radiolucency is indicative of loosening. The prosthesis has also sunk deeper into the femur with the flange of the prosthesis now sitting closer to the lesser trochanter. The bone proximally in the fenestration of the Moore prosthesis has been eroded, also indicative of the sinking of the prosthesis.

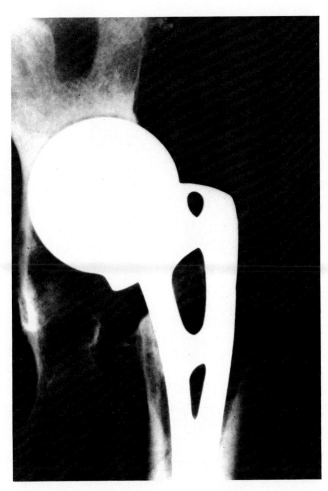

Figure 3-5. Surgically proven, firmly seated Austin-Moore prosthesis with marked resorption of the femoral neck. Resorption of the femoral neck is a normal finding following prosthetic replacement of the femoral neck.

shortening of the effective length of the glutei, surgeons may transplant the greater trochanter distally to bring the gluteal muscles to their most effective length. Failure to maintain the appropriate distance may result in weakness, which could result in a limp, subluxation, or dislocation.

The direction of pull of the iliopsoas muscle is an important factor in maintaining reduction of the hip. To maintain reduction, the articular surface of the femoral head should be medial to the iliopsoas tendon; the more medial it lies, the more stable the hip will be. Should the head be lateral (which occurs with marked valgus of the hip), the partially medially directed vector of force of the iliopsoas on the femoral head is lost, lessening the stability of the hip. This is of greatest importance in the patient with paralytic hip disease whose gluteal muscles are also weak and is discussed more extensively in Chapter 5.

Although only a few of the factors predisposing to subluxation and dislocation can be evaluated on the radiograph, the detection of abnormal alignment or of muscle abnormalities permits the addition of external support until soft-tissue and fascial healing has occurred. Once healed, the added support of the soft tissues and fascial planes will often prevent subsequent subluxation and dislocation.

LOOSENING

An appliance that is loose at its contact with bone can often be recognized because its motion changes the stress applied to the bone and causes osteoclastic resorption of bone. When this stress is applied to medullary bone, a large amount must be resorbed before the bone loss becomes detectable. Cortical resorption commonly occurs around loose screws; it is uncommon with intramedullary prostheses, but when it occurs it is easily recognizable (Figure 3-2a,b,c). In those cases in which the body has surrounded the prosthesis or its methacrylate with a thin rim of sclerotic bone, this sclerotic medullary bone will also be affected by the loosening and may either be destroyed or migrate away from the appliance (Figure 3-3a,b,c,d). Although a 1-mm radiolucent separation between the appliance and the bone is common, occasionally even 2 to 3 mm may be normal. If serial films demonstrate a progressive widening of the band of radiolucency, loosening is almost certain. One must be careful however, not to confuse the initial development of bands of radiolucency and sclerosis in the 12 months following surgery with its displacement. The etiology of the common and asymptomatic 1 mm of radiolucency is uncertain. The zone is composed of fibrous tissue filling a space which may result from minimal motion or from differences in the elasticity of the bone and the appliance.

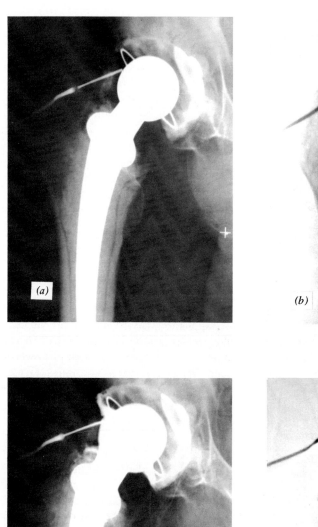

(a)

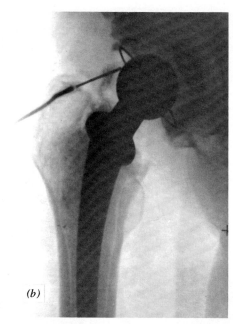

(b)

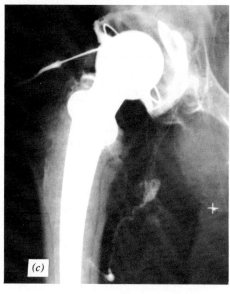

(c)

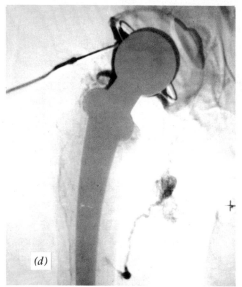

(d)

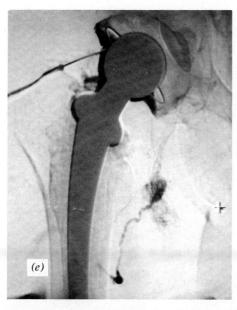

(e)

Figure 3-6. Arthrogram in a patient with loosening of the femoral component of a Charnley-Muller total hip prosthesis. (*a*) Scout film. (*b*) Reversal film of Scout. (*c*) Film following injection of contrast material. Lymphatic filling is present. A very thin band of contrast material outlines the lateral femoral-methacrylate junction. (*d*) This tracking of contrast material around the methacrylate is confirmed on the subtraction view, confirming the loosening. (*e*) A slight malalignment of the reversal film (*b*) and the arthrogram film (*c*) results in a false black line adjacent to the lateral margin of the metal prosthesis. The malalignment can be recognized by the white line along the opposite (medial) margin of the prosthesis.

Some femoral prostheses, when they are loose, settle deeper into the femoral shaft (Figures 3-3*c,d* and 3-4*a,b*). Occasionally, this settling results in better impaction of the prosthesis or methacrylate into the medullary bone, and the prosthesis becomes firmly fixed again. Because the medial femoral neck remnant often resorbs following surgery (Figure 3-5), it is important to judge the position of the prosthesis against a fixed structure such as the lesser trochanter, rather than to judge it in relation to the femoral neck.

Although loosening may be painful it need not be, and indeed many patients with radiographic signs of minimal loosening have minimal or no symptoms and do not require additional surgery.

Loosening can be confirmed by arthrography; while this technique has false negatives and some reported false positives, it is still very useful. When radiopaque barium-methacrylate has been used, subtraction technique can be helpful. In the subtraction technique, the leg is immobilized. A reversal of the scout film (Figure 3-6*a,b*) is made (since the scout or plain film is a standard radiograph, it is a negative—thus the reversal image is a positive). A film from the arthrogram, taken in the same position (Figure 3-6*c*), is then laid on top of this reversed (positive) scout film. The combination is printed, and, if done accurately, only the contrast material shows (Figure 3-6*d*). It is important to be certain that the alignment of the positive scout and the arthrogram film be perfect. If the alignment is off, the subtraction film will demonstrate a false-positive contrast adjacent to the prosthesis—but only on one side of the prosthesis (Figure 3-6*e*). In the false positive, the prosthesis will have a white line on one side and a black line on the other. In the true positive, only the black line of the contrast will show, and no white lines will be apparent.

INFECTION

Infection following surgery on the hip may present either early in the postoperative period or after a delay of several years. With some infections, the radiographs appear completely normal, both in the early and late infections. Because of this, if infection is suspected of if there is unexplained postoperative pain, it is important to obtain a hip-joint aspiration for culture. It is necessary to culture for both aerobic and anaerobic organisms. The author and his orthopedic colleagues prefer to do the aspiration under fluoroscopic control. If no fluid is obtained it is helpful then to perform an arthrogram to be certain that the needle was truly in the hip joint. Because of the thick pseudocapsule following surgery, the needle may be extra-articular when it feels intra-articular. Arthrographic signs

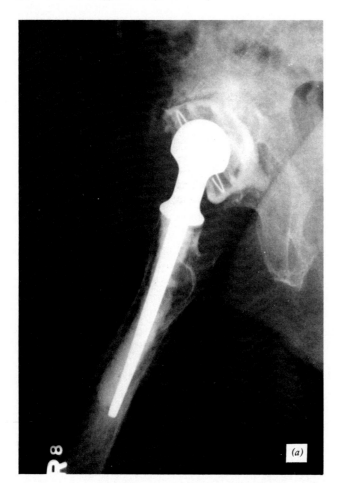
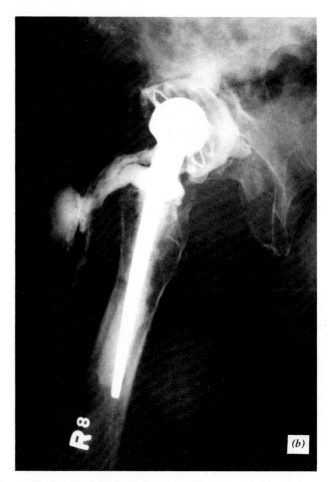

Figure 3-7. An infected Charnley-Muller total hip prosthesis with a large sinus tract. (*a*) Scout film. (*b*) Sinogram.

of infection include sinus tracts in soft tissue (Figure 3-7*a,b*) or in bone and evidence of partial or complete loosening of the prosthesis. Differentiation between loosening and infection may not be possible by radiographs.

Although aspiration of the hip and arthrography are the best methods of diagnosing a hip infection, several radiologic signs are also quite helpful; for example, classical permeative lytic destruction may be seen in the acetabulum (Figure 3-8) or femur (Figure 3-9). Since the infections usually involve intra-articular bone (which lacks perios-

teum), periosteal reaction is usually absent. In addition, focal resorption around an appliance that is not loose or in a pattern incompatible in shape with movement around a prosthesis—for example, irregular cavities or uneven resorption (Figure 3-10)—is highly suggestive of infection.

Occasionally, the only manifestation of infection is marked ectopic bone formation around the joint (Figure 3-11); whenever this is seen, infection should be ruled out, even though most cases of ectopic bone formation will not be associated with infection.

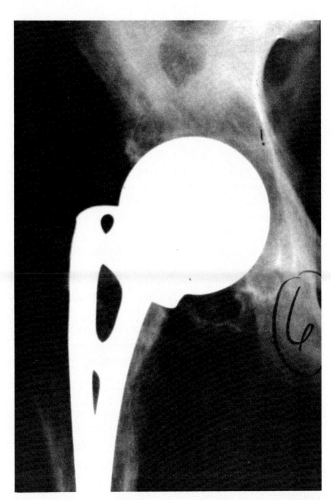

Figure 3-8. Permeative lysis of the acetabular roof is secondary to a pseudomonas infection of the hip joint.

UNEXPLAINED PAIN

Unexplained pain has many potential causes. Pain may be referred or radiated from the back. Trochanteric bursitis is common and should be searched for clinically; radiographically soft-tissue calcification, either lateral to or superior to the greater trochanter, may be seen. Stress fractures can occur both in the inner wall of the acetabulum or in the ischium. Femoral stress fractures can

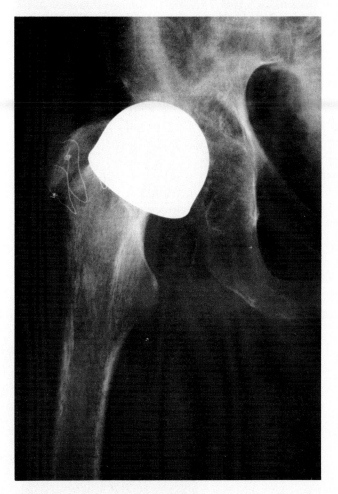

Figure 3-9. Permeative lysis of the femoral shaft following a cup mold arthroplasty was secondary to a Klebsiella-aerobacter infection of the hip joint.

ECTOPIC BONE FORMATION

Ectopic bone frequently forms lateral and anterior to the hip joint following hip surgery. In general it is a self-limited process that does not result in limitation of motion. In an occasional patient, extensive ectopic bone forms, limiting motion at the hip. When ectopic bone is extensive, infection may be present and should be ruled out.

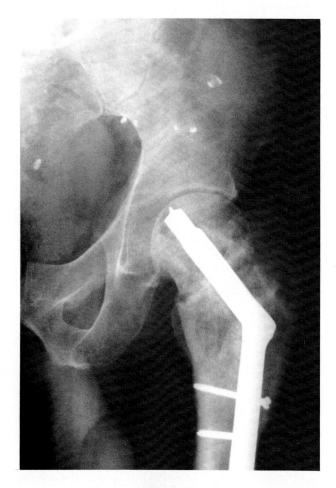

occur but are rare. Patients with significant unexplained pain should have a hip aspiration and culture with an arthrogram.

COMMUNICATION WITH THE ORTHOPEDIST

Because there are many factors involved in the management of the patient with a problem hip, the radiologist should not be too presumptuous in his written report. If he is strongly concerned that complications may be occurring, it is best to discuss this with the surgeon and thereby learn more about the patient. At the same time it is important not to lose objectivity. A physician who operates on a patient has invested a great deal of emotion in the successful result, and it is often very difficult for the surgeon to accept even the thought of possible failure until he or she has been made aware of the unequivocal clinical or radiographic changes.

Subsequent chapters deal with the treatment of specific diseases. In those chapters, the general approach given above will be expanded and exceptions stated.

Figure 3-10. Irregular resorption around the stem and nail portions of a Ken nail is indicative of infection. Culture grew staphylococcus epidermitis.

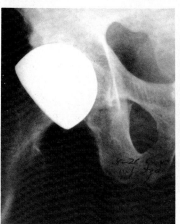
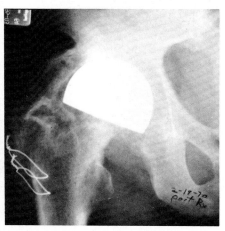

Figure 3-11. Extensive ectopic bone formation has enveloped this infected cup mold arthroplasty. (Reprinted by permission, *Radiologic Clinics of North America,* April 75, p. 55).

Part 1

THE CHILD'S HIP

4
Congenital Displacement of the Hip

Dislocation and subluxation of the hip are common neonatal diseases. Their early diagnosis (before 18 months of age) permits closed or open surgical reduction, allowing soft-tissue repair to be accomplished without the need for bone realignment (2,15,18,26,33,45,46). Because of muscular and ligamentous changes and progressive bone deformity, surgical bony reconstruction is usually necessary when the initial treatment is begun after 18 months of age. The prognosis of congenital dislocation is somewhat different from that of the congenitally subluxing hip. The prognosis of untreated congenital dislocation of the hip is poor, with a delay in walking, progressing to an awkward, mechanically inefficient gait, resulting eventually in low back and hip pain. An untreated subluxing hip often presents with painful degenerative arthritis, usually developing in the teenage years. Subclinical displacement of the hip is thought to be a common precursor of adult degenerative arthritis (32). Early diagnosis and treatment is the key to a good prognosis.

THE RECOGNITION OF THE DISPLACED FEMORAL HEAD

Clinical and radiologic methods are used for the diagnosis of congenital displacement of the hip. In the newborn period, physical examination is the best method for the detection of hip instability. Radiographs may demonstrate the displacement of the femoral head from the acetabulum, but they often appear normal. Two physical examiniation tests are common: the Ortolani and the Barlow maneuvers. Both tests can demonstrate dislocation; Barlow's test also shows instability.

The Ortolani test (24,36,40,42) is performed with the infant supine. The hips are flexed to 90° and the knees are flexed. The hip is slowly abducted. If the hip is dislocated, somewhere in the 90° arc of abduction, the femoral head will slip back into the acetabulum with a visible and palpable, but not audible, click. The test may be falsely negative if full abduction of the hip is not possible (40) and may be negative if the joint capsule is very lax (42). If the test is negative, it should be repeated at four to six weeks and at six months to detect the occasional patient whose hip instability is missed in the newborn period (24,40,42).

The Barlow test (2,40,42) is performed with the infant supine. The hips and knees are flexed with the calf within the webspace between the thumb and index finger. The thumb is placed along the medial thigh near the lesser trochanter, and the middle finger is placed near the greater trochanter. The hips are placed in midabduction. Pressure is applied on the greater trochanter directed towards the symphysis pubis. If the femoral head slips into the acetabulum, the hip was subluxed or dislocated.

Pressure is then applied to the lesser trochanter directed posterolaterally by the thumb. If the femoral head slips from the acetabulum, the hip is unstable.

When the presence of instability is uncertain, the pelvis can be stabilized with the other hand by placing the thumb on the pubic symphysis and the fingers on the sacrum and then proceeding with the test as described.

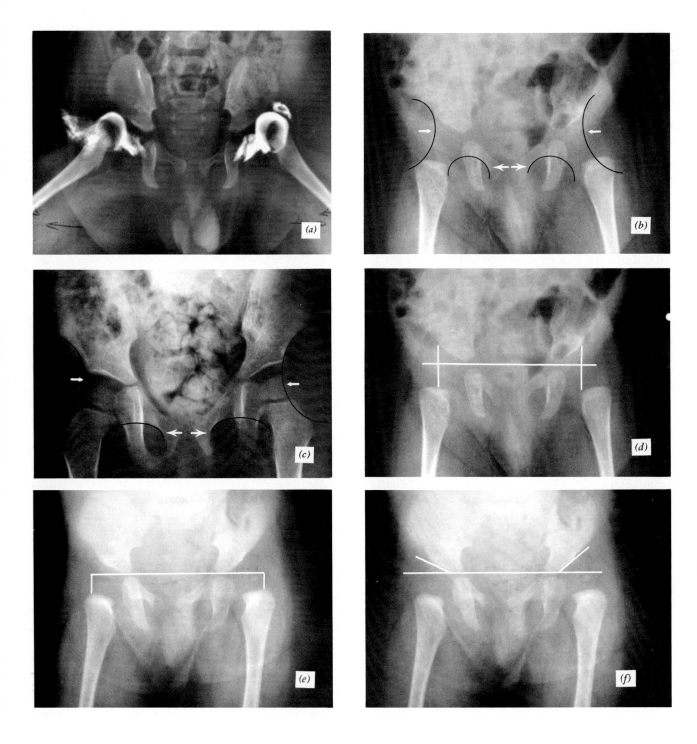

THE ROLE OF RADIOLOGY IN THE EARLY DETECTION OF CONGENITAL DISPLACEMENT OF THE HIP

The initial screening for hip dislocation should be clinical. Radiographs play no role in screening for the early detection of hip dislocation (17,32,40,42). The clinical tests are more sensitive and, when properly performed, only rarely miss hip instability. Radiographs are often normal in the newborn with hip instability.

Radiographs can be used to confirm the presence of dislocation and are useful in confirming the success of reduction. The most useful view in the newborn period is the Andrén-von Rosen view (2,36,40) (Figure 4-1a). This is taken with the hips extended and the thighs abducted 45° with medial rotation. This view should be taken when the hip is clinically dislocated. When dislocation is present, a line drawn along the shaft of the femur points towards the anterior-superior iliac spine and crosses the lumbar spine above the lumbosacral junction.

The view obtained with the legs extended and parallel may also be useful, though its interpretation may be more difficult (32). On this view, several lines may be drawn to detect femoral-head subluxation or dislocation.

Shenton's line is a curved line along the roof of the obturator foramen that in the normal hip extends in a smooth arc into the curve of the medial portion of the femoral neck (Figure 4-1b,c).

A second line, (Figure 4-1b,c) described by Simon (40), curves along the lateral margin of the ilium and forms a continuous curve with the lateral portion of the femoral neck.

The normal location for the still unossified proximal femoral epiphysis can be judged by pinpointing its predicted epiphyseal location by a line drawn between the Y cartilages of the two acetabula and a vertical line drawn from the edge of the ossified acetabulum (Figure 4-1d). The normal epiphysis should lie within the inner inferior quadrant. Epiphyses estimated to lie within the lower lateral quadrant are subluxed; those in the upper lateral quadrant are dislocated.

The distance of the metaphysis from the Y-Y line should be symmetrical and is decreased with subluxation or dislocation (Figure 4-1e).

The acetabular angle (Figure 4-1f), the angle between the Y-Y line and a line drawn along the ossified superior acetabular roof, is used as an estimate of acetabular disease. While subject to much controversy (25,32), this angle is of use in evaluating unilateral hip displacement (40).

The ossified acetabular roof does not represent the actual margin of the acetabulum, which is still cartilaginous, but reflects a delay in its ossification. Since ossification of this lateral margin is inhibited by abnormal stress, its ossification is delayed in the subluxing hip. Accurate measurement of this angle is difficult, as it is affected by the centering of the x-ray beam and by the degree of lordosis and rotation of the pelvis (25,32). If no rotation is present, the acetabular angles of the two hips can be compared. Absolute measurements of the angle are of less use

Figure 4-1. Radiographic techniques for the recognition of the displaced hip. (a) The Andrén-von Rosen view. Bilateral hip dislocation. The legs are abducted 45° and internally rotated. This view is obtained when the hips are clinically dislocated. When normal, a line drawn along the femoral shaft should intersect the acetabulum. With dislocation, the line is directed superior to the acetabulum. In this radiograph, the arthrographic contrast media confirms the dislocation of the femoral head. (b,c) Anteroposterior view with the legs in neutral position. Shenton line (large arrows) and Simon's line (small arrows) (see text) confirm the left hip subluxation. (b) Newborn. (c) Age two years with minimal residual subluxation. (d) Anteroposterior view with legs in neutral position. While the epiphyses are not yet ossified, the estimated position for them would be in the lower inner quadrant on the right (normal) and in the lower outer quadrant on the left (subluxed). See text. (e) The left hip is subluxed. The distance from the metaphysis to the Y-Y line is decreased on the left. (f) Acetabular angle. Left hip subluxation. The left acetabular angle is increased compared to the right.

because of the difficulties in standardizing the view, a subject extensively reviewed in an excellent article by R. D. Laurenson (25).

THE ROLE OF ARTHROGRAPHY

Hip arthrograms can be used to evaluate for hip dislocation and subluxation, since they clearly demonstrate the acetabulum and femoral head. Their greatest usefulness is in the child in whom the clinical signs of instability are unclear or in the child in whom the success of reduction is uncertain (21,29,43). Hip arthrograms are used by many surgeons as a key factor in deciding upon a closed or open reduction.

THE NORMAL ARTHROGRAM (Figure 4-2a)

The relation of the femoral head to the acetabulum and the position and shape of the acetabulum must both be studied. The femoral head should be nearly spherical and more than one-half of its superior surface should be covered by the acetabulum. The head should be deeply seated within the acetabulum and only minimal contrast should collect medial to the femoral head. The free edge of the acetabular labrum, the limbus, should be identified superolateral to the femoral head, and this limbus should lie at or inferior to the Y-Y line (21,26,29).

Subluxation and dislocation can be recognized by decreased coverage of the femoral head and by the presence of increased contrast within the depths of the acetabulum (Figure 4-2b).

In the patient whose femoral head cannot be reduced, blocks to reduction include inversion of the limbus (Figure 4-2c), constriction of the joint capsule (creating an hourglass deformity, Figure 4-2d), and occasionally, increased soft tissue within the depths of the acetabulum (29,40).

THE TREATMENT OF CONGENITAL DISPLACEMENT OF THE HIP

The treatment of congenital displacement of the hip varies with the age of the patient and the ability to obtain reduc-

tion. The older child may have acetabular or femoral deformity or contractures of the soft tissues that require different methods of treatment than the younger child without deformity whose tissues remain malleable.

THE TREATMENT OF CONGENITAL DISPLACEMENT OF THE HIP FROM 0 TO 18 MONTHS

When instability of the hip is detected in the newborn, correction and stabilization will occur without specific therapy in more than 50% of the patients in the first few days of life (12,42). With reduction and sustained abduction almost all of these patients will have a stable hip within three months (2,36,37). Although the appropriate therapy of the patient whose hip spontaneously stabilizes in the first few days is often debated (some physicians will treat these patients, while others will follow their progress for any evidence of subsequent hip instability), those hip displacements that do not correct in the first few days are treated until stability can be demonstrated. Protective bracing (usually at night) is then usually continued for several more months.

Those children in whom hip instabilities are recognized after the newborn period may have already sustained soft-tissue contractures and adhesions. If reduction can be achieved, sustained abduction until the hip is stable (usually about three months) will usually assure a stable hip. In those hips which cannot be reduced, surgery coupled with arthrography will probably be necessary to remove the block to reduction.

One of the common blocks to reduction is the infolding of the free edge of the superolateral or posterior acetabular labrum, or limbus (Figure 4-2c); adhesions between the labrum and the joint capsule will be present. Constriction of the waist of the joint capsule (an hourglass deformity) may be present but is more frequent in the older child (Figure 4-2d) (40). Enlargement of the Haversian fibro-fatty pad may partially fill the acetabulum. When these blocks are present, surgical repair is often indicated, though some feel that these blocks will atrophy when subjected to the pressure of a femoral head pointed into the acetabulum (34).

Once reduced, the displaced hip is usually found to be most stable in abduction. Depending on the degree of in-

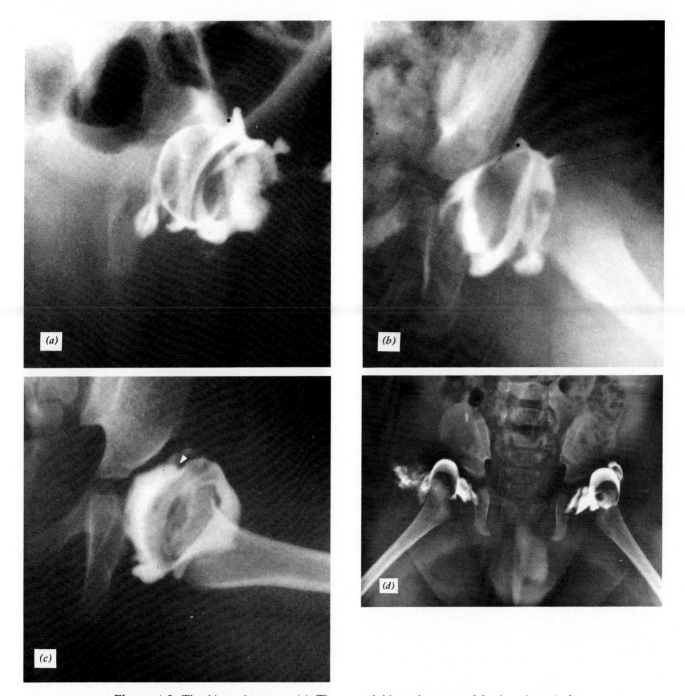

Figure 4-2. The hip arthrogram. (*a*) The normal hip arthrogram, abduction view. A dot identifies the limbus. (*b*) The subluxed hip. There is decreased acetabular coverage of the acetabulum. A dot marks the limbus. (*c*) A dislocated hip with an inverted limbus (arrow). There is increased contrast within the medial portion of the acetabulum. (*d*) An hourglass constriction of the joint capsule. Dislocated hip, five months.

stability, abduction can be maintained by the use of tripled diapers (three diapers thick), by the Frejka pillow (34) (a pillow between the legs that sustains abduction), by braces, and for the most unstable hip, a short leg spica cast (34).

Adductor tightness may accompany hip displacement, and adductor tenotomy (cutting of the adductor tendons permitting them to heal with a longer length) may be required (34).

Example 4-1. At age 3 months, during a well-baby examination, a left Ortolani hip click was detected. Asymmetric buttock skin folds were present and a diagnosis of displacement of the left hip was made. Radiographs at that time demonstrated the lateral subluxation of the left hip, which failed to reduce with abduction (Figure 4-3*a,b*).

One week later, in the orthopedic clinic, reduction was easily achieved with abduction (Figure 4-3*c*). Treatment was sustained by abduction maintained with a Frejka pillow (Figure 4-3*d*). This was later changed to a von Rosen splint (Figure 4-3*e*).

After five months of treatment, the splints were only used at night, and after nine months of use were discontinued.

At follow-up, at age three years, the hips were clinically and radiographically normal and further follow-up was considered unnecessary (Figure 4-3*f*).

Not all patients respond as readily. Careful follow-up is necessary to assure that femoral-head displacement does not recur.

Example 4-2. Dislocation of the left hip was detected during a routine newborn physical exam shortly after birth. Closed reduction was easily accomplished and the patient was treated with tripled diapers. Follow-up exams in the newborn nursery disclosed an occasional click with full abduction. At discharge, left hip abduction was minimally decreased.

One month after birth, displacement of the left hip was again detected (Figure 4-4*a,b*), and several days later an arthrogram (Figure 4-4*c,d*) demonstrated a lax capsule. No block to reduction was present; a closed reduction was accomplished and held in an abduction cast (Figure 4-4*e*).

Following removal of the cast, the hip remained located for two years. A mild adduction contracture was present.

At 27 months of age, the adduction contracture had increased and the hip had resubluxed (Figure 4-4*f*). Treatment consisted of an adductor tenotomy, with correction of the contracture and of the subluxation.

THE TREATMENT OF CONGENITAL DISPLACEMENT OF THE HIP PERSISTING TO AGE 18 MONTHS TO 3 YEARS

With early detection and treatment, very few patients will be seen in this category. Occasionally, a patient will be missed in initial screening, and sometimes a patient will fail to respond to the simpler and earlier treatments. After the age of 18 months, closed or open reduction will usually not result in a stable hip (30) due to fixed distortion in the soft tissues and the cartilaginous and bony structures. Soft-tissue repairs, coupled with operative bony realignment, will usually be required to correct the increased anterior and lateral opening of the acetabulum and the increased anteversion of the proximal femur.

The two realignments commonly used are a proximal femoral varus and derotational osteotomy to decrease anteversion and valgus deformity, and the Salter pelvic innominate bone osteotomy (Figure 4-5). The varus derotational osteotomy directs the femoral head more directly and forcefully into the acetabulum (22) and helps to mold the acetabular cartilage to a more normal shape (6,7,31,38,43). In the Salter procedure an osteotomy is cut through the supraacetabular portion of the ilium. Rotation through the symphysis pubis and ischiopubic synchrondrosis permits the reorientation of the acetabulum downward, with less opening of the acetabulum anterior and laterally. This procedure provides better coverage for the femoral head, greatly decreasing the possibility of dislocation or subluxation. Repair of the joint capsule and tenotomies to correct adduction and flexion contractures are important to the success of the procedure (38).

The results of the Salter innominate pelvic osteotomy are most successful if the femoral head is brought down to the level of the acetabulum by preoperative traction to gain adequate muscle length (muscles under tension result in too great a force on the bone of the femoral head, perhaps inducing a predisposition to Legg Perthes disease and stiffness) (38,47). Many surgeons combine the Salter

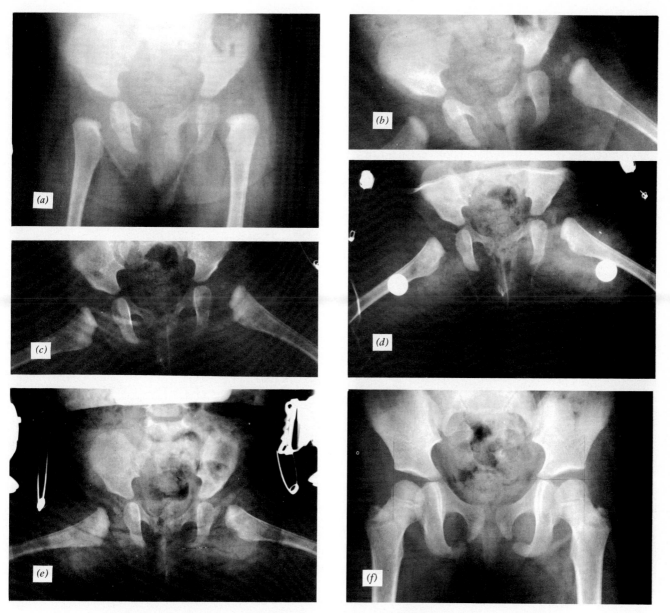

Figure 4-3. Example 4-1. Early detection and successful treatment of hip subluxation by sustained abduction. (*a*) Neutral view of the hips. The left his is subluxed. Shenton and Simons lines are broken; the minimally ossified epiphysis is displaced laterally and superiorly. (*b*) An abduction view. On this view a line drawn along the shaft of the femur should intersect the acetabulum. In this case, the line points to the iliac spine. This view differs from the von Rosen view in that the femur is externally rotated in this case, but in the von Rosen view it would be internally rotated. (*c*) Reduction in abduction. A line drawn along the femoral shaft now intersects the acetabulum. (*d*) Abduction maintained by a Frejka pillow. (*e*) Abduction maintained by a von Rosen splint. The degree of abduction is greater with the splint. (*f*) At age 3, the hips appear normal. The epiphyses lie within the inner inferior quadrant. Shenton and Simon lines are intact.

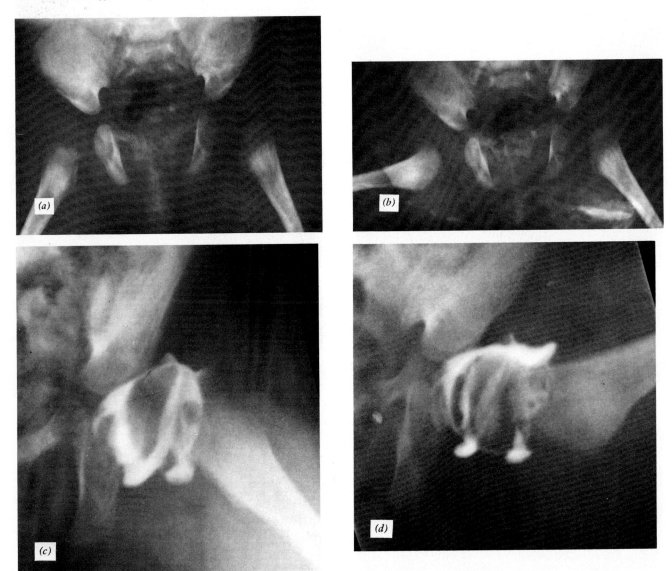

osteotomy with a proximal femoral varus derotational osteotomy to provide better coverage for the femoral head and better molding of the acetabulum and to lessen the muscle pull across the joint (6,13,38,47).

The Salter procedure often results in a minor increase in leg length. Occasionally this increase causes an excessive leg length discrepancy, resulting in a limp. Varus osteotomy combined with the Salter procedure may prevent or correct such a leg length discrepancy.

Over the age of 6 years, the cartilage of the symphysis pubis and ischiopubic synchondrosis may not permit rotation of the acetabulum. In this situation Steel's modification (44) of the Salter osteotomy can be used. Steel performs a triple osteotomy through the pubic bone, ischium, and supraacetabular portion of the ilium.

Example 4-3. This child is the daughter of a class A diabetic mother who was on Mysoline and Dilantin for

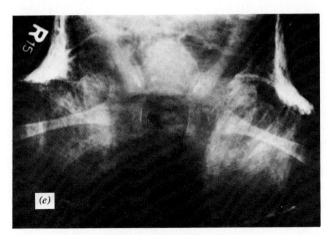

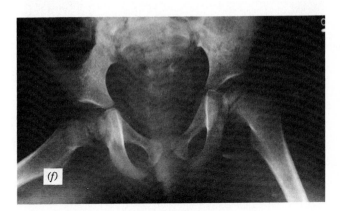

Figure 4-4. Example 4-2. Hip dislocation treated with reduction and sustained abduction. Adduction deformity with late recurrence of subluxation. (*a*) At 1 month of age, the proximal left femur is displaced laterally and sueriorly. Shenton and Simon lines are interrupted. Minimal lateral subluxation of the right hip may also be present. (*b*) The abduction view demonstrates left adduction deformity. The right hip is located; the left hip remains subluxed. (*c*) Left hip arthrogram. Joint laxity is present. The femoral head is subluxed laterally: increased contrast media is present in the medial portion of the acetabulum. The limbus is normal. (*d*) Following reduction in abduction, the femoral head is well centered within the acetabulum. The limbus is normal. (*e*) Treated in an abduction cast. The hips are located. If hip anatomy cannot be seen adequately through the cast, a single tomographic sectional view may be helpful. (*f*) Patient at 27 months of age; an abduction view demonstrates adduction deformity of the left femur. The slope of the left acetabular roof is increased.

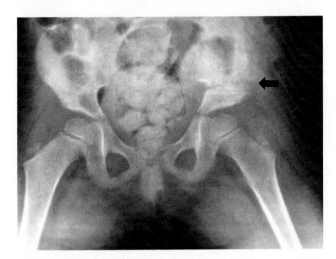

Figure 4-5. Salter osteotomy left ilium, used for treatment of a congenitally subluxing hip. Wedge-shaped bone graft (arrow) has been placed within the iliac osteotomy to redirect the acetabulum downward and anteriorly.

seizure disorder (birth weight of child: 2,960 grams with an Apgar of 9). At birth there was no evidence of hip dislocation or Ortolani click. The child was in the third percentile and was followed closely for complaints of failure to thrive. It was eventually decided that this was a small child who was the daughter of a small mother and small father and otherwise normal; however in the third month, during a follow-up visit, the child was noted to have a trace of adductor spasm, and by 4 months she exhibited a right Ortolani click with slight asymmetry of the posterior skin folds of the buttock. This condition was treated by an abduction brace for 1 year. Follow-up was continued, and at the age of 3 years, because of complaints of occasional pain in the left hip and a radiograph showing continued subluxation (Figure 4-6*a,b*), the patient was admitted for surgical treatment. Hip motion was equal bilaterally and was normal. An arthrogram (Figure 4-6*c*) performed at the time of surgery revealed borderline cartilaginous coverage of the left femoral head, of a type that

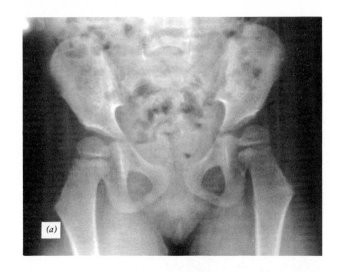

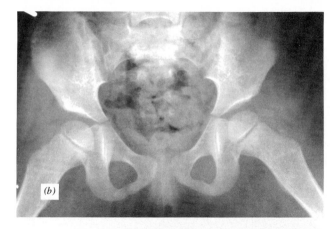

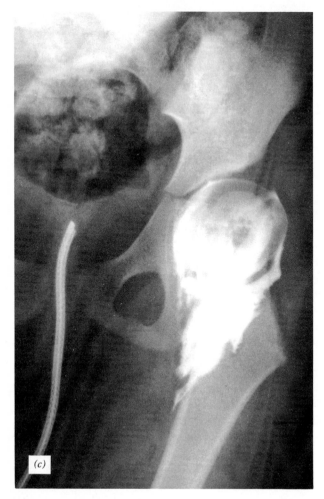

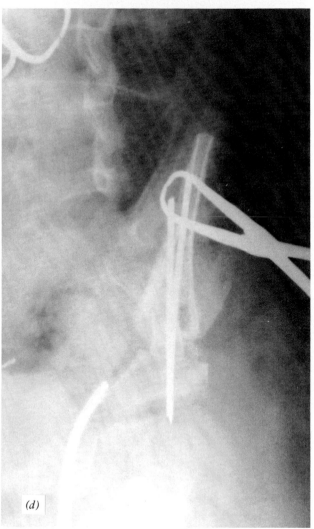

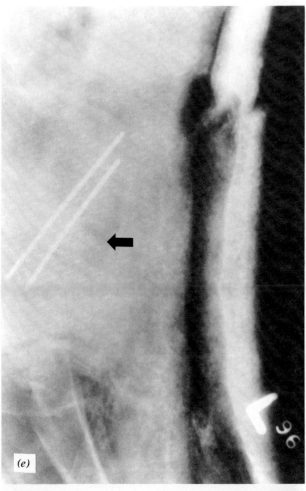

(e)

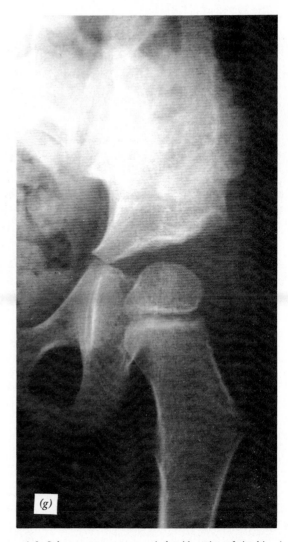

(g)

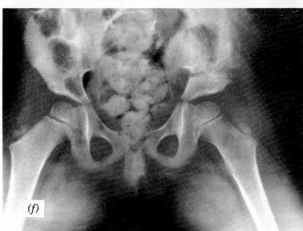

(f)

Figure 4-6. Salter osteotomy, congenital subluxation of the hip. (*a,b*) Appearance of hips at age 3. The left femoral head is minimally laterally and superiorly subluxed with a slightly increased acetabular angle. Shenton line is disrupted. (*c*) Intraoperative arthrogram disclosing slight lateral uncovering of the femoral head. (*d*) Intraoperative lateral view of the acetabulum demonstrates two K wires holding the wedge-shaped bone graft (arrow) and the redirected acetabulum. (*e*) Postoperative view in plaster demonstrates the two K wires holding the bone graft (arrow) and the acetabulum in the desired positions. (*f*) View one month following surgery demonstrates the improvement of the left acetabular angle. (*g*) Three-month postoperative view demonstrates the healed Salter osteotomy with its resulting deformity of the ilium.

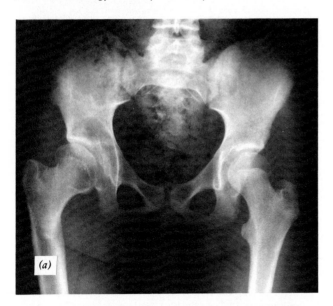

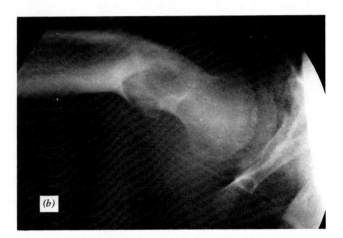

Figure 4-7. Patient at age 15; the residua of the right femoral varus derotational osteotomy and right Salter osteotomy can be recognized. (*a*) The right acetabulum remains shallow, with a minimally upwardly sloping roof. Minimal elongation of the femoral head is apparent. (*b*) The lateral view demonstrates probable retroversion of the proximal femur used to achieve better placement of the femoral head within the acetabulum.

would probably be improved by a Salter osteotomy. The Salter osteotomy was performed (Figure 4-6*d,e*), and the child was doing well first at 1 month and then at 3 months postsurgery (Figure 4-6*f,g*).

The Salter innominate osteotomy is most successful when the acetabulum and femoral head are no more than minimally deformed, limiting its use to the younger child (47). Continual subluxation of the hip will usually result in widening of the acetabulum with distortion of its superolateral rim (28). Eventually, the lateral rim will slope superiorly, resulting in a smooth, gliding surface for subluxation. Occasionally, a pseudoacetabulum is formed superior and posterior to the true acetabulum. A Salter osteotomy performed once deformity is present will usually fail to restore normal joint mechanics. Figure 4-7*a,b* is of a patient, age 15 years, who had had a varus osteotomy at age 4 and a Salter osteotomy at age 6, by which time acetabular deformity was presumably present. At age 15, acetabular deformity with a sloping roof and elongation of

the femoral head are present. Despite the slight deformity of the acetabulum, the function of the two hips is considered normal.

This patient's Salter osteotomy was performed at age 6, presumably following the development of deformity of the acetabulum. The residual deformity would be expected in future years to predispose the development of degenerative arthritis. The Salter osteotomy is best limited to patients whose acetabulum is of near normal appearance.

TREATMENT, AGE 3 AND UP

Acetabuloplasty

When there is deformity with enlargement of the acetabulum, several alternative procedures are available in which the acetabulum is reformed—the acetabuloplasty (4,5,9,10,15,27). Under the age of 4, restoration of joint congruence may result in acceptable remodeling of the acetabulum without acetabuloplasty (22). Above the age of 4, spontaneous remodeling to a congruent shape may not occur and it may be necessary to perform an acetabuloplasty. The eventual prognosis of the hip in a patient with a shallow acetabulum is closely related to the degree of acetabular coverage of the lateral portion of the femoral head. The less the degree of coverage, the greater the chance of degenerative arthritis. This may be measured by Wiberg's center-edge angle, which is further discussed in Chapter 6, page 99. The acetabuloplasty increases the lateral coverage of the femoral head by reshaping the acetabulum. The procedure currently in widest use is the Pemberton acetabuloplasty (33,46,47,16). (See Figure 4-8a,b,c). In this procedure, the bone just superior to the acetabulum is cut, with the osteotomy reaching to the Y cartilage in the medial acetabulum. This thin shelf of bone is then shaped to fit the size of the femoral head closely and is then held in place by bone graft. Although some skill is required to form an acetabulum of the proper size, the results are usually quite good, with bony growth and remodeling correcting the minor irregularities frequently seen on the initial postoperative films. The deformed acetabulum is too open laterally and anteriorly, thereby permitting subluxation; the Pemberton procedure wraps the acetabulum around the femoral head, decreasing the chance of subluxation.

The Pemberton acetabuloplasty depends on the flexibility of the Y cartilage of the acetabulum and of the supraacetabular bone. Prior to age 3, the bone is too soft (16), and after age 7 the acetabular cartilage lacks sufficient flexibility to be bent to the shape of the femoral head. Femoral-head deformity is a contraindication for this procedure, and this deformity is frequently present after the age of 7. Because of this situation, one of several other procedures may be needed after the age of seven.

The Colonna Procedure

In those patients with a shallow acetabulum, the Colonna capsular arthroplasty can be used to provide a deep acetabulum (9,10,40) (Figure 4-9). In this procedure, traction is used to bring the femoral head to the level of the acetabulum. The acetabulum is then curetted to form a deep and adequate acetabulum. The joint capsule is then placed over the femoral head and the hip reduced. The patient is casted for four weeks, followed by active rehabilitation in order to restore joint motion. This is a form of fascial interposition arthroplasty, which historically is a forerunner of the cup-mold arthroplasty discussed in Chapter 13.

The Chiari Osteotomy

The Chiari osteotomy (8) (Figure 4-10a,b) is a medial displacement osteotomy of the acetabulum, or pseudoacetabulum, which can be used successfully for many types of hip problems from about age 5 into adulthood (6,11,30,39,46,47). This procedure is designed to deepen the acetabulum by forming a bony buttress over the more lateral aspect of the joint capsule. This is accomplished by cutting the bone just superior to the capsular attachment, along the superior aspect of the acetabulum, and extending this osteotomy medially across the ilium entering the pelvis. This permits the medial displacement of the acetabulum by 1 to 3 cm, thus providing a bony support over the more lateral aspect of the joint capsule. In addition to providing coverage for the femoral head, this medial displacement also corrects the lateral drift of the femoral head resulting from the congenital displacement, thus reducing the force across the hip on weight bearing (8,47). It is important that the amount of displacement be sufficient to give good coverage of the femoral head. It is better to have too much rather than too little displacement.

The Chiari osteotomy requires careful postsurgical rehabilitation, (47) but when this is done, the new acetabulum with its lateral support will frequently become smooth. It is thought that the joint capsule subjected to the stress of weight bearing undergoes metaplasia into a firm fibrous tissue, resulting in a smooth articular surface.

The Chiari osteotomy is most suited for unilateral problems, as there is the potential danger that bilateral procedures in females may narrow the birth canal sufficiently to cause dystocia. There have been, however, two cases reported of successful vaginal delivery following bilateral Chiari osteotomy. The use of the procedure is described in Example 5-4, a patient with cerebral palsy.

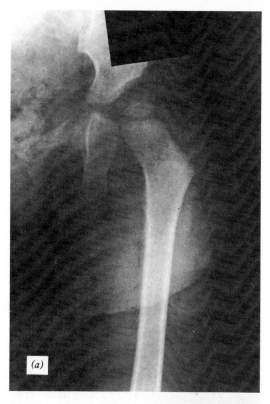

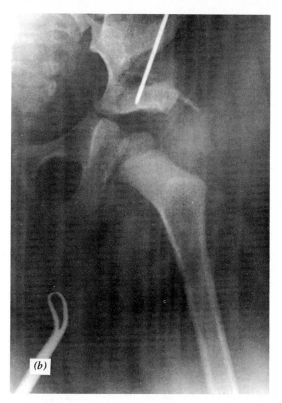

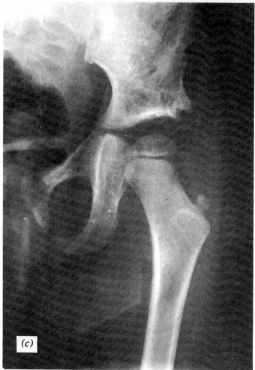

Figure 4-8. The Pemberton acetabuloplasty. (*a*) Preoperative view. There is increased slope to the acetabular roof. The femoral head is displaced superolaterally. (*b*) Early postoperative view. The acetabular roof has been molded around the femoral head. (*c*) A late postoperative view. Good coverage of the femoral head is present. Only minimal lateral displacement of the femoral head is present. (Case courtesy of Dr. Lynn Staheli, Seattle).

TREATMENT FROM LATE CHILDHOOD INTO ADULTHOOD

The Shelf Procedure

Beyond the age of 3, the hip muscles of a dislocated hip are shortened, and the initial lengthening of the hip muscles prior to surgery becomes progressively more difficult. Occasionally, despite several months of preoperative traction, reduction is not possible.

Many procedures have been devised to form a bony shelf above an irreducibly dislocated hip. These procedures are most helpful in cases where the femoral head cannot be brought down opposite the acetabulum by preoperative

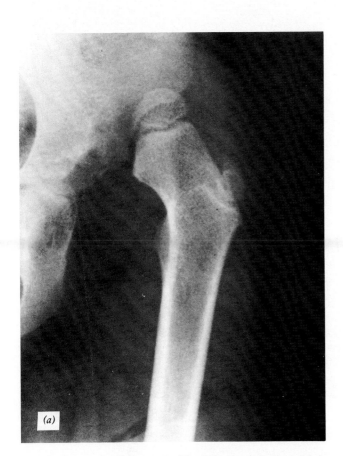

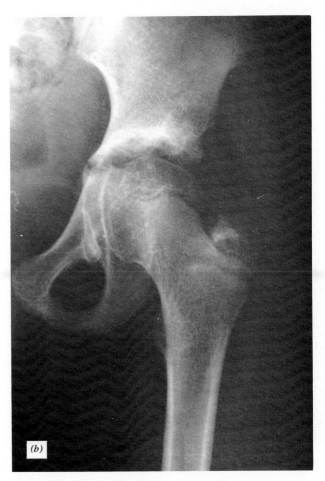

Figure 4-9. The Colonna procedure. (*a*) A preoperative view. The femur is dislocated and riding high. The femoral head articulates with a pseudoacetabulum on the iliac crest. (*b*) A late postoperative view. Following traction to bring the femoral head to the level of the true acetabulum and reaming of the acetabulum to deepen it, the joint capsule was interposed in the hip joint; following extensive rehabilitation and growth, the femoral head lies within a well-formed acetabulum. It is well covered and is not subluxed. (Case courtesy of Dr. Lynn Staheli, Seattle).

traction and in the older child or adolescent whose acetabulum can no longer be easily reshaped by the previously described methods (50). In these situations, it is possible to create a shelf of bone just superior to the best obtainable position of the femoral head to prevent subluxation (1,3,4,5,12,14,20,23,27,48,50) (Figures 4-11 and 4-12). Although these procedures do not give as good results as those previously described, they still are occa-

sionally necessary. Though the result may not be ideal, it is often a useful intermediate step, permitting a delay in the need for total hip-joint replacement prosthesis or other arthroplasty.

Example 4-4. This 60-year-old woman presented with degenerative arthritis of the right hip. The patient's history is of bilateral congenital dislocation of the hip,

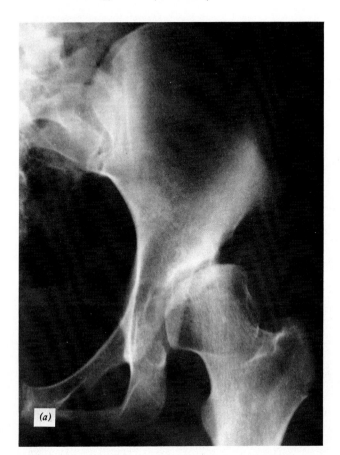 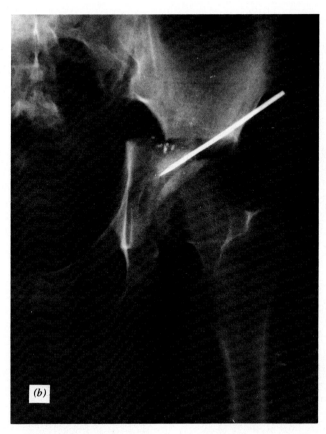

Figure 4-10. The Chiari osteotomy. (*a*) Preoperative view. The sloping of the acetabulum and the flattening of the femoral head are secondary to a chronically subluxing hip. (*b*) Postoperative view. The supra-acetabular osteotomy has been transfixed with a K wire following medial displacement of the acetabulum. Following this displacement, the coverage of the femoral head is highly improved.

unresponsive to initial therapy, with persisting subluxation. In her teenage years she developed increasing pain in both hips, and at that age of 19 she had a shelf operation performed on the right hip. A different surgical procedure (a Girdlestone arthroplasty, Chapter 15) was used on the left hip. She did well for many years, but at age 60 required treatment for right hip pain. A total hip arthroplasty was performed. The radiographs (Figure 4-11) demonstrate displacement of the femoral head superolaterally. The femoral head no longer articulates with the original acetabulum but lies in a pseudoacetabulum. The

lateral aspect of the pseudoacetabulum is covered by a shelf of bone, which consists of bone graft taken from the lateral aspect of the iliac crest. The cartilage between the pseudoacetabulum and the femoral head was found to be worn through in several areas, a manifestation of degenerative arthritis.

Shelf operations are occasionally used to deepen a shallow acetabulum.

Example 4-5. The clinical history of this 23-year-old man is vague because of mental retardation due to a severe head

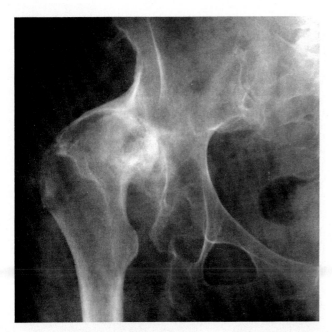

Figure 4-11. Example 4-3. Forty-one years after a shelf arthroplasty for a congenitally dislocated hip. The femoral head articulates with the operative shelf of bone superior to it. This shelf has been placed superior to the pseudoacetabulum. Marked cartilage narrowing, moderate sclerosis, and medially placed femoral head osteophytes are indicative of secondary degenerative arthritis.

injury at age 15. The history available indicates that surgery had been performed for a partial dislocation of the right hip. The age at the time of the operation is uncertain. The radiograph (Figure 4-12) demonstrates a shelf of bone graft incorporated into the normal acetabulum, deepening it. The source of the bone graft is the lateral aspect of the right ilium.

Shelf procedures are uncommon now because of their high rate of failure. The bone graft either may not grow or may resorb, often resulting in a recurrence of the disability (5,48). In addition, because of the shortening involved in the maintenance of the pseudoacetabulum, gait is often awkward (14). For these reasons, it has been recommended that nothing be done for these patients until pain is sufficient to warrant hip replacement (46); however, a successful shelf procedure is useful in the management of selected patients (48,50).

The Subtrochanteric Angulation Osteotomy

The case of the patient with untreated bilateral hip dislocation presenting in late childhood or teenage years is frequently not amenable to the previously described methods of treatment. Pain may be no problem even into the fifth or sixth decade; however, fatigue is common. Each step may be difficult, with the femur gliding along the ilium until the femoral shaft shifts against the ilium and becomes stabilized. These patients tire quickly because of the marked muscular exertion involved. One method of ameliorating this mechanical inefficiency is the Schanz angulation osteotomy (19,35). In this procedure, a valgus osteotomy is performed at the level of the ischial ramus, which changes the ilium from a gliding surface into a relatively fixed weight-bearing surface. Mechanical efficiency

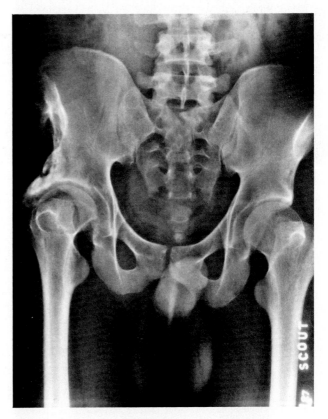

Figure 4-12. A right shelf arthroplasty performed to deepen a shallow acetabulum to prevent hip subluxation.

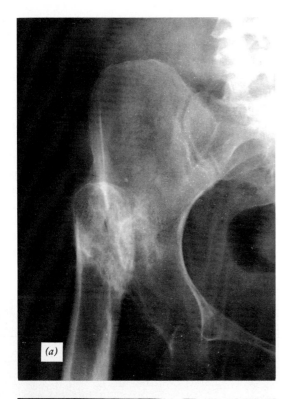

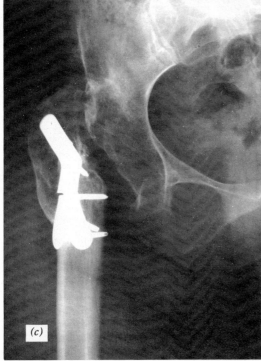

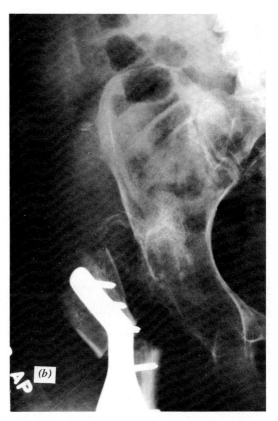

Figure 4-13. Milch osteotomy for late deformity of congenitally dislocated hip. (*a*) Age 43. The femoral head is flattened and merges with the neck. The femur articulates with a verticle pseudoacetabulum. The minimal sclerosis may reflect the degenerative arthritis found at surgery. (*b*) At 43. One month following surgery. The valgus osteotomy held by a Batchelor plate can be seen. There is minimal ectopic bone formation superior to the pseudoacetabulum. (*c*) Age 53. The healed valgus osteotomy can be seen. The Batchelor plate has broken.

is improved, and although gait is still awkward, the distance the patient can walk without fatigue or pain is much increased.

Batchelor and Milch also used a simlar valgus angulation arthroplasty combined with the Girdlestone resection of the femoral head and neck (Figure 4-13*b*). This technique is usually used in adults as a salvage procedure (Chapter 15, page 291). The valgus osteotomy permits a transfer of force from the sloping lateral wall of the pelvis to the now-angled proximal femur.

Example 4-6. This 51-year-old woman was first diagnosed as having a dislocated right hip at age 2 years. An open reduction at that time was of limited success, and at age 8 she had severe right hip pain. When seen again at age 39, the pain was severe and a grinding sensation could be felt on examination. At age 43 (Figure 4-13*a*), the femoral head is so flattened that it is unidentifiable and a vertical femoral-pseudoacetabular articulation is present. A pelvic-support osteotomy was performed (Milch osteotomy), with resection of a very deformed femoral head and with a valgus subtrochanteric osteotomy (Figure 4-13*b*). Six months postoperatively, the patient was dancing at a wedding and developed sudden, but transitory, pain (probably associated with the breakage of the metal plate). When seen at age 53 (Figure 4-13*c*), the patient had free motion of the right hip with no pain and no crepitus.

SUMMARY

Surgical treatment of congenital displacement of the hip varies with the age of diagnosis and the degree of deformity present. The most common procedures are closed reduction or open soft-tissue repairs in the first 18 months of life. From 18 months to 3 years of age, one of two surgical procedures are most likely to be of greatest usefulness. If the acetabulum and femoral head are of normal shape, varus derotational osteotomy and/or the Salter pelvic innominate osteotomy are useful. If the acetabulum is misshapen, an acetabuloplasty permits correction of this deformity. Beyond the age of 3 years, the choice of procedure becomes greater, and the quality of results of each procedure becomes poorer. The Colonna arthroplasty and the Pemberton acetabuloplasty may be used to age 6. Beyond this age, the Chiari medial displacement osteotomy and the shelf procedures are available. By late childhood and teenage years, some patients will be seen who are not suitable for the Chiari osteotomy. In these patients, the valgus angulation osteotomy may be effective for symptomatic relief of marked fatigue in walking;

however, a markedly abnormal gait will persist, and most of these patients will be considered candidates for total hip replacement (see Example 14-11).

REFERENCES

1. Anderson ME, Bickel Wm.: Shelf operation for congenital subluxation and dislocation of the hip. *J Bone Joint Surg* 33A:87–102, 1951.
2. Barlow TG: Early diagnosis and treatment of congenital dislocation of the hip. *J Bone Joint Surg* 44B:292–301, 1962.
3. Bickel Wm, et al: Shelf operation for congenital subluxation and dislocation of the hip. *Clin Orthop* 106:27–34, 1975.
4. Bosworth D, et al: Hip shelves in children. *J Bone Joint Surg* 42A:1223–1238, 1960.
5. Chapchral G: Indications for the various types of pelvic osteotomies. *Clin Orthop* 98:111–115, 1974.
6. Chapchral G: The intertrochanteric osteotomy in the treatment of congenital dysplasia of the hip. *Clin Orthop* 119:54–59, 1976.
7. Chiari, K: Medial displacement osteotomy of the pelvis. *Clin Orthop* 98:55–71, 1974.
8. Colonna PC: Arthroplasty of the hip joint for congenital dislocation in children. *J Bone Joint Surg* 29:711–721, 1947.
9. Colonna PC: Capsular arthroplasty for CDH. *J Bone Joint Surg* 35A:179–197, 1953.
10. Colton CL: Chiari osteotomy for acetabular dysplasic in young subjects. *J Bone Joint Surg* 54B:578–589, 1972.
11. Compere E, Phemister D: The tibial peg in CDH. *J Bone Joint Surg* 17:60–72, 1935.
12. Crellin RQ: Innominate osteotomy for congenital dislocation and subluxation of the hip. *Clin Orthop* 98:171–177, 1974.
13. Dickson F: The shelf operation in treatment of congenital dislocation of the hip. *J Bone Joint Surg* 17:43–47, 1935.
14. Eyre-Brook AL: Treatment of congenital dislocation or subluxation of the hip in children over the age of three years. *J Bone Joint Surg* 48B:682–692, 1966.
15. Eyre-Brook AL, Jones DA, Harris FC: Pemberton's acetabuloplasty for congenital dislocation or subluxation of the hip. *J Bone Joint Surg* 60B:18–24, 1978.
16. Finlay HVL, et al: Dislocatable hip and dislocated hip in the newborn infant. *Br Med J* IV:377–381, 1967.
17. Fredensborg N: The results of early treatment of typical congenital dislocation of the hip in malmo. *J Bone Joint Surg* 58B:272–278, 1976.
18. Gaenshen FJ: The Schanz subtrochanteric osteotomy for irriducible dislocation of the hip. *J Bone Joint Surg* 17:76–87, 1935.

19. Ghormley RK: Use of the anterior superior spine and crest of ilium in surgery of the hip joint. *J Bone Joint Surg* 13:784–798, 1931.

20. Gill AB: Plastic construction of an acetabulum in congenital dislocation of the hip—The shelf operation. *J Bone Joint Surg* 17:48–59, 1935.

21. Grech P: *Hip Arthrography*. Philadelphia, JB Lippincott Company, 1977.

22. Harris NH, Lloyd-Roberts GC, Gallien R: Acetabular development in congenital dislocation of the hip with special reference to the indications for acetabuloplasty and pelvic or femoral realignment osteotomy. *J Bone Joint Surg* 57B:46–52, 1975.

23. Heyman C: Long-term results following a bone-shelf operation for congenital and some other dislocations of the hip in children. *J Bone Joint Surg* 45A:1113–1146, 1963.

24. Hiertonn, T, James U: Congential dislocation of the hip: Experiences of early diagnosis and treatment. *J Bone Joint Surg* 50B:542–545, 1968.

25. Laurenson RD: The acetabular index: A critical review. *J Bone Joint Surg* 41B:702–710, 1959.

26. Laurenson RD: Development of the acetabular roof in the fetal hip. *J Bone Joint Surg* 47A:975–983, 1965.

27. Massie Wm K, Howorth MB: Congenital dislocation of the hip. Part II. Results of open reduction as seen in the early adult period. *J Bone Joint Surg* 33A:171–190, 1951.

28. Massie Wm K, Howorth MB: Congenital dislocation of the hip. Part III. Pathogenesis. *J Bone Joint Surg* 33A:190–198, 1951.

29. Mitchell GP: Arthrography in congenital displacement of the hip. *J Bone Joint Surg* 45B:88–95, 1963.

30. Mitchell GP: Chiari medial displacement osteotomy. *Clin Orthop* 98:146–150, 1974.

31. Monticelli G: Intertrochanteric femoral osteotomy with concentric reduction of the femoral head in treatment of residual congenital acetabular dysplasia. *Clin Orthop* 119:48–53, 1976.

32. Palmen K: Preluxation of the hip joint. *Acta Paediatrica* 50(Suppl 129), 1975.

33. Pemberton PA: Pericapsular osteotomy of the ilium for the treatment of congenitally dislocated hips. *Clin Orthop* 98:41–54, 1974.

34. Ponseti IV: Non-surgical treatment of congenital dislocation of the hip. *J Bone Joint Surg* 48A:1392–1403, 1966.

35. Ring PA: The treatment of irreduced congenital dislocation of the hip in adults. *J Bone Joint Surg* 41B:299–313, 1959.

36. Rosen S von: Diagnosis and treatment of congenital dislocation of the hip in the newborn. *J Bone Joint Surg* 44B:284–291, 1962.

37. Rosen S von: Further experience with congenital dislocation of the hip in the newborn. *J Bone Joint Surg* 50B:538–545, 1968.

38. Salter RB: Ostetomy of the pelvis—editorial comment. *Clin Orthop* 98:2–4, 1974.

39. Salvati E, Wilson PD: Treatment of irreducible hip subluxation by Chiari's iliac osteotomy. *Clin Orthop* 98:151–161, 1974.

40. Sharrad WJW: *Paediatric Orthopaedics and Fractures*. Oxford and Edinburgh, Blackwell Scientific Publications, 1971, pp 148–186.

41. Simon G: *Principles of Bone X-ray Diagnosis*. Washington, Butterworths, 1965, pp 25–27.

42. Smaill GB: Congenital dislocation of the hip in the newborn. *J Bone Joint Surg* 50B:524–536, 1968.

43. Somerville EW: A Long-term follow-up of congenital dislocation of the hip. *J Bone Joint Surg* 60B:25–30, 1978.

44. Steel HH: Triple osteotomy of the innominate bone. *J Bone Joint Surg* 55A:343–350, 1973.

45. Stewart SF: Congenital dislocation of the hip. *J Bone Joint Surg* 17:11–17, 1935.

46. Tachdjian M: *Pediatric Orthopedics*. Philadelphia, W B Saunders, 1972, pp 135, 160–167, 228–230.

47. Utterback T, MacEwen GD: Comparison of pelvic osteotomies for the surgical correction of the congenital hip. *Clin Orthop* 98:104–110, 1974.

48. Wainwright D: The shelf operation for hip dysplasis in adolescence, abstracted. *J Bone Joint Surg* 56B:563, 1974.

49. Wedge JH Salter RB: Innominate osteotomy: Its role in the arrest of secondary degenerative arthritis of the hip in the adult. *Clin Orthop* 98:214–224, 1974.

50. Wilson JC: Surgical treatment of the dysplastic acetabulum in the adolescent. *Clin Orthop* 98:137–145, 1974.

5
Surgery in Neurogenic Dysfunction of the Hip

Normal motion of the hip and the absence of dislocation and subluxation depend on a balance of muscular forces around the hip, as well as on a relatively normal configuration of the femur and acetabulum. Surgery for neurogenic dysfunction may therefore involve both muscle-transfer operations and operations to improve the shape and depth of the acetabulum or to change the orientation of the femoral neck; these latter operations are those used in congenital displacement of the hip.

Surgical correction of the hip for neurogenic dysfunction is now most commonly seen in the treatment of myelomeningocele patients and is less often necessary in patients with cerebral palsy.

MENINGOMYELOCELE PATIENTS

Correction of the hip subluxation and dislocation is important in myelomeningocele patients in order to improve their ambulation and to increase the percentage of time spent in the upright position. Enabling these children to assume an upright posture promotes urinary drainage, decreases the incidence of bedsores, and is often of psychological benefit.

Meningomyelocele patients can be subdivided according to the level of neurologic impairment (9,12). In Sharrard's

(12) report of 183 children with myelomeningocele, the incidence of hip abnormality and the choice of a method for treatment depended on the level of innervation. Since the innervation of each of the hips in a child may be at different levels, different treatments may be used on each side.

T-12 Level

In children with normal innervation only to the T-12 level, the hip muscles are flaccid. In Sharrard's group of 65 hips, there were no hip dislocations, but 10 of 65 hips did sublux. Thirty-two of the 65 developed valgus femoral necks. Surgical correction of the hip was usually not necessary.

L1-L2 Level

Those children with an L1 or L2 level demonstrated weak abductors. In Sharrard's series, 8 of 60 hips had dislocated and 38 of 60 hips had subluxed. Valgus deformity was common. These children's hips usually respond quite well to varus osteotomy and adductor tenotomy (cutting of the adductor tendons).

Varus osteotomy (Figure 5-1b) of the femur is important in the correction of the hip displaced by neuro-

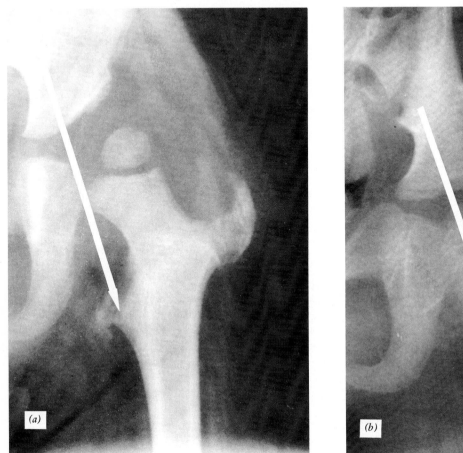
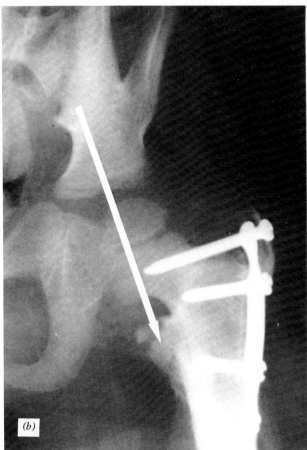

Figure 5-1. (*a*) Valgus deformity of the proximal femur with arrows indicating the path of the iliopsoas tendon. With a valgus proximal femur, the iliopsoas tendon lies medial to the femoral head and fails to act as a hip stabilizer. (*b*) Following varus derotational osteotomy, the iliopsoas tendon (arrows indicate its location) now provides a medially directed force across the hip, helping to stabilize it.

genic dysfunction. During growth, patients lacking pull on the greater trochanter tend to develop a valgus femoral neck, usually with increased anteversion. Both the valgus and the anteversion deformities increase the chance of subluxation and dislocation, because they redirect the pull of the psoas muscle. With normal alignment, the psoas muscle tendon crosses the femoral neck lateral to the femoral head, and its pull helps to hold the femoral head reduced (Figure 5-2). With the development of valgus de-

formity, as the neck-shaft angle approaches 180°, the psoas tendon will cross medial to the center of the femoral head and will tend to pull the head superiorly and laterally (Figure 5-1*a,b*). In the myelodysplastic child with weak gluteal muscles, the iliopsoas may be the only active muscle pulling the femoral head into the acetabulum; its maldirection will therefore lead to subluxation and dislocation of the femoral head. In these patients, a varus osteotomy will redirect the psoas pull medially across the hip joint (Figure 5-1b). Similarly, the increasing anteversion of the femoral neck may bring the center of the femoral head anterior to the psoas tendon, changing it from a posteriorly directed reducing force on the hip to an anteriorly directed subluxing force. A combined varus and derotational osteotomy can be used to correct these abnormal alignments (14,15).

Hip dislocation may also occur in the myelodysplastic child with a short limb and a pelvic tilt. When the femoral neck-pelvic Y-Y cartilage line angle approaches 90°, the psoas tendon alignment is shifted so that it is directed medially to the center of the femoral head. If the glutei are weak, subluxations and dislocations may occur. Treatment

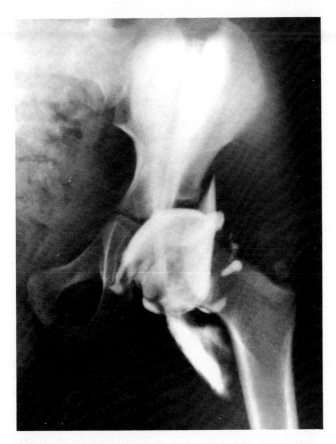

Figure 5-2. An accidental injection of contrast material into psoas tendon sheath demonstrates its position. (Performed in a patient with Legg-Perthes disease).

with a shoe lift may be successful, but in some patients a varus osteotomy is needed (14,15).

L3-L4 Level

Normal innervation of the L3 or L4 level results in near normal innervation of the hip flexors and adductors, with weak or absent hip extensors and abductors. In Sharrard's series, 72 of the 85 hips with an L3-L4 level were dislocated, and the remaining hips were subluxed. These patients have valgus femoral necks and benefit from varus osteotomies and adductor tenotomies; the benefit is, however, usually shortlived and redislocation is common 2 to 4 years following surgery, due to recurrence of the valgus deformity.

Correction of the muscle imbalance is necessary to prevent recurrent valgus. This correction could be achieved by increasing the force on the greater trochanter or by decreasing the force on the lesser trochanter. In 1952, W. T. Mustard (7) described a transfer operation of the iliopsoas tendon from its normal insertion on the lesser trochanter anterolaterally through a notch or hole cut in the iliac crest to insert on the greater trochanter (Figure 5-3a,b). This operation (usually performed by Mustard for the treatment of patients with poliomyelitis) changed the function of the iliopsoas muscle from a hip flexor to a weak hip abductor. By doing this, Dr. Mustard removed a deforming force across the hip and used it to substitute for the absent hip abductors. He later extended the use of this operation to patients with myelomeningocele (8).

In 1959, W. J. W. Sharrard modified Mustard's approach by transferring the iliopsoas tendon posterolaterally through a hole cut in the iliac crest to insert on the posterior aspect of the greater trochanter of the femur (13), providing greater replacement for the stabilizing function of the weak gluteal maximus (Figure 5-4c). While this approach is theoretically superior to Mustard's approach, each procedure has its advocates (1,2,3,6,13,15), and the few statistical comparisons seem to disclose no significant difference in the eventual degree of hip disability or complications (6,10).

The Mustard and Sharrard procedures are effective in myelomeningocele patients with an L3 or L4 level both because they remove the deforming flexion force of the psoas

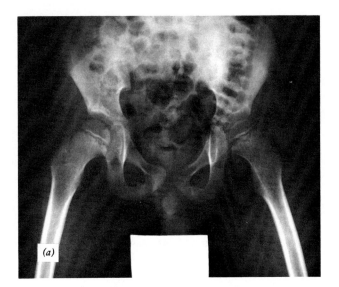 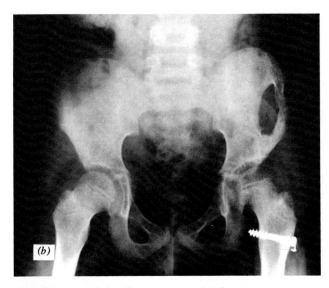

Figure 5-3. Mustard procedure. The hole in the lateral aspect of the iliac crest permits the iliopsoas tendon to pass anterolaterally to its new insertion on the greater trochanter.

muscle and because they form an active tenodesis, replacing the weak or absent abductors. These procedures usually do not result in active abduction, but they do allow support of the pelvis during ambulation, preventing a Trendelenburg gait by the active contraction of the iliopsoas. Hence it is termed an active tenodesis—"active" referring to the muscular activity and "tenodesis" referring to a type of operation in which a tendon is used to substitute for a ligament holding the two sides of a joint together (1,13).

The Sharrard and Mustard procedures are best limited to those patients with an L3 or L4 level, as their effective functioning depends on the presence of an adequate sartorius muscle (hip flexor) to preserve hip flexion (7,13,15). Sartorius muscle function is limited in children who have an L1 or L2 level. Its presence in children with an L3 or L4 level permits success with the Sharrard procedures.

The complications of the Sharrard and Mustard iliopsoas muscle transfers are similar, with a 20 to 30% incidence of pathologic fractures of the femur, most occurring at the time of the removal of the cast, and a 10 to 25% incidence of avascular necrosis of the femoral head (1,3,6,9,10). The transferred tendon can become detached

and, if marked with a metal suture, can be identified. Reoperation may or may not be indicated (9).

Occasionally, the Sharrard and Mustard procedures are combined with acetabular reshaping or redirecting procedures that are discussed in the chapter on the treatment of congenital displacement of the hip (1,2,5,6,15).

Example 5-1. This 7-year-old boy's problem started at birth, at which time he was noted to have a meningomyelocele and hydrocephalus. He had a motor level at L2-L3 and L3-L4 and a sensory level at T12. A ventriculoperitoneal shunt was performed for hydrocephalus. His dislocation was noted at 1 day of age and was treated with temporary success by leg casts for six weeks. By 1 year of age subluxation of the left hip had recurred, with minimal lateral displacement of the femoral-head epiphysis (Figure 5-4a). By 3 years of age (Figure 5-4b), the child had recurrent marked subluxations of the left hip, and later that same year the left hip dislocated and could not be reduced by closed methods. At this time the child was found to have functioning adductors, a functioning psoas muscle, and equivocal poor function of the quadriceps. Minimal hamstring function was also present. Evaluation was compatible with a level between L2-3 and L3-4. He had a left Sharrard transfer and was placed in long leg braces (Figure 5-4c). By 4½ years of age, the left hip was again beginning to sublux (Figure 5-4d). There was valgus deformity of the proximal femur. This was treated supportively until the child was 5 years of age, at which time a varus osteotomy was performed (Figure 5-4e). At the child's last visit at the age of 5, physical examination demonstrated a 30° flexion contracture of the right knee. The right leg was 2 cm shorter than the left. The child is ambulatory using quad-canes, with a reciprocal trunk gait. The child's ileal loop is functioning well and there have been no recent urinary-tract infections.

L-5 Level

Seven of 27 hip cases with an L5 level in Sharrard's series had dislocated hips, and 12 of 27 had subluxated hips. Patients with this level still show muscle imbalance with normal hip flexors, opposed by poor to good hip extensors and abductors. They usually respond well to varus osteotomy of the proximal femur (13,15).

It is uncommon for patients with lower levels of neurologic impairment to have significant hip disability.

POLIOMYELITIS

Fortunately poliomyelitis is now rarely seen. The flaccid paralysis of specific muscle groups, however, respond well to selected muscle transfer operations, including the Mustard and Sharrard procedures (7,8,13,15), as well as the procedures used for congenital displacement of the hip.

Example 5-2. The patient is a 63-year-old woman who had poliomyelitis affecting the right leg at age 2 years. In addition she had a history of dislocation of the right hip, either a congenital dislocation of the hip or one associated with the muscle weakness of poliomyelitis. Between the ages of 2 and 6, several tendon transfers were performed on the right leg. By age 19, because of continued subluxation of the right hip, a shelf of bone was placed above the dislocated right hip. At age 46, the patient had a distal femoral osteotomy for degenerative arthritis of the knee. At

age 63 (Figure 5-5), she presented with increasing pain and disability from her right hip. At the time of surgery it was found that there was no cartilage between the head of the femur and the bony shelf. A total hip replacement was performed with good results.

CEREBRAL PALSY

Hip dislocation in spastic paresis usually will respond to adductor tenotomy and selected nerve sectioning. In many patients with spastic paresis, additional surgery is not necessary. Occasionally a Salter or a Sharrard procedure is helpful (4). In one series (11) of very severely affected, chronically hospitalized patients, however, the incidence of subluxation and dislocation was 28%; and in this severely affected group, soft-tissue release and varus derotational osteotomies were helpful in decreasing the incidence of femoral fractures, in decreasing pain, and in improving sitting balance and the level of activity.

Example 5-3. This 5-year-old girl was first evaluated at age 16 months. At birth there was evidence of fetal distress with precipitous delivery. An Apgar of 1 was assessed at 1 minute and an Apgar of 4 at 5 minutes after birth. Resuscitation was difficult. Seizures started at 4 hours of age and on analysis were though to be due to neonatal asphyxia. Height and weight have remained below the third percentile. The child is microcephalic. Aminoacidurea of uncertain etiology is also present. At age 16 months the child was found to be severely retarded with an estimated IQ of 25. The child is living at home. Hip x-rays demonstrated early dislocation of the right hip (Figure 5-6a). At the age of 3 years, because of continued hip problems, an intraoperative hip arthrogram and a closing-wedge varus derotational osteotomy were peformed with an increase in varus of 25° and a derotation of 20° (Figure 5-6b). Arthrogram revealed fairly good coverage of the head. Two years later the plate was removed and the patient had an obturator neurectomy. On evaluation at that time there was a 60° flexion contracture of the right hip and an adductor contracture. The child was unable to walk or talk and was still in diapers.

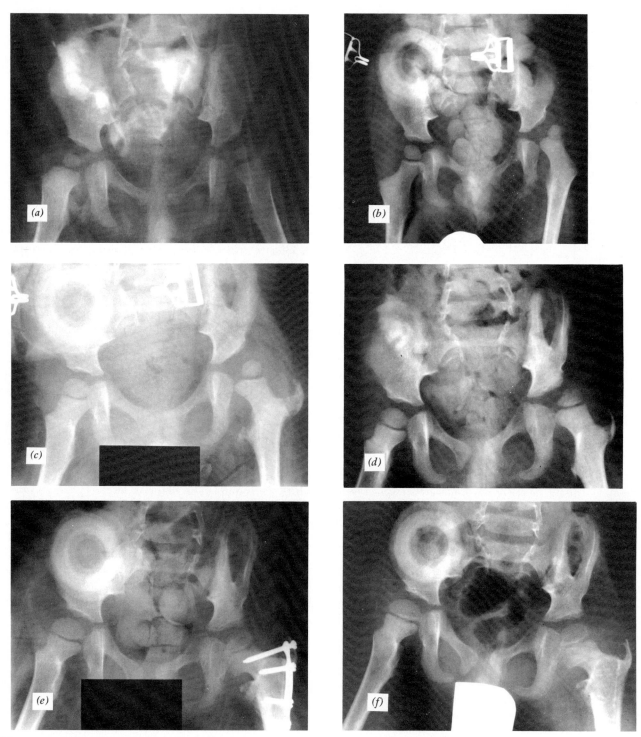

84

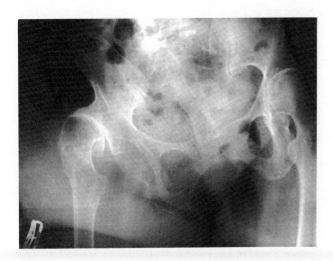

Figure 5-5. Shelf procedure for hip subluxation due to poliomyelitis. A 63-year-old woman who had poliomyelitis in childhood with right leg paresis. Chronic dislocation of the right hip is present. The femoral head lies superior to the true acetabulum and articulates with an operative bony shelf. No cartilage space remains at this articulation. Forty-four years following the shelf procedure, a total hip replacement was used as treatment for degenerative arthritis.

Example 5-4. This 12½-year-old boy suffered cerebral anoxia during a difficult delivery in a primigravida. He demonstrated moderate to marked mental retardation associated with marked spasticity. The patient had a chronically subluxing right hip. The child had not walked by the age of 2 years; however by the age of 5 years he was standing and walking with difficulty. He walked with assistance on his toes with minimal to no scissoring. He was able to sit by himself. At age 10½ (Figure 5-7a), because of increasing problems with the right hip leading to loss of the ability to ambulate (with the patient confined to a wheelchair), plans were made for surgical correction of the bilateral hip problems. The patient at that time had hyperactive, lower extremity deep-tendon reflexes, with hip flexion contractures of 15 to 20° bilaterally. There was limited abduction. At 11 years of age, he had a right Salter osteotomy (Figure 5-7b), which improved the coverage of the right femoral head and prevented subluxation. Following healing of the Salter osteotomy the child was able to ambulate independently without support. He was able to rise and sit without assistance. He walked with his knees together and his hips and knees flexed approximately 20°. At age 13 (Figure 5-7c), because of increasing problems with the left hip, a Chiari pelvic osteotomy (Figure 5-7d,e) was performed, improving coverage of the left femoral head. This healed well.

Figure 5-4. The Sharrard procedure. Patient at one year of age; the left hip is minimally subluxed laterally. The interpedicular widening of the vertebrae is associated with the meningomyelocele. The contrast material in the lower abdomen is in the ileal-loop urinary diversion. Film was taken during an intravenous urogram. (b) By age 3 years, in this patient marked subluxation of the left hip is present. The slope of the left acetabular roof is increased. A urinary collection bag covers the right lower portion of the abdomen. (c) Age 3½. The patient is now post-Sharrard procedure. The hip remains minimally subluxed, the acetabular roof slope remains increased. The hole in the left ilium permits the iliopsoas tendon to be attached to the greater trochanter. The deformity of the greater trochanter is commonly seen following the tendon re-attachment. (d) Patient age 4½ year. The subluxation of the left hip has increased. The enlargement of the hole in the ilium is a common sequella of the Sharrard procedure and is of no clinical significance. (e) Patient age 5. An intertrochanteric osteotomy with varus repositioning has supplemented the Sharrard procedure, adequately reducing the hip. The metal plate is used to hold the desired position until bony union has occurred. (f) Following bony union, the plate is removed. Plates and appliances used in children are often removed after bony union has occurred.

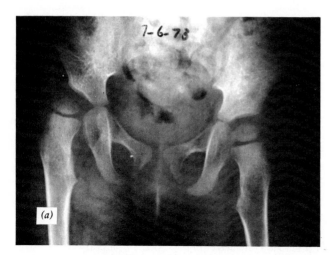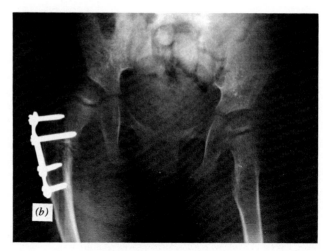

Figure 5-6. Varus osteotomy in cerebral palsy. (*a*) Patient at age 18 months. Moderate lateral subluxation of the right hip is present, with an increased slope of the acetabular roof. Valgus deformity of both proximal femurs is present. (*b*) Following an intertrochanteric varus derotational osteotomy, the hip is less subluxed.

Figure 5-7. Cerebral palsy. Salter and Chiari procedures. (*a*) Age 10½. Moderate subluxation of the right hip is present. The acetabulum is deformed, with a moderate increase in the slope of its roof. (*b*) Age 11. Shortly following a right Salter innominate bone osteotomy. Bone graft (held with a K wire) has been placed to redirect the acetabulum so that it is less open anteriorly and laterally, providing better coverage for the femoral head. (*c*) Age 13. Increasing subluxation of the left hip is present. The right Salter osteotomy has now healed, with improved coverage of the right femoral head. The right hip is no longer subluxed. (*d*) The Chiari supra-acetabular osteotomy with medial displacement of the acetabulum is seen in plaster. (*e*) This view of the partially healed Chiari osteotomy out of plaster better demonstrates the acetabular displacement and the improved coverage which it gives to the femoral head.

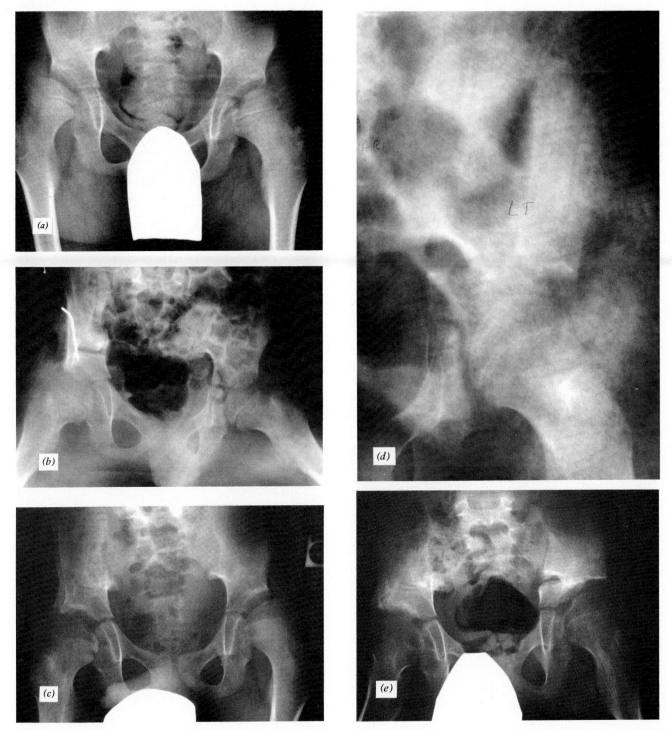

SUMMARY

The patient with abnormal muscle balance around the hip joint will frequently require surgery for correction of valgus deformity or for the correction of muscle imbalance. Commonly performed procedures include varus osteotomies and the Sharrard and Mustard muscle transfer procedures. In appropriately selected patients these procedures permit better stance and better ambulation, thus improving both the patient's appearance and mobility.

REFERENCES

1. Carroll MC, and Sharrard WJW: Long-term follow-up of posterior iliopsoas transplantation for paralytic dislocation of the hip. *J Bone Joint Surg* 54A:551–560, 1972.

2. Cruess RL, Turner MS: Paralysis of hip abductor muscles in spine bifida. *J Bone Joint Surg* 52A:1364–1372, 1970.

3. Freehafer AA, Vessely JC, and Mack R: Iliopsoas muscle transfer in the treatment of myelomeningocele patients with paralytic hip deformities. *J Bone Joint Surg* 54A:1715–1729, 1972.

4. Freiberg AH: Congential luxation of the hip. *J Bone Joint Surg* 17:1–10, 1935.

5. Gill AB: Plastic reconstruction of an acetabulum in congenital dislocation of the hip. *J Bone Joint Surg* 17:48–59, 1935.

6. Menelaus MB: Dislocation and deformity of the hip in children with spina bifida cystica. *J Bone Joint Surg* 51B:238–251, 1969.

7. Mustard WT: Iliopsoas transfer for weakness of hip abductors. A preliminary report. *J Bone Joint Surg* 34A:647–650, 1952.

8. Mustard WT: A follow-up study of iliopsoas transfer for hip instability. *J Bone Joint Surg* 41B:289–298, 1959.

9. Parker B, Walker G: Posterior psoas transfer and hip instability in lumbar myelomeningocele. *J Bone Joint Surg* 57B:53–58, 1975.

10. Rueda J, Carroll MC: Hip instability in patients with myelomeningocele. *J Bone Joint Surg* 54B:422–431, 1972.

11. Samilson RL, et al: Dislocation and subluxation of the hip in cerebral palsy. *J Bone Joint Surg* 54A:863–873, 1972.

12. Sharrard WTW: Posterior iliopsoas transplantation in the treatment of paralytic dislocation of the hip. *J Bone Joint Surg* 46B:426–444, 1964.

13. Somerville EW: Paralytic dislocation of the hip. *J Bone Joint Surg* 41B:279–288, 1959.

14. Tachdjian M: *Pediatric Orthopedics.* Saunders, Philadelphia, 1972, pp 905–916.

15. Tachdjian M: *Pediatric Orthopedics.* Saunders, Philadelphia, 1972, pp 964–967.

6
Legg-Calvé-Perthes Disease

Waldenstrom-Calvé-Legg-Perthes disease is a common affliction of children, occurring with an incidence of about 1 in every 750 boys and 1 in every 3,700 girls (18). It is the result of ischemia of the femoral head. Its prognosis depends on the degree of deformity that occurs during the body's repair of the ischemic area. The ischemia itself is frequently painful in the early stages and can present with hip pain or a limp. On occasion it follows transient synovitis of the hip, a disease in which the hip is painful and has a joint effusion, but usually there is no history of previous hip symptomatology. Early diagnosis depends on having a high index of suspicion, as the initial films are frequently normal and it is only on follow-up radiographs that the lack of growth of the bony epiphysis or its resorption and reconstitution can be detected.

Example 6-1. At age 3, this boy presented with right hip pain and a limp, considered to be transient synovitis of the hip. Radiographs were normal (Figure 6-1a). The symptoms resolved, only to recur two months later. A diagnosis of Legg-Perthes disease was made, though the radiographs remained normal. Treatment was initially in "broomstick" plasters—a cast on each leg with a wooden bar holding the casts and the hips in abduction and internal rotation (Figure 6-1b). These were later replaced by abduction splints.

At three months, minimal sclerosis and partial collapse of the anterolateral segment were present (Figure 6-1c,d). Progressive sclerosis then appeared (Figure 6-1e).

Progressive resorption of the ossific nucleus of the epiphysis followed, associated with lateral extrusion of the epiphyseal fragments (Figure 6-1f,g,h). Because of the lateral uncovering, an arthrogram (Figure 6-1i) was performed, which demonstrated good acetabular coverage of the femoral head in abduction. A 20° closing-wedge varus and 10° lateral rotation subtrochanteric osteotomy was performed, providing good coverage for the involved portion of the femoral head (Figure 6-1j).

Five years following surgery (Figure 6-1k), the femoral head is nearly normal, with only minimal increased width of the epiphysis.

THE STAGES OF PERTHES DISEASE

The progression of the changes of Perthes disease can be divided into phases (17): the phase of ischemia, the phase of absorption (or resorption), and the phase of reconstitution or reossification. In the ischemia phase, growth of the ossific nucleus of the femoral head ceases; in the resorption phase, the damaged portion of bone is removed; and during the reconstitution phase, new bone is laid down to replace that previously resorbed.

Phase I—The Phase of Ischemia

During the ischemia phase, the involved portion of the ossified femoral-head epiphysis ceases to grow. The cartilagenous portion is frequently unaffected. Initially, the epiphysis will appear normal (Figure 6-1a), and the diagnosis must be made clinically. It is with the passage of time that an asymmetry between the two femoral-head

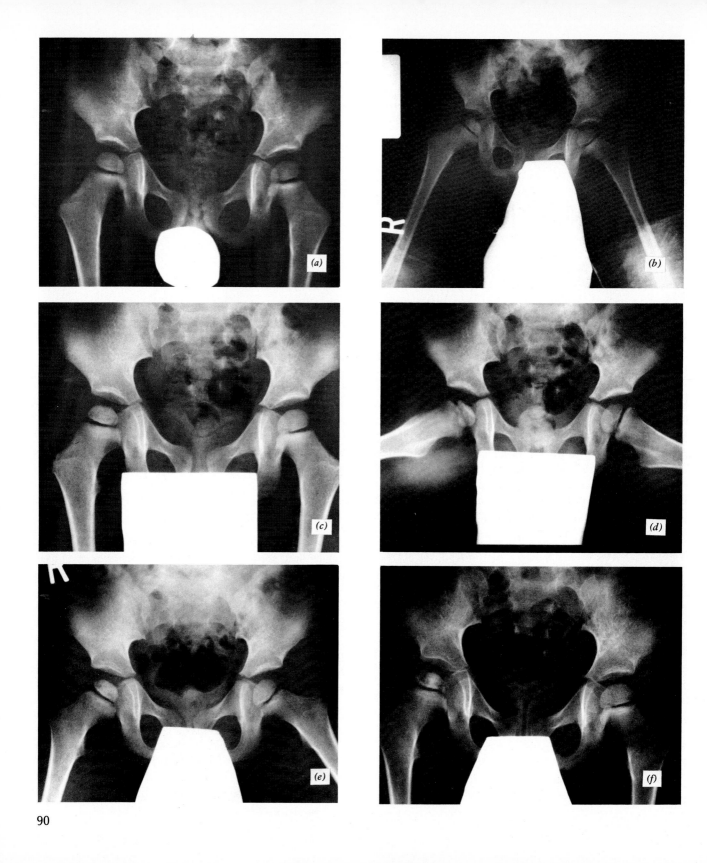

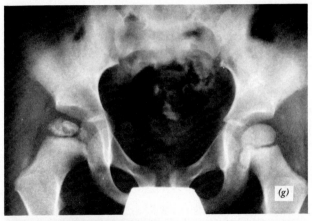

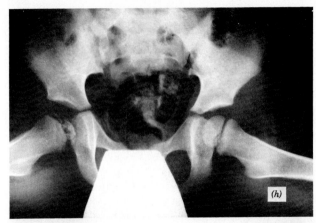

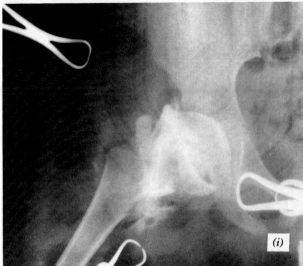

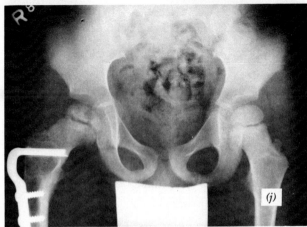

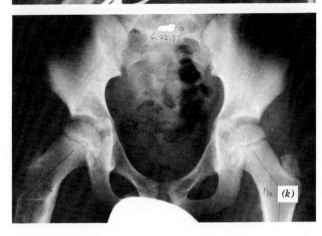

Figure 6-1. Example 6-1. Stages of Legg-Perthes disease. Varus osteotomy. (*a*) At age 3, the hips appear normal. (*b*) Treatment was by a broomstick plaster with casts on each leg. A wooden bar holds the legs apart and the hips in abduction and internal rotation. This position of the femurs gives good coverage of the femoral heads by the acetabulum. (*c*) At 4 months the right femoral head is smaller than the left. Minimal sclerosis is present. (*d*) The epiphysis is thinner anteriorly, probably representing partial collapse. (*e*) The sclerosis of the right femoral head has increased. (*f*) Minimal resorption is now present laterally. Only the central portion of the epiphysis remains radiodense. (*g,h*) Spotty resorption of the bone of the entire epiphysis is now present. The lateral portion of the femoral head is now partially uncovered. (*i*) Arthrography shows a smooth femoral head cartilage surface with good coverage when the femur is abducted. (*j*) One year following a varus and lateral rotation osteotomy, the coverage of the femoral head is good, with the leg in neutral position. Reossification is occuring. (*k*) Five years following the osteotomy, the femoral head is reformed. The width of the epiphyseal plate is slightly increased.

91

epiphyses can be recognized: a difference in size between the epiphyses and an increased distance from the superior and medial margins of the acetabulum (Figure 6-1c). It is only after several months that the radiographs can confirm the clinical diagnosis. Ossification of the epiphysis is also delayed in patients with congenital displacement of the hip without concurrent ischemia.

In many patients, the ischemia is limited to the anterior and lateral portions of the bony epiphysis and, in these patients, the disease may be most easily recognized on the lateral view (Figure 6-1d). Occasionally, the anterior view will remain totally normal during the course of the disease, and lateral views are therefore essential for diagnosis and for following the stages of the disease.

Isolated segmental involvement of the anterolateral portions of the femoral head is due to the selective involvement of one of the two vascular groups serving the femoral head at this age: the lateral epiphyseal vessels serve the anterolateral and the medial metaphyseal vessels serve the posteromedial segments of the ossific femoral head (17,19). Ligamentum teres vessels are absent or serve only a limited portion of the femoral head near the fovea centralis at this time (19). In the older child, the medial metaphyseal vessels are absent and total involvement of the femoral head is more likely.

Legg-Perthes disease may be unilateral or bilateral. When bilateral it may be synchronous or asynchoronous.

Late in the ischemia phase, the nongrowing epiphysis may become slightly radiodense prior to the start of resorption (Figure 6-1c,e). The etiology of this radiodensity is uncertain.

Phase Two—The Phase of Resorption

During the resorption phase, vascular ingrowth occurs, permitting the resorption of the dead bone (Figure 6-1f,g,h). As the bone is resorbed, its absence weakens the femoral head, permitting its deformation. The resorption may be diffuse, with a spotted appearance, or more focal, with a few lytic areas appearing and then progressively coalescing. The ossification of repair bone usually does not begin until resorption is complete.

Phase Three—The Phase of Reconstitution

During the phase of reconstitution and reossification, fiber bone is produced, which is progressively replaced by mature lamellar bone (Figure 6-1j,k). Robert Salter (13,14) has studied this process in pigs and has shown that, during this remodeling of the fiber bone, the epiphysis can be deformed by focal pressure. It is during this reconstitution of the femoral bony epiphysis that the deformity becomes recognizable.

THE NATURE OF THE DEFORMITY

The characteristic deformity of Legg-Perthes disease is a groove in the anterior and lateral margins of the femoral head, close to the edge of the acetabular margin with the hip in neutral position. This groove is visible during arthrography (Figure 6-2c,d,e and Figure 6-9d) and can be confirmed at surgery. Because it is adjacent to the edge of the acetabulum, it is probable that pressure from this bony and cartilagenous rim deforms the weakened femoral head.

Associated with this groove, the height of the epiphysis is often decreased and its width increased. The widened cartilagenous epiphysis is often supported by a widened femoral metaphysis.

Example 6-2. This child was initially diagnosed as having Legg-Perthes disease of the left hip at age 9. He was treated with nonweight bearing for one year (though he may not have complied with this proscription).

At age 10, the child had a limp. Radiographs at this time revealed deformity with partial resorption of the anterolateral portion of the bony epiphysis (Figure 6-2a,b). A few flecks of calcium are seen lateral to the main portion of the epiphysis, indicative of minimal lateral extrusion.

An arthrogram (Figure 6-2c,d,e) performed at this time demonstrated deformity of the femoral epiphysis with anterior and lateral grooves within the cartilage surface corresponding to those portions normally in contact with the edge of the acetabulum.

The patient was treated with a varus derotational osteotomy that placed the femoral head within the acetabulum. One year following surgery, the hip functioned normally (Figure 6-2f). One centimeter of shortening was present, which was treated with a shoe lift.

Four and one-half years following surgery (Figure 6-2g), the femoral head is reconstituted, with a flattened and broadened epiphysis. The hip is asymptomatic at this time. The long-term prognosis is uncertain.

THE RECOGNITION OF THE DEFORMITY

Two different problems are met in the recognition of the deformity of Legg-Perthes disease: the more difficult is the recognition of the deformity prior to reossification of the bony epiphysis: the second is its evaluation following reossification.

Example 6-3. At presentation at age 4 with Legg-Perthes disease, this child's radiographs were abnormal only on the lateral view (Figure 6-3a,b): the anterior portion of the right femoral epiphysis was growing less than the posterior portion. After six months, the entire right epiphysis was smaller than the left and sclerotic (Figure 6-3c). At the end of nine months, a notch was seen in the lateral portion of the epiphysis, with minimal adjacent metaphyseal irregularity (Gage's sign) (Figure 6-3d). This is indicative of widening of the epiphysis and indicates that the head is at risk for further deformity.

Thirteen months following the initial diagnosis (Figure 6-3e), the epiphysis was in the resorption phase. Faint calcification is present lateral to the main portion of the epiphysis. This is also a sign of widening of the epiphysis and is a second sign that the head is at risk for further deformity.

At the end of eighteen months, an arthrogram was performed, disclosing moderate lateral uncovering of the cartilagenous epiphysis with a lateral bulge of the cartilage (Figure 6-3f).

A varus osteotomy was performed to place the femoral head well within the mold of the acetabulum (Figure 6-3g,h). Serial films demonstrate the reforming of the epiphysis with moderate flattening (Figure 6-3i). The head appears congruous with the acetabulum; 1½ cm of shortening is present. The long-term prognosis is uncertain.

Recognition of the deformity prior to reossification depends on the observation of subtle signs of epiphyseal and epiphyseal-plate widening and of femoral-head flattening (4). The widening of the epiphyseal plate has both direct and indirect signs. Indirectly, the widening of the epiphyseal plate results in a widening of the metaphysis and can be detected by comparison with the opposite side (Figure 6-3e). More directly, lateral extrusion of the cartilagenous epiphysis may be recognized by the presence of faint flecks of calcium just lateral to the ossified epiphysis (Figure 6-3e, Figure 6-10b). Lateral displacement of the ossific nucleus probably reflects widening of the cartilage medially and is usually associated with concurrent flattening of the epiphysis. Gage's sign (4,5), a radiolucent notch in the lateral portion of the ossified nucleus and adjacent metaphysis, probably represents lateral extrusion of a portion of the bony epiphysis (Figure 6-3d, Figure 6-4).

Recognition of the loss of height of the epiphysis is an important early sign of poor prognosis; comparative measurements of the distance of the epiphyseal plate from the roof of the acetabulum aid in the diagnosis of this deformity. When epiphyseal height loss occurs early in the phase of resorption, results are usually poor.

The signs described above are used to detect the head at risk for deformity (4,7), thereby helping to select those who might benefit from treatment for the prevention of additional deformity.

Catterall (4) used these signs of the head at risk to divide femoral heads with Legg-Perthes disease into four groups. His grouping is commonly used to compare results among different series.

CATTERALL'S GROUPS

Catterall's Group 1

Involvement of the ossific nucleus is limited to the anterior portion. No collapse of height of the epiphysis occurs.

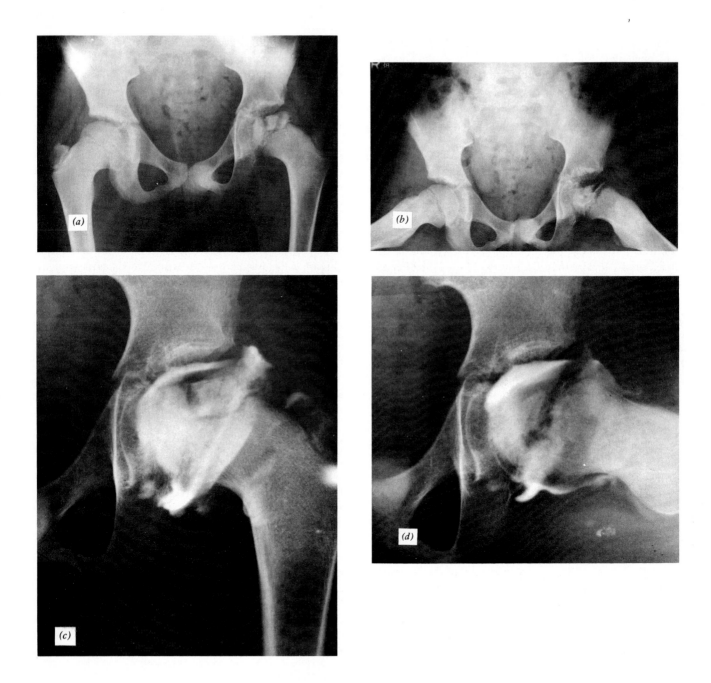

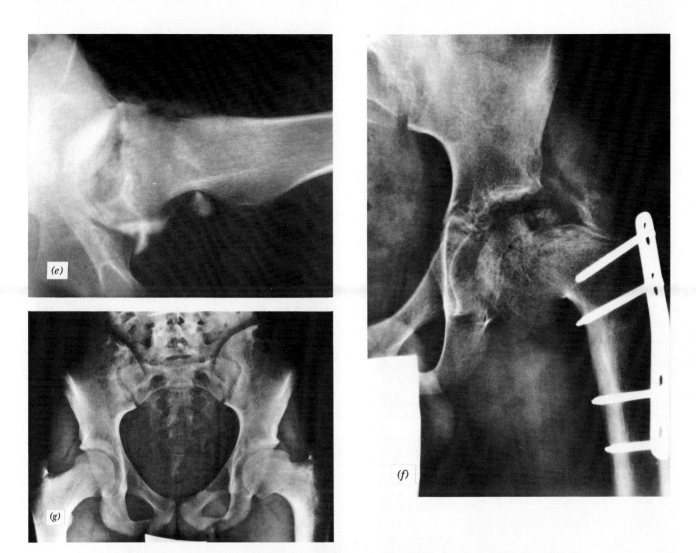

Figure 6-2. Deformity resulting from Legg-Perthes disease. (*a*) At age 10, one year after clinical onset, radiographs disclose flattening and fragmentation of the mid and lateral portions of the left femoral head. A few faint flecks of calcium are present lateral to the main portion of the epiphysis, due to minimal lateral extrusion. (*b*) The lateral view demonstrates flattening of the anterior portion of the femoral head. (*c*) Arthrography demonstrates a broad depression near the lateral margin of the femoral head, with lateral extrusion of part of the epiphyseal cartilage. (*d*) The abduction lateral demonstrates anterior flattening. (*e*) The true lateral view demonstrates that this anterior flattening is adjacent to the anterior lip of the acetabulum. (*f*) One year following the varus osteotomy, the femoral head is reossifying and is contained within the acetabulum. The epiphysis is flattened. The acetabulum is deformed; its superior margin is displaced superiorly and its lateral lip is flattened. (*g*) Four and one-half years following surgery, the femoral head is flattened and broadened. The acetabulum is enlarged.

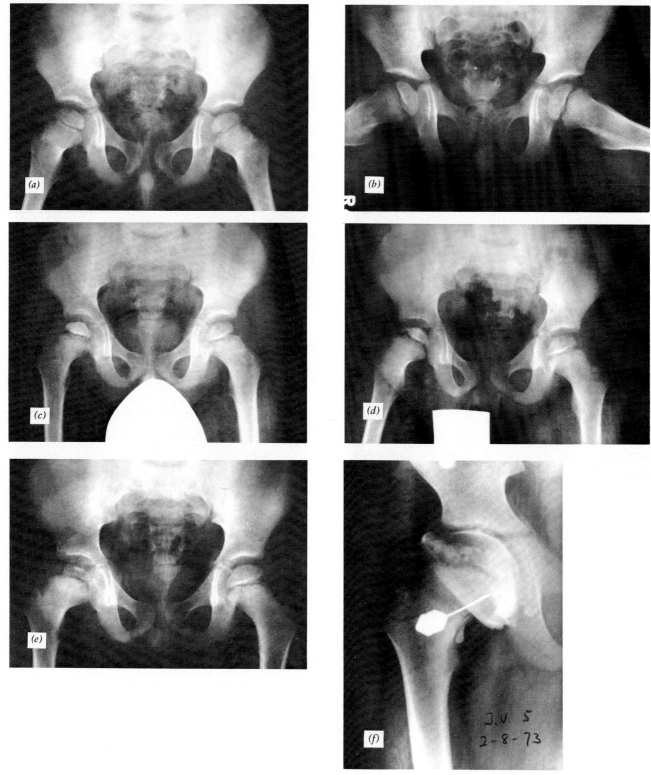

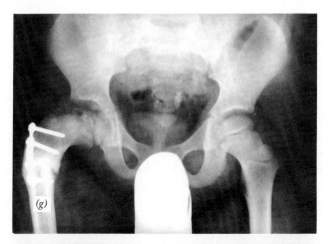

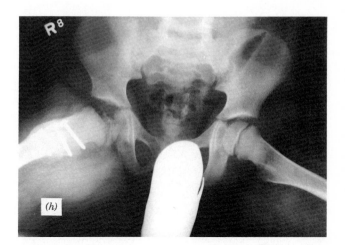

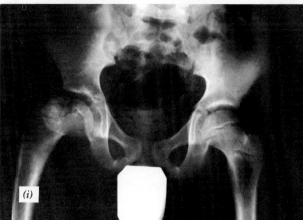

Figure 6-3. Example 6-3. Legg-Perthes disease with early signs of deformity. (*a*) Age 4. The hips are normal on this frontal view. (*b*) The lateral view demonstrates less growth of the anterior portion of the right femoral head: the phase of ischemia is affecting the anterolateral portion of the femoral epiphysis. (*c*) Six months after the patient's first examination, the right femoral head is smaller than the left and is moderately sclerotic. The epiphysis is late in the phase of the ischemia. (*d*) A notch is now present in the lateral portion of the epiphysis (Gage's sign). Resorption is now occurring. (*e*) Thirteen months following initial examination, further resorption has taken place. Faint calcification is present lateral to the ossified epiphysis, indicating widening of the epiphysis. Widening of the metaphysis is also present and indicates epiphyseal plate widening. (*f*) At 18 months, there is lateral uncovering of the cartilagenous epiphysis with a small lateral bulge of the cartilage. (*g*) Following varus osteotomy, the femoral head is well contained within the acetabulum. The lateral portion of the epiphysis is in the resorption phase. (*h*) The lateral view following osteotomy demonstrates the high degree of anterior resorption. (*i*) Five years after the patient first came for treatment and 3 years following osteotomy, the right femoral head has largely reossified, with moderate flattening of the epiphysis and deformity of the lateral lip of the acetabulum.

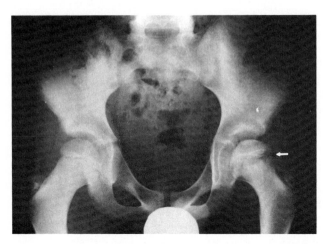

Figure 6-4. Gage's sign. Resorption of the lateral portion of the epiphysis with adjacent metaphyseal irregularity. Left femoral epiphysis.

Complete absorption of the segment occurs without sequestrum. The results are good without any treatment being given.

Catterall's Group 2

More of the anterior portion is involved with collapse to a dense sequestrum. This sequestrum is then resorbed. A transient metaphyseal cyst may occur. The epiphyseal height is maintained by the noninvolved areas. In those patients under the age of 4, results are good; over the age of 4 weight-bearing relief improves results (See Example 6-1).

Catterall's Group 3

Only a small portion of the femoral head is not involved. One may see flecks of calcium lateral to the epiphysis, outside of the acetabulum, reflecting collapse and lateral displacement. The femoral neck may be widened. Two-thirds of these patients end up with a fair or poor result (see Example 6-6). Nonweight bearing does not affect results under age 4 and may affect them after that. Brotherton (2), treating patients with 26 months of bed rest with legs

in wide abduction with internal rotation, demonstrated good results in 44% compared to Catterall's 20%.

Catterall's Group 4

The whole epiphysis is sequestered, with total collapse and early loss of height of the epiphysis. Extensive metaphyseal changes are present (see Example 6-2). These hips have a poor prognosis without treatment. Brotherton reports 50% good results with 26 months of best rest with legs in wide abduction with internal rotation.

Thus, treatment may benefit those patients with signs of their femoral head being at risk in Catterall's groups 2 and 3 and with certain methods of treatment in Catterall's group 4.

THE END POINT—THE GOOD HIP

The final desired result of treatment for Legg-Perthes disease is a functional, pain-free hip lasting to old age. With most methods for treatment of Legg-Perthes disease, the period of follow-up is far too short; in most articles the follow-up is less than 10 years.

Snyder (16) reports a series with follow-up averaging 10 years (with variable methods of treatment). O'Hara (11) reports follow-up of 10 to 43 years in patients treated with an ischial weight-bearing brace; and Brotherton (2) gives follow-up averaging 17 years in patients treated in bed with wide abduction and medial rotation casts. The operative techniques have not been used long enough for long-term follow-up of their results. For this reason, several techniques of assessing results based only on radiologic criteria have evolved. While we will discuss these shortly, it is of value to note here that both Drs. Snyder (16) and O'Hara (11) found a poor correlation of the radiographic appearance with the functional end result.

One of the radiographic indicators is the Mose (10,15) sphericity gauge (Figure 6-5a,b), a thin plastic sheet on which concentric circles are engraved 2 mm apart. A spherical femoral head constitutes a good result and is identified by the femoral head being congruent with the same circle on both frontal and lateral views. A fair result

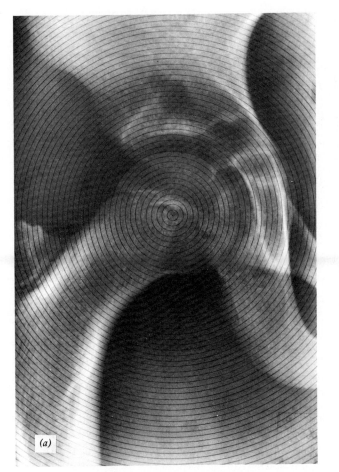
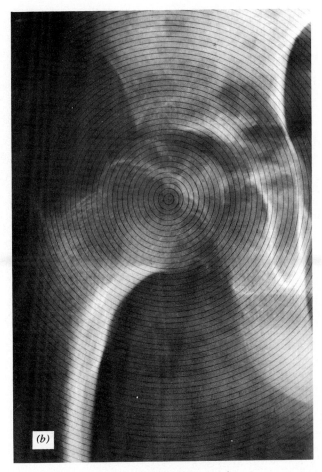

Figure 6-5. The use of the Mose sphericity gauge. A thin plastic sheet on which are engraved concentric circles 2 mm apart is placed over the femoral head. (*a*) Good result—deviation is less than 1 mm. (*b*) Poor result—deviation is greater than 2 mm.

can be seen with two different patterns: a spherical head aligned with the same circle on both views, but with decreased height of the epiphysis, or a non-spherical head with deviation of its shape from a circle by less than 2 mm. The result is considered poor if different circles are aligned with the femoral head on the frontal and lateral views, or when the head is non-spherical (10,11,15,16).

Another radiographic indicator is the CE (center edge) angle of Wiberg (11)—Figure 6-6 (17). This is the angle between two lines, one drawn from the edge of the

acetabulum to the center of the femoral head, and the second drawn as a vertical line through the center of the femoral head. When this angle is greater than 20°, the result is good; 15 to 20° is considered a fair result (this measurement reflects lateral uncovering of the femoral head and the shallowness of the acetabulum).

Catterall (4) uses a more complex set of criteria: Acetabular containment with no adaptive changes indicates a good result (Figure 6-7*a*). Loss of epiphyseal height with a round femoral head often not completely within the

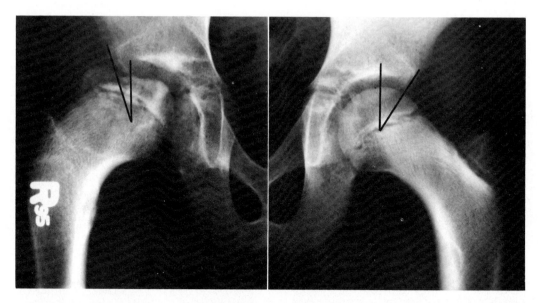

Figure 6-6. Wiberg's center edge angle.

acetabulum indicates a fair result (Figure 6-7*b*). Restriction of motion and a flattened femoral head at least one-fifth uncovered indicate a poor result (Figure 6-7*c*).

METHODS FOR THE PREVENTION OF DEFORMITY

Although the available studies fail to show that the long-term prognosis is related to the degree of deformity, the aim of treatment is the prevention of deformity. The deformity results from asymmetric pressure on the femoral head during the phases of resorption and remodeling and occurs at the edge of anterior and lateral lips of the acetabulum when this is in contact with the damaged portion of the femoral head. Deformity therefore should be preventable by decreasing the forces across the hip joint or by the containment of the involved portion of the femoral head well within the acetabulum, placing the edge of the acetabulum adjacent to normal bone (2,6,7,11,12, 13,14,17,18).

METHODS OF DECREASING THE FORCE APPLIED TO THE DAMAGED PORTION OF THE FEMORAL HEAD

When the area of involvement of the femoral head is limited in extent, the surrounding, more normal bone can provide adequate support for the transfer of the force of weight bearing, and no treatment may be necessary.

In the child under the age of 5, the prognosis for the hip involved with Legg-Perthes disease is very good; one of the proposed reasons for this is that the thick cartilage present at this age distributes the force of weight bearing and prevents deformity. The child at this age is also relatively small and has less muscle power than at a later age; thus, less stress is placed across the joint in these younger children (6).

With more than minimal areas of involvement, or in the child over the age of 5, the forces across the hip can be reduced by strict bed rest and by braces; but even with these methods, muscular activity around the hip will persist and can be a significant deforming force. For this reason, the methods of decreasing force across the hip are

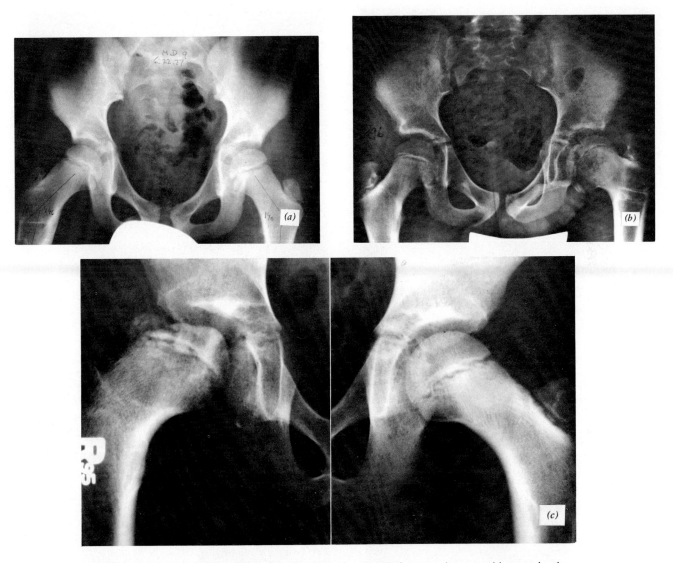

Figure 6-7. Catterall's critera. (*a*) Good result. Acetabular containment with no adaptive change. (*b*) Fair result. Loss of epiphyseal height with a round femoral head, often not completely within the acetabulum. (*c*) Poor result. A flattened femoral head at least one-fifth uncovered.

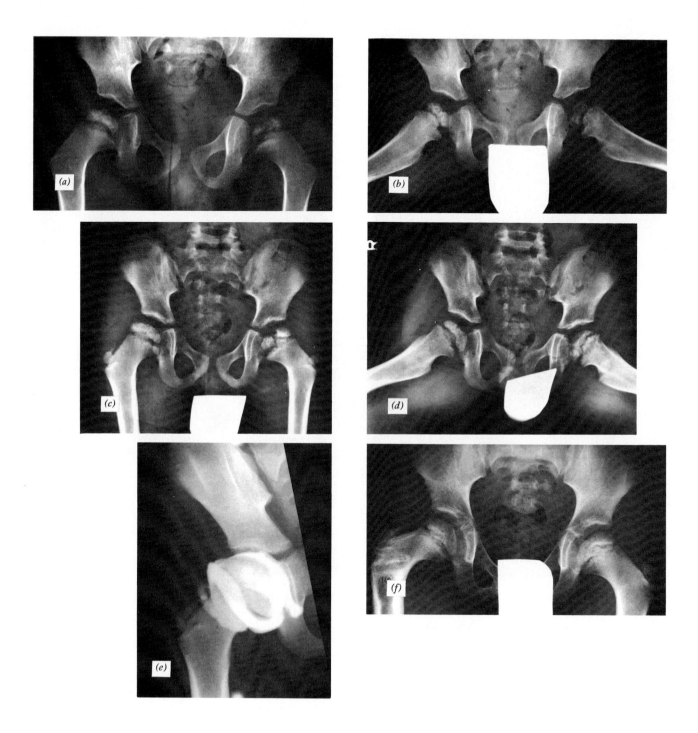

usually combined with methods for the containment of the femoral head within the acetabulum.

METHODS TO CONTAIN THE DAMAGED PORTION OF THE FEMORAL HEAD WITHIN THE ACETABULUM

The deformity of the femoral head usually occurs where the involved portion of the femoral head is in contact with the anterior and lateral margins of the acetabulum. Once this deformity develops, abduction and flexion become painful and limited because of the incongruity. The methods of containment aim either to prevent the deformity completely by placing normal bone adjacent to this deforming acetabular margin, or to have the resultant deformity occur far anteriorly and far laterally on the femoral head, so that the resultant deformity will not interfere with the usual motions of the hip when normal alignment is restored. The use of the acetabulum as a mold should help assure the eventual congruity of the femoral head with the acetabulum. Operative and nonoperative methods of achieving femoral head-acetabular containment are used.

NONSURGICAL METHODS OF CONTAINMENT

Abduction with internal rotation can be maintained by plaster casts on each leg, held apart by a piece of wood (a "broomstick plaster") (6,12,18). Braces can also be used to hold this position (11). Radiographs are obtained to assure containment of the involved portion of the femoral

head and to follow the progress of the repair. Patients treated by these methods may be kept nonweight bearing for two to three years or may be permitted up on crutches (8,12). These methods markedly limit the motor and social activities of these patients (2).

THE SURGICAL METHODS OF CONTAINMENT

Coverage of the involved portion of the femoral head by the acetabulum can be achieved surgically either by redirecting the proximal femur or by redirecting the acetabulum.

Varus, derotational, and extension proximal femoral osteotomies improve the femoral-head coverage and decrease muscle forces across the hip, but result in a slightly short lower extremity (1,7,17). The Salter pelvic osteotomy (described in Chapter 4) redirects the acetabulum anteriorly and laterally downward, covering the femoral head better (3); however, this technique results in a slightly long lower extremity. Each of these methods permits the patient to be up, with full weight bearing, after several months, usually with no restriction of activity. Early radiographic and clinical results with these techniqes are good, but the long-term prognosis is still uncertain.

Example 6-4. At age 3, this boy started to limp and was diagnosed as having bilateral Legg-Perthes disease. He was treated elsewhere for 15 months at bed rest, at which point his parents sought another opinion. Review of the radiographs (Figure 6-8a,b) at that time disclosed bilateral

Figure 6-8. Bilateral Legg-Perthes disease treated by varus osteotomy. (a) Age 4½ years. Anteroposterior view 15 months after initial treatment. Bilateral Legg-Perthes disease is present. Both epiphyses are in the resorption stage. The left epiphysis is well covered by the acetabulum. the right epiphysis is minimally uncovered laterally. (b) Abduction confirms the total epiphyseal involvement. (c) Age 7. The lateral uncovering of the right epiphysis has increased, with minimal lateral displacement of the ossific nucleus. (d) Age 7, abduction lateral view. (e) Arthrogram view demonstrating the lateral uncovering of the femoral head cartilage and the slight flattening of the epiphysis. The lateral shift of the bony epiphysis is due to epiphyseal widening. (f) Age 9. Two years following the varus osteotomy of the right femur. The right femoral head is reconstituted, with minimal loss of height. The left femoral head is healing, with minimal loss of height and sphericity. The left acetabulum is slightly enlarged.

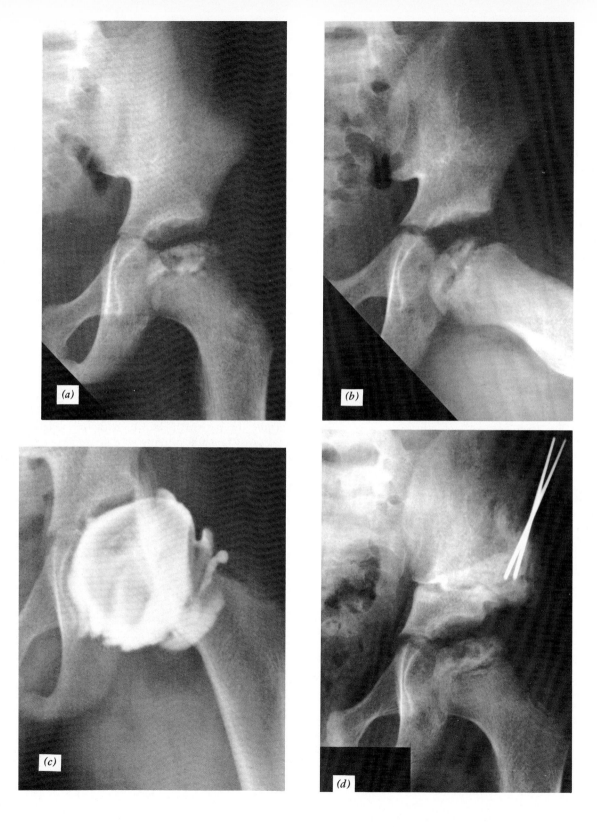

104

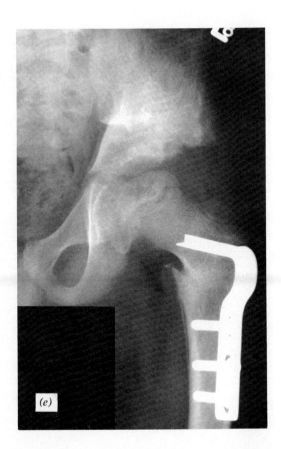
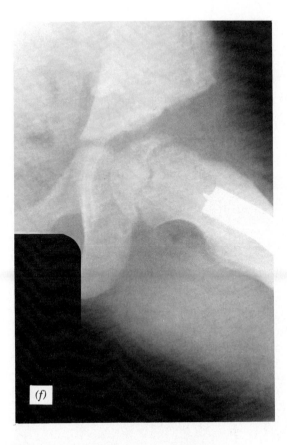

Figure 6-9. Example 6-5. Legg-Perthes disease treated by Salter and varus osteotomies. Age 6½, when the patient was first examined for a limp. The left hip demonstrates femoral epiphyseal flattening with sclerosis. Small focal lytic areas represent areas of bone resorption. (*a*) Frontal view, (*b*) Abduction lateral view. (*c*) The arthrogram demonstrates lateral uncovering of the femoral head cartilage with a slight lateral bulge of the epiphyseal cartilage. (*d*) Following the Salter osteotomy, the lateral coverage of the femoral head remains incomplete. Following the additional procedure, a varus osteotomy, the coverage of the femoral head is improved. Reossification of the femoral head is occurring and a near spherical head has been achieved. (*e*) Frontal view, (*f*) Lateral view.

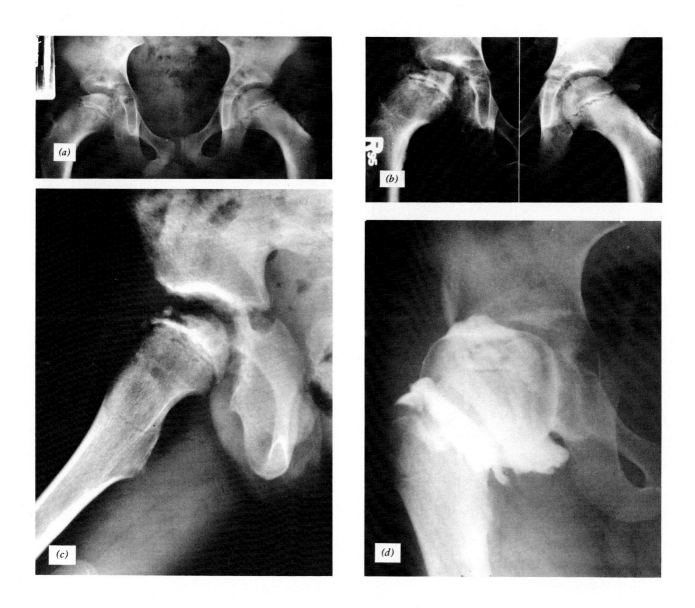

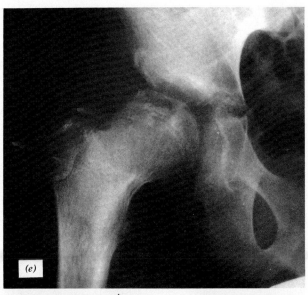

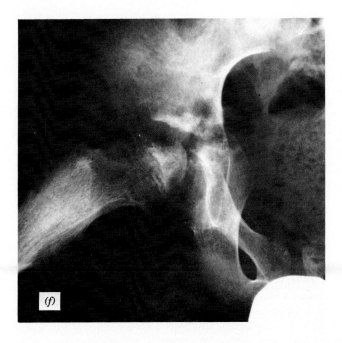

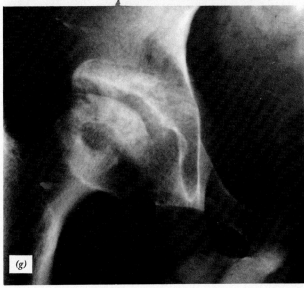

Figure 6-10. Example 6-6. An 11-year-old boy with femoral head deformity from Legg-Perthes disease, showing removal of bony and cartilagenous lateral and anterior bumps. (*a*) Patient at age 11. The femoral head is in the phase of ischemia. The entire epiphysis is smaller than the left, with increased space from the acetabulum to the femoral epiphyseal ossification center. The flattening is more pronounced laterally. Nine months following diagnosis, the anterolateral portion is in the resorption phase; the posteromedial portion is still in the ischemia phase and is not growing. There is faint calcification lateral to the main portion of the ossified epiphysis, indicating a lateral bulge of the epiphysis. The distance between the epiphysis and the medial wall of the acetabulum has increased. The metaphysis has widened, indicating widening of the epiphysis. (*b*) Frontal view, (*c*) Lateral view. (*d*) This internal rotation view from the arthrogram demonstrates the superolateral groove in the cartilagenous epiphysis. Views after the resection of the extra bone and cartilage, showing smoothing of the femoral head; the lateral bony excrescence is removed. Because part of the head is still in the phase of resorption, the degree of congruence achieved cannot be ascertained from the films. (*e*) Frontal view, (*f*) Lateral view shows the marked anterior resorption. (*g*) Three years following surgery there is mild flattening of the femoral head. The medial portion of the femoral head is now in the resorption phase. A cyst is present in the metaphysis, which was later reamed and filled with bone graft.

Legg-Perthes disease. The left hip was in the phase of resorption and was well covered by the acetabulum. The right hip was in the early resorption phase. The right hip was minimally laterally uncovered by the acetabulum.

At age 7, the lateral uncovering of the femoral head had increased (Figure 6-8c,d), and an arthrogram and varus osteotomy were advised. The arthrogram confirmed the lateral uncovering of the femoral head (Figure 6-8e) and the improved position with abduction. A varus osteotomy was performed. One year following surgery the plate was removed. Two years following surgery (Figure 6-8f), the femoral head on the right had reformed. The left femoral head is now almost completely healed, with minimal loss of height of the epiphysis and minimal enlargement of the acetabulum.

Example 6-5. This 8-year-old child with sickle thalassemia was first evaluated at the age of 1 year with acute poststreptococcal glomerulonephritis. At age 6½, the child came to the Orthopedic Clinic with a history of limp for 3 weeks. Diagnosis at that time was early aseptic necrosis (Figure 6-9a,b). The patient's case was followed for four months, at which time an arthrogram (Figure 6-9c), followed by a Salter osteotomy, was performed. Although the Salter osteotomy improved coverage of the head anteriorly, the coverage laterally was incomplete (Figure 6-9d). For this reason, the Salter osteotomy was followed three months later by a varus derotational osteotomy (Figure 6-9e,f). The combination of the two procedures resulted in improved coverage of the femoral head. At follow-up, the acetabululm and femoral head were near congruent.

TREATMENT OF THE DEFORMED FEMORAL HEAD

When early management of Legg-Perthes disease fails to prevent deformity of the femoral head, patients may return in their early teenage years into adulthood with pain or limitation of motion. To a variable extent, the younger patient may self-remodel the deformed femoral head to a more congruent joint (18). Snyder (16) suggests it is this long period of time available for remodeling that gives the child under 5 with Legg-Perthes disease such a good prognosis.

Attempts can be made in the teenager to assist in the remodeling of the femoral head by the resection of the areas of femoral-head incongruity (9). Although rehabilitation following this surgery is prolonged and difficult, it may be of help in selected patients. Alternatively, the methods of arthroplasty discussed in subsequent chapters for the adult patient can be used.

Example 6-6. This 11-year-old boy presented with right groin pain and a limp and was diagnosed as having Legg-Perthes disease of the right hip. He was treated for six months in a hip spica and was then changed to an ischial weight-bearing brace. Radiographs at that time (Figure 6-10a) disclosed that the head was in the ischemia phase, with a smaller epiphysis than that of the left head.

At this time, 9 months after diagnosis (Figure 6-10b,c), flattening of the right femoral epiphysis is present with a lateral bump that impinges on the acetabulum in abduction, thereby limiting abduction. The deformity of the cartilagenous epiphysis was confirmed by arthrography (Figure 6-10d). Following the arthrographic confirmation, a bumpectomy was performed, and sufficient bone and cartilage was removed to make the femoral head congruous with the acetabulum (Figure 6-10e,f). Much of the hyaline cartilage had to be removed during this procedure, and the postoperative rehabilitation was difficult. There was a moderate initial loss of motion, which was eventually regained. Three years following surgery (Figure 6-10g), the patient walked without a limp, but he had occasional pain when the weather changed. The long-term prognosis is uncertain.

SUMMARY

The etiology of the ischemia that initiates Legg-Perthes disease is uncertain, but the deformity that develops from the body's repair of this ischemic bone has been well studied. Treatment aims to prevent deformity and consists of decreasing the stress placed on the remodeling femoral head and placing the damaged portion of the femoral head within the acetabulum, so that the acetabulum can serve as a mold to achieve acetabular-femoral congruence. Operative and nonoperative methods are available. Surgery may be used to redirect the proximal femur or to redirect the acetabulum. The long-term prognoses of these surgical methods are uncertain.

REFERENCES

1. Axer A: Subtrochanteric osteotomy in the treatment of Perthes disease. *J Bone Joint Surg* 47B:489–499, 1965.

2. Brotherton BJ, McKibbirn B: Perthes disease treated by prolonged recumbency and femoral head containment: A Long-term appraisal. *J Bone Joint Surg* 59B:8–14, 1977.

3. Canale ST, D'Anca AF, Cotler JM, Snedden HE: Innominate osteotomy in Legg-Calve-Perthes' disease. *J Bone Joint Surg* 54A:25–40, 1972.

4. Catterall A: The natural history of Perthes' Disease. *J Bone Joint Surg* 53B:37–53, 1971.

5. Gage HC: A possible early sign of Perthes' disease. *Br J Radiol* 6:295–297, 1933.

6. Harrison MHM, Menon MPA: Legg-Calve-Perthes disease. *J Bone Joint Surg* 48A:1301–1318, 1966.

7. Lloyd-Roberts GC, Catterall A, Salmon P: A controlled study of the indications for and the results of femoral osteotomy in Perthes disease. *J Bone Joint Surg* 58B:31–36, 1976.

8. Marklund T, Bengt T: Coxa plana: A radiological comparison of the rate of healing with conservative measures and after osteotomy. *J Bone Joint Surg* 58B:25–30, 1976.

9. McKay DW: Cheilectomy in Perthes disease. Lecture in disease of the hip in child and adult. Durham, North Carolina, Nov. 5, 1973.

10. Mose K: *Legg-Calve-Perthes disease,* thesis, Copenhagen, 1964.

11. O'Hara JP, et al: Long-term follow-up of Perthes disease treated nonoperatively. *Clin Orthop* 125:49–56, 1977.

12. Petrie JG, Bitenc I: The abduction weight-bearing treatment in Legg-Perthes disease. *J Bone Joint Surg* 53B:54–62, 1971.

13. Salter RB: Experimental and clinical aspects of Perthes disease, abstracted. *J Bone Joint Surg* 48B:393–394, 1966.

14. Salter RB, Bell M: The pathogenesis of deformity in Legg-Calve-Perthes disease, Abstracted. *J Bone Joint Surg* 50B:436, 1968.

15. Sanders JA, MacEwen GD: A long-term follow-up on coxa plana at the Alfred I. DuPont Institute. *South Med J* 62:1042–1047, 1969.

16. Snyder CR: Legg-Perthes disease in the young hip—does it necessarily do well? *J Bone Joint Surg* 57A:751–758, 1975.

17. Somerville EW: Perthes disease of the hip. *J Bone Joint Surg* 53B:639–649, 1971.

18. Tachdjian M: *Pediatric Orthopedics.* Philadelphia, Saunders, 1972, pp 384–406.

19. Trueta J: The normal vascular anatomy of the human femoral head during growth. *J Bone Joint Surg* 39B:358–394, 1957.

7
Slipped Capital Femoral Epiphysis

SLIPPED CAPITAL FEMORAL EPIPHYSIS

Slippage of the capital femoral epiphysis is a common disease occurring in adolescent boys 13–16 years of age and in girls 11–14 years of age. It is two to five times more common in boys (17). Once the epiphysis has slipped, there is a good probability that it will slip further if untreated (7). Marked slippage predisposes boy or girl to early osteoarthritis (14,17). Treated or untreated, there is a substantial incidence of cartilage degeneration and a lesser incidence of avascular necrosis of the femoral head (4,9,10,13,14). In one series, reported by Orofino (13), the hips of more than half the patients were causing severe, incapacitating pain by age 18 years (including 20 untreated patients). For this reason, surgery is common. The most desirable type of surgery is, however, strongly debated. Most series lack long-term follow-up, and most procedures are reported to be highly satisfactory in the hands of their proponents; when others attempt these procedures, the results are often poorer. Clearly, a number of years will have to elapse before definite judgments of preferred type of procedure can be made.

Teleologically, it seems apparent that restoring normal anatomy is the most desirable procedure (2). Closed manipulation, followed by transfixing the epiphyseal plate with a nail or pins, is widely practiced. There is a danger however, that overreduction may place sufficient traction on the blood vessels to result in ischemia (5,17). Often, by the time the slip is recognized, callus will have formed on the inferior aspect of the femoral neck, rendering reduction difficult (vessels would have to be stretched over the callus

(8). The duration of the slip can be judged by the presence or absence of femoral neck callus (1). Open reduction is usually reserved for those patients with an acute slip, with no callus (Figure 7-1*a,b).*

Example 7-1. This 5′1″, 135-lb 11-year-old girl had a two-week history of pain in her right hip. On the day of her admission, she slipped on the ice and was then unable to walk because of severe pain in her right hip. Examination in the emergency room of the hospital disclosed pain on movement of the extremity. Radiographs disclosed a marked slip of the capital femoral epiphysis (Figure 7-2*a,b).* The following day the patient was taken to the operating room, where a closed manipulation by internal rotation and gentle abduction reduced the deformity. Open surgery was then performed using Knowles pin fixation (Figure 7-2*c).* The patient has done well postoperatively, with only short-term follow-up available. Hip motion is normal, except that internal rotation is limited to 30° (Figure 7-2*d,e).*

In open reduction, performed with care to preserve the blood vessels and with resection of any callus that might prevent accurate reduction, good results can be achieved by experienced surgeons (2). However, because of the skill necessary to prevent vascular damage, this operation is not widely performed. On occasion, the reduction is limited by contracture of the retinacular vessels supplying the femoral head. In these patients, a portion of the distal femoral metaphysis can be resected to compensate for the decreased length of the vessels (2). Skill and experience are required

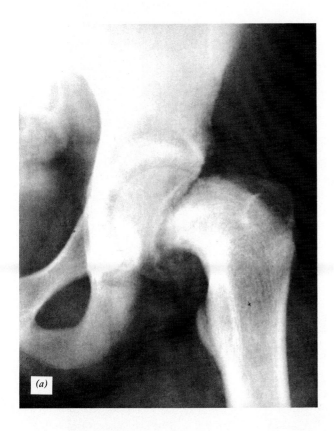

(a)

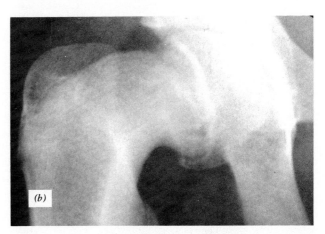

(b)

Figure 7-1. (a) An acutely slipped capital femoral epiphysis. The epiphysis is displaced inferiorly. No callus is seen at the base of the femoral neck. Reduction should not subject the vessels to stretching. (b) A chronic slip of the capital femoral epiphysis. Callus is seen along the inferomedial portion of the femoral neck. Any attempt at reduction is likely to stretch the retinacular vessels and could result in ischemia of the femoral head.

for this difficult procedure. On short-term follow-up, the results appear excellent.

The patient with slipped capital femoral epiphysis may develop limitation of abduction and internal rotation because of the resultant deformity of the femoral head. It can be demonstrated that this bump can impinge on the acetabulum in abduction or internal rotation (2,7). An osteoplastic resection of the bump can markedly improve motion of the hip (17).

Probably the most important aspect of the treatment of slipped capital femoral epiphyses is the prevention of additional slippage. For this reason, orthopedists may fuse across the epiphyseal plate or place a nail or several pins across it without attempting reduction (3,7,16,17). If the extent of displacement is less than one-third to one-half, results of fixation in situ are good on short-term follow up (17). Long-term results are uncertain. Usually extensive remodeling of the femoral neck takes place over several

years following the slip, and thus some surgeons argue that reduction is not necessary.

Example 7-2. This 14-year-old male had a one-month history of intermittent pain in his left hip. The pain sometimes occurred while exercising and sometimes while at rest. He was aware of limitation of motion during this time, and his grandmother, with whom he resided, noted that he leaned to the left side when he walked with what appeared to be a painful limp. X-rays demonstrated a left femoral capital epiphysis slip (Figure 7-3a,b). Examination disclosed full range of motion of both hips but with pain on external and internal rotation of the left hip. A Knowles pinning of the left hip was performed without any attempt at reduction. Two months later there was no residual pain and essentially normal joint motion. Follow-ups at 9 months (Figure 7-3c,d) and 18 months (Figure 7-3e) postsurgery demonstrated full range of motion without

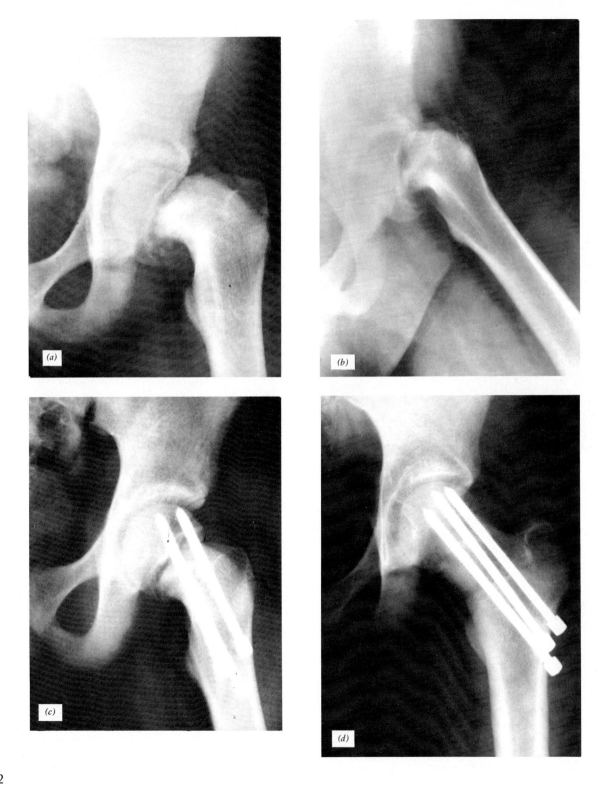

112

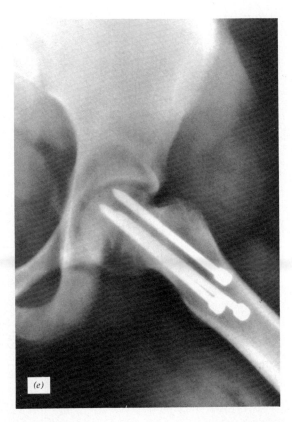

(e)

Figure 7-2. (a) Acute slip of the proximal femoral epiphysis. Frontal view discloses the inferior displacement of the epiphysis: little or no callus is present. (b) Abduction lateral demonstrates the posterior slip of the epiphysis. (c) Open reduction with Knowles pin fixation has restored near anatomic alignment. The epiphyseal plate has now fused. Alignment is anatomic. (d) Frontal view, (e) Lateral view.

any symptoms in the operated hip. The opposite hip was also normal on physical examination and x-ray evaluation.

Any surgery on the femoral neck, whether this is open or closed reduction or simply the placing of the pins across it, carries a significant incidence of avascular necrosis. In order to avoid this problem, partial correction of the deformity can be achieved by base of the neck, inter-trochanteric, and subtrochanteric osteotomies (5,8,14, 16,17). These partially correct the deformity and have good short-term results. Long-term results are more un-

certain; one series of 25 patients, 1 to 40 years post-osteotomy (average $8\frac{1}{2}$ years), demonstrated a high and progressive incidence of degenerative arthritis 8 to 15 years postosteotomy, the incidence equaling those treated without surgery (14).

Example 7-3. The patient is a 9-year-old girl who fell on her right leg $2\frac{1}{2}$ months prior to admission and has been limping since then. At the time of the initial injury, her right knee was swollen, and when she arrived at the emergency room, she was complaining of pain in her right knee. On physical examination she was noted to be obese and short in stature. She walked with an abductor lurch on the left side. There were no joint effusions palpable. There was limitation of motion and pain in the knee on external rotation of the right leg. X-ray demonstrated a clear slip of the right capital femoral epiphysis (Figure 7-4a,b). The patient was admitted to Orthopedics for treatment by valgus osteotomy (Figure 7-4c). The osteotomy healed without incident and the hip was asymptomatic on follow-up (Figure 7-4d,e). The patient is in the seventy-fifth percentile for height and well above the ninety-seventh percentile for weight.

METABOLIC DISTURBANCES IN SLIPPAGE OF THE CAPITAL FEMORAL EPIPHYSIS

There are three groups of patients who sustain slippage of the capital femoral epiphysis. In one group, slippage occurs following significant trauma with a true fracture through the epiphyseal plate (11). In a second group, slippage occurs following degenerative changes in the epiphyseal cartilage (1)—the so-called idiopathic slip. Most patients who develop this are short and overweight and are entering their pubertal growth spurt. These patients may also have an altered immunologic state with alterations of complement C3 and immunoglobulins. Whether this is the primary defect or secondary to the slip is uncertain. The third group in which slippage occurs includes children with acquired hypothyroidism (12) and children with hypopituitarism secondary to intracranial tumors (6).

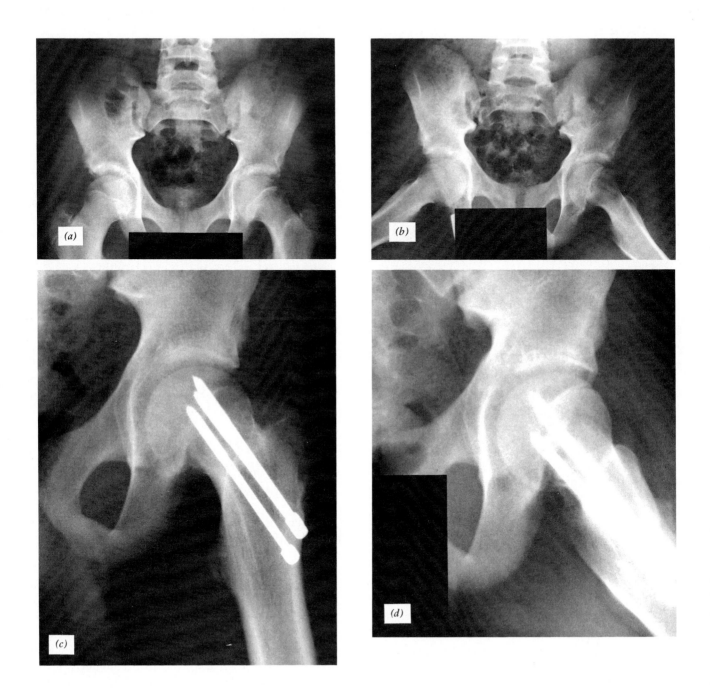

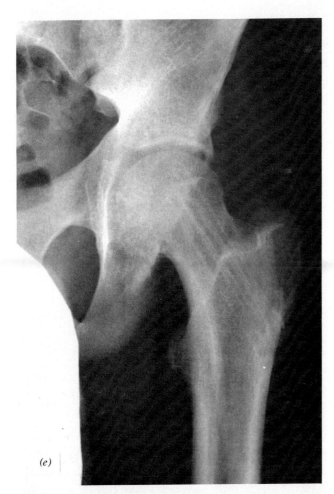

(e)

Figure 7-3. Minimal and subacute slip of the proximal femoral epiphysis. (*a*) The minimal slip of the left capital femoral epiphysis demonstrated by the slightly decreased height of the femoral epiphysis and by the slight medial shift of the epiphysis. (A line drawn along the superior aspect of the femoral neck should intersect a small portion of the epiphysis. It does so on the right, but not on the left.) (*b*) Abduction lateral demonstrates the posterior slip to better advantage. A small amount of callus is seen along the posterior-inferior portion of the femoral neck. The slipped capital epiphysis was pinned with three Knowles pins without reduction. (*c*) Frontal view, (*d*) Lateral view. (*e*) Following fusion of the epiphyseal plate, the pins were removed.

COMPLICATIONS OF SLIPPED CAPITAL FEMORAL EPIPHYSIS AND SURGERY FOR ITS CORRECTION

The two main complications of slippage are avascular necrosis (1,10,17) of the femoral head, occurring in from 5 to 35% of patients, and acute cartilage necrosis (9,10,13,14) occurring in perhaps 15% of patients (14). A minor degree of shortening of the femoral neck may be seen, but is of no clinical importance (2,3,7,17).

Acute cartilage necrosis is a commonly occurring degeneration and narrowing of the articular cartilage of the femoral head following epiphyseal slippage. It is occasionally seen following other types of hip trauma (15) and, rarely, it appears spontaneously (18). Acute cartilage necrosis appears to be much more common in adolescents with Hawaiian or Negro ancestry (10,13) and may be related to preoperative traction and postoperative immobilization. Initially, it often is only mildly painful, and the patient is aware of minimal limitation of motion. The cartilage narrowing can be detected radiologically four to six weeks following surgery. The cartilage necrosis usually progresses, resulting in severe pain with severe degenerative arthritis, often within the first year following the epiphyseal slip (10,13). Fibrous ankylosis can occur; occasionally, severe arthritic change may ensue, but this is unusual. Cartilage necrosis is usually unassociated with avascular necrosis of the femoral head, infection, or sickle-cell disease (10). Clinically and radiologically, differentiation from a joint-space infection is important. The absence of bone destruction is helpful; however, fluoroscopically controlled joint aspiration and culture are frequently necessary.

Example 7-4. This 13-year-old Negro girl presented with left hip and thigh pain, which was found to be due to a moderate epiphyseal slip (Figure 7-5*a*). This was pinned in situ with three Knowles pins. The patient did well postoperatively for about three months; at that time, restriction of motion started to develop and then a mild ache in the hip. Progressive dissolution of joint cartilage was noted on x-rays (Figure 7-5*b*). Aspiration of the hip was performed with culture and was negative. During the year following surgery, the pain in the hip increased and the range of motion of the hip decreased. When last seen,

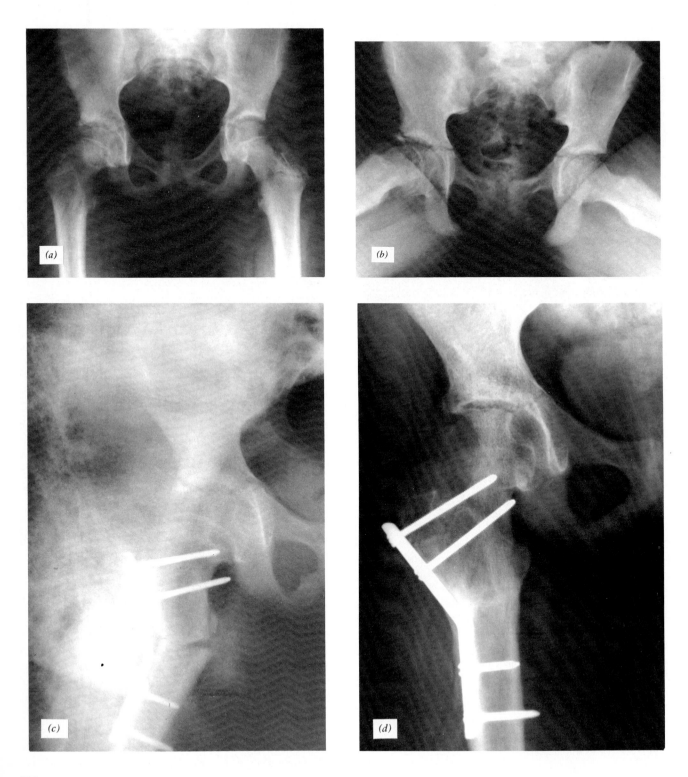

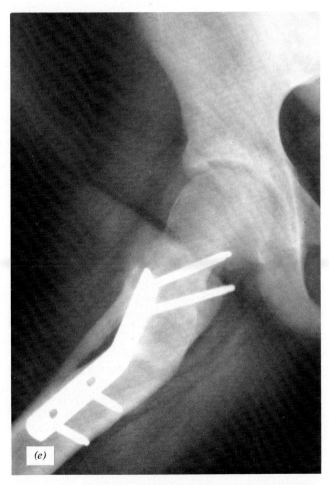

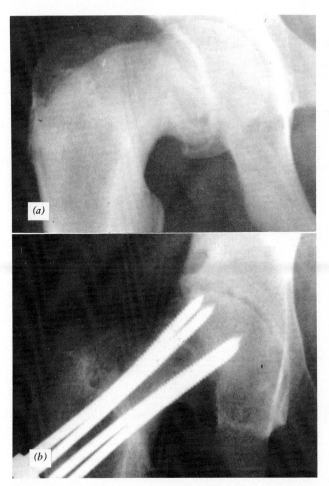

Figure 7-4. Chronic slip of the proximal femoral epiphysis treated by valgus subtrochanteric osteotomy. (*a*) The height of the right femoral epiphysis is less than that on the left, suggesting of a posterior slip of the epiphysis. (*b*) The abduction lateral confirms the moderate posterior slip. Callus is present along posteroinferior aspect of the femoral neck indicating the chronicity of the slip. The left hip is normal. (*c*) A subtrochanteric valgus and flexion osteotomy was performed to decrease the shear forces across the epiphyseal plate. The desired position is maintained by a metal plate. Following healing of the osteotomy and fusion of the epiphyseal plate, the redirection of the proximal fragment is apparent. The flexion and valgus repositioning changed the alignment of the epiphyseal plate so that it was almost parallel to the ground. (*d*) Frontal view, (*e*) Lateral view.

Figure 7-5. Chronic epiphyseal slip with Knowles pinning. Complication: acute cartilage necrosis. (*a*) When first seen, the moderate slip was apparent. Callus lies along the inferomedial portion of the femoral neck. The thickness of the joint cartilage is normal. (*b*) Following treatment by Knowles pinning without reduction, moderate narrowing of the articular cartilage has occurred. This is compatible with acute cartilage necrosis and is usually (as in this case) unassociated with infection.

the patient was being considered for cup arthroplasty or possibly for total hip replacement.

SUMMARY

The patient with slippage of the capital femoral epiphysis may be treated by a wide variety of surgical procedures to prevent additional deformity and hopefully to prevent the development of early degenerative arthritis in the second and third decade of life. Depending on the surgeon and his or her experience, the surgical procedure may range from pin fixation or epiphyseal fusion in situ to careful open reduction of the displacement. Frequently, the surgical correction is performed on the intertrochanteric or subtrochanteric region, thus realigning the hip joint. Unfortunately, most of the procedures now used are of recent formulation, and long-term results are not yet available. Short-term results are good, though the two major complications of avascular necrosis and acute cartilage necrosis seem to occur with all procedures (and even with no treatment) and may result in major disability.

REFERENCES

1. Aadalen R, et al: Acute slipped capital femoral epiphysis. *J Bone Joint Surg* 56A:1473–1487, 1974.
2. Dunn DM: The treatment of adolescent slipping of the upper femoral epiphysis. *J Bone Joint Surg* 46B:621–629, 1964.
3. Fairbank TJ: Manipulative reduction in slipped upper femoral epiphysis. *J Bone Joint Surg* 51B:252–262, 1969.
4. Frymoyer JW: Chondrolysis of the hip following Southwick osteotomy for severe slipped capital femoral epiphysis. *Clin Orthop* 99:120–124, 1974.
5. Gibson DA: Slipped upper femoral epiphyses: Review of the late results of subtrochanteric osteotomy. *Can J Surg* 9:153–158, 1966.
6. Heatley FW, Greenwood RH, Boase DL: Slipping of the upper femoral epiphyses in patients with intracranial tumors causing hypopituitarism and chiasmal compression. *J Bone Joint Surg* 58B:169–175, 1976.
7. Herndon CH, Heyman CH, Bell DM: Treatment of slipped capital femoral epiphysis by epiphysiodesis and osteoplasty of the femoral neck. *J Bone Joint Surg* 45A:999–1012, 1963.
8. Kramer WG, William C, Stanford N: Compensatory osteotomy at the base of the femoral neck for slipped capital femoral epiphysis. *J Bone Joint Surg* 58A:796–800, 1976.
9. Lowe HG: Necrosis of articular cartilage after slipping of the capital femoral epiphysis. *J Bone Joint Surg* 52B:108–118, 1970.
10. Maurer R, Irar L: Acute necrosis of cartilage in slipped capital femoral epiphysis. *J Bone Joint Surg* 52A:39–50, 1970.
11. Milgram JW, Lyne ED: Epiphysiolysis of the proximal femur in very young children. *Clin Orthop* 110:146–153, 1975.
12. Moorefield Wm G, Urbaniak JR, Ogden Wm S, Frank JL: Acquired hypothyroidism in slipped capital femoral epiphysis. *J Bone Joint Surg* 58A:705–708, 1976.
13. Orofino C, Innis JJ, Lowrey CW: Slipped capital femoral epiphysis in Negroes, a study of 95 cases. *J Bone Joint Surg* 42A:1079–1083, 1960.
14. Pearson JR, Riddell DM: Subtrochanteric osteotomy in the treatment of slipped upper femoral epiphysis. *J Bone Joint Surg* 46B:155, 1964.
15. Salvati E, Wilson PD: Treatment of irreducible hip subluxation by Chiari's iliac osteotomy. *Clin Orthop* 98:151–161, 1974.
16. Salemins P, Kivilaakso R: Results of treatment in slipped femoral epiphysis. *J Bone Joint Surg* 50B:221–222, 1968.
17. Tachdjian M: *Pediatric Orthopedics*. Philadelphia, Saunders, 1972, vol 1, 463–491.
18. Wenger DR, Mickelson MR, Ponseti IV: Idiopathic chondrolysis of the hip. Report of two cases. *J Bone Joint Surg* 57A:268–270, 1975.

Conclusion

The aim of surgery on the hip in childhood is to produce a pain-free, stable, mobile, cosmetically acceptable hip joint. Surgery is often required for congenital displacement of the hip, Legg-Calvé-Perthes disease, paralytic dislocation of the hip, and for slippage of the capital femoral epiphysis. Patients with congenital dislocation of the hip may be treated by soft-tissue repair with no plain film radiologic change. On occasion, femoral osteotomies or pelvic osteotomies are required. Reshaping of the acetabulum may be performed to improve the congruence of the femoral head and acetabulum. Rarely, a shelf is placed above the femoral head to form a new acetabulum.

For a paralytic dislocation of the hip the same types of procedures performed for congenital dislocation can be done; however in addition there are two specific transfers of the iliopsoas tendon, the Sharrard and Mustard procedures. The characteristic x-ray appearances of these procedures have been described.

In patients with Legg-Calvé-Perthes disease, prevention of the late deformity may require osteotomies of either the pelvis or the femoral neck, as well as an occasional procedure of modeling of the femoral head with resection of excessive bone.

The treatment of slippage of the capital femoral epiphysis may involve osteotomies of the subtrochanteric portion of the femur, the intertrochanteric portion of the femur, or the femoral neck. Usually the procedure performed consists simply of fusing across the epiphyseal plate either by open epiphysiodesis (removal of the epiphyseal plate) or by the placement of a nail or several pins across the capital femoral epiphysis to prevent further deformity. Major complications of slippage of the capital femoral epiphysis, with or without treatment, are necrosis of the joint cartilage and avascular necrosis of the femoral head.

Part 2

THE ADULT'S HIP

Section A: Fractures
of the Proximal Femur

8
Fractures of
the Femoral Neck

Femoral neck fractures are a common problem in elderly patients. They are seen at all ages but are much more common in the osteoporotic adult. There are several methods of treatment, including bed rest without surgery (2), assorted methods of internal fixation, and prosthetic replacement. Subcapital fractures (those without any femoral neck attached to the proximal fragment) are difficult to treat by internal fixation (16), and most surgeons prefer to treat them by prosthetic replacement. Subcapital fractures have a higher incidence of avascular necrosis than neck fractures. Those surgeons who use internal fixation for subcapital fractures use techniques similar to those described in this chapter for internal fixation of transcervical fractures (9).

Treatment by prosthetic replacement will be covered in the chapters dealing with femoral head replacements and total hip replacements.

Any fracture in an elderly patient may be of serious consequence: in one series of institutionalized elderly patients, the mortality rate of femoral neck fractures varied from 18 to 55%, depending on the method of treatment (21). While this group of patients was more debilitated than most, the mortality rate of femoral neck fractures remains high.

Fractures of the femoral neck are prone to nonunion and avascular necrosis with all methods of treatment, and therefore there are many methods of treatment, each claiming superiority in its results. This is not the proper place for such arguments; of more importance to us as radiologists are the fundamental principles that guide the orthopedist in his choice of proper reduction and fixation.

THE PROPER REDUCTION

For most fractures, an anatomic reduction is best (Figure 8-1a,b). This is also true of the femoral neck fracture, but it is often difficult to keep an anatomic reduction from slipping into an unsatisfactory position. The cortices of the femoral neck are quite thin, and during fixation and impaction these cortices may fragment, permitting a shift in the position of the fragments. The strongest portion of the femoral neck is the medially and inferiorly placed portion of the femoral neck—often called the calcar femoralis. Most surgeons writing on femoral neck fractures propose using the calcar as a buttress against weight-bearing stress by either achieving anatomic reduction or by placing the inferior cortex of the proximal fragment superior to the inferior cortex of the distal fragment, as shown in Figure 8-1c) (15). When this form of reduction is impacted, it will usually shift into a slight valgus position (because of fragmentation of the thinner bone of the superior portion of the femoral neck). Thus, many surgeons prefer the slight valgus position for fixation of femoral neck fractures (14).

Massie (15) and Garden (11) have appropriately pointed out that in the initial postoperative period, when the patient is still in bed, the force placed on the hip is largely that of external rotation. This external rotational force stresses the posterior portion of the femoral neck, an area commonly fragmented by the initial fracture. Awareness of the reduction in the lateral view thus also becomes of major importance. On the lateral view, the anatomic position is preferred (Figure 8-1b). If this position cannot

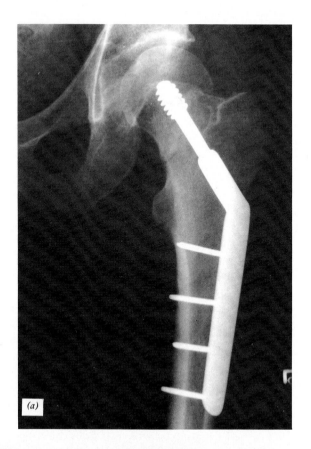

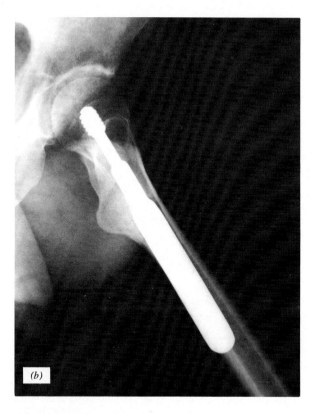

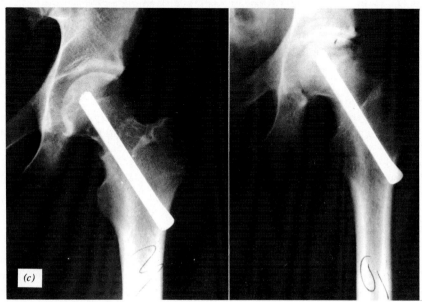

Figure 8-1. Proper position of the femoral neck cortices for stable reduction. (*a,b*) Anatomic reduction of inferior and posterior cortices of the femoral neck (compression screw fixation). (*a*) Frontal view, (*b*) Lateral view. (*c*) Proximal inferior cortex slightly superior to distal cortex. Minimal valgus angulation (Smith-Petersen nail).

be achieved, the posterior cortex of the proximal fragment should be anterior to the posterior cortex of the distal fragment (7). This is to permit the impaction of a beak of bone attached to the posterior portion of the proximal fragment into the medullary bone of the distal fragment, thus stabilizing the reduction (17). Several surgeons even advise the placement of bone graft posteriorly to help support this posterior cortex against this external rotational force; they also advocate the placement of their fixation device in the posteroinferior quadrant of the femoral neck to help guard against posterior femoral neck collapse (19). The bone graft is also thought to provide some blood supply to the femoral head (20). The proper positioning of the cortices on the frontal as well as on the lateral view is probably the prime factor for improving the prognosis of this sometimes treacherous fracture.

Proper reduction is also of major importance in preventing the two major complications of femoral neck fractures, those of avascular necrosis and of nonunion.

AVASCULAR NECROSIS

Example 8-1. This 60-year-old woman tripped and fell down several steps, sustaining an impacted proximal femoral neck fracture (Figure 8-2a). A Ken sliding nail was inserted to hold the position, which was shifted by the surgery into moderate valgus (Figure 8.2b,c). Views obtained over the subsequent year disclosed progressive changes of avascular necrosis with superior segment collapse (Figure 8-2d,e,f).

Avascular necrosis occurs in different series of femoral neck fractures in from 5 to 85% of patients. Those patients who develop collapse of the femoral head following neck fracture often demonstrate failure of adequate reduction on the initial radiographs. The usual position leading to avascular necrosis is that of marked valgus position. The proposed etiologies for this are of interest. Smith (22), in the examination of femoral head fragments at the time of reconstructive surgery, studied the bleeding which occurred from the femoral head fragment when held in various positions. He noted that any position, pushed to its extremes, diminished bleeding from the raw, bony surface of the femoral head fragment, but that moderate valgus

position completely stopped the bleeding (probably because of the stretch or compression of the ligamentum teres and its vessels).

Mary Catto (4,5) in her fascinating histologic studies of the femoral head following fracture, noted an interesting pattern in the vascularity of the femoral head following femoral neck fractures. Almost all femoral heads became ischemic at the time of the initial fracture (1,4,5), but in those heads with intact ligamentum teres vessels a new blood supply across the femoral fracture site was rapidly established. In these cases the bone became revascularized and no problem occurred. In those heads where the artery of the ligamentum teres was not patent, this vascular ingrowth across the fracture site was much more limited and avascular changes were more marked. Femoral heads with avascular necrosis and collapse removed several years following the fracture showed an additional finding: although the femoral heads showed progressive revascularization, this was not uniform across the femoral head. Interestingly, the area for normal weight bearing tended to be revascularized, while an area superior to the fovea remained infarcted. When the hip is in valgus position, this area of dead bone near the fovea centralis shifts into the position of weight bearing. In many of Catto's cases of ischemic collapse, the reduction had been in a valgus position. Thus, although minimal valgus is a desirable position, more than minimal valgus predisposes to avascular necrosis.

Garden (10,12) has even more precisely defined the limits of a good reduction by relating an angle of the alignment of the trabecular pattern in the femoral head with the alignment of the shaft of the femur in both frontal and lateral views. He gave limits for the AP view of 155 to 180° and 180 to 155° on the lateral view (Figure 8-3a,b). When these limits were exceeded, avascular necrosis was common, whereas it was rare when within these limits.

NONUNION

Example 8-2. This 61-year-old woman fell on her way to the bathroom and developed severe right hip pain. The clinical impression of a high femoral-neck fracture was confirmed by the radiographs (Figure 8-4a). Marked

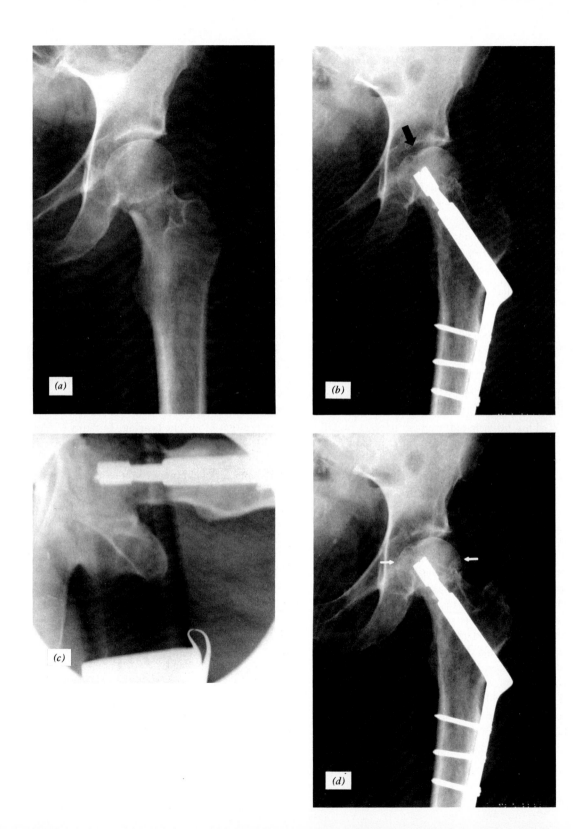

126

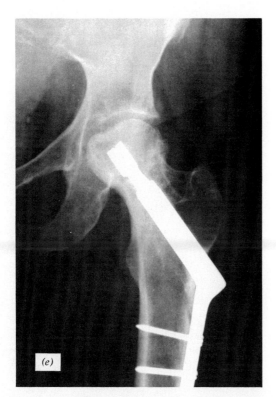
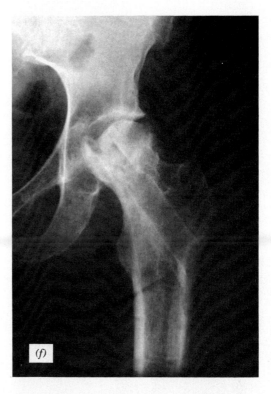

Figure 8-2. High (or proximal) femoral neck fracture, valgus malreduction with subsequent avascular necrosis. A 60-year-old woman who tripped and fell down several steps. (*a*) The initial film demonstrates the proximal femoral neck fracture with mild valgus alignment. The band of density at the fracture line is indicative of probable impaction. (*b*) Two months following fixation with a Ken sliding nail and operative impaction, the femoral head has shifted into greater valgus, with the fovea centralis (arrow) shifted superiorly to lie along the weight-bearing surface. (*c*) The lateral view demonstrates comminution of the anterior cortex. The nail is placed anteriorly, which would help to support the fragmented cortex. Increased lucency is seen in the subarticular-subchondral bone medially and laterally, reflecting focal osteoporosis. This becomes clearer on subsequent studies. (*d*) Three months following surgery, the superior quadrant appears radio-dense compared to the more osteoporotic bone surrounding it, suggesting avascular necrosis. The subchondral bone resorption (arrows) is more apparent, and its failure to develop along the superior aspect of the femoral head increases the likelihood that avascular necrosis is present. (*e*) One year following surgery, partial collapse of the superior segment of the femoral head has occurred. The areas that showed subchondral osteoporosis are spared by the process. (*f*) Fourteen months following surgery, the nail has been removed: the collapse of the superior segment has progressed. When this patient was seen three years following surgery, she had only limited pain in the hip.

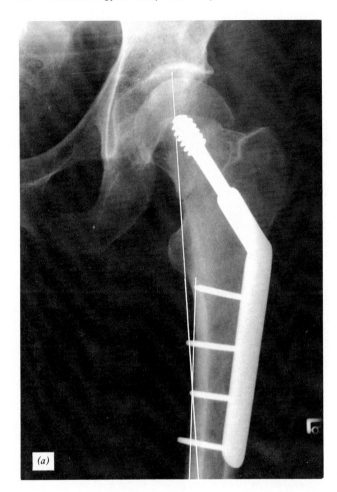

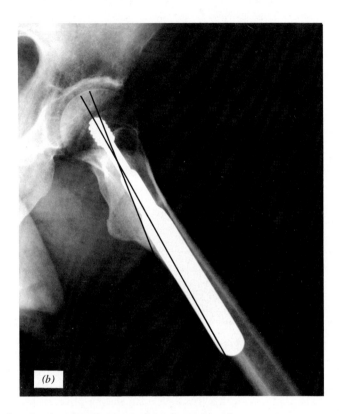

Figure 8-3. Demonstration of Garden's method of evaluating the alignment of the femoral head and neck. (*a*) On the frontal view, the first line is drawn through the median trabeculae of the femoral head. The second line is drawn parallel to the medial femoral cortex. The angle between them should be approximately 160°, with a range of 155 to 180°. (*b*) On the lateral view, the first line is drawn through the median trabecula of the femoral head. The second line is drawn through the axis of the femoral neck. The angle of these lines is usually 180°, with a range of 180 to 155° posterior angulation of the femoral neck-head alignment.

external rotation of the femoral shaft can be recognized by the position of the lesser and greater trochanters.

Intra-operative films (Figure 8-4*b*) demonstrate the placement of a Ken sliding nail with approximately 1 cm between the fins and the barrel—to allow for up to 1 cm of shortening. On the intra-operative film, the head is in

moderate valgus and the region of the inferior femoral neck is slightly distracted. On the lateral view (Figure 8-4*c*), the comminution of the anterior portion of the femoral neck can also be identified.

Two and three weeks following the surgery (Figure 8-4*d,e*), films demonstrate the progressive loss of reduction, with the femoral head shifting posteriorly and the femoral shaft shifting superiorly. This is probably the result of the femoral neck comminution and the failure of adequate impaction at the time of initial reduction. Ectopic bone formation is present.

The patient was nonambulatory at her most recent evaluation, four years following the fracture (Figure 8-4f).

Nonunion is a common complication of femoral neck fracture and is probably due to continued motion at the fracture site, perhaps associated with malreduction. For this reason, firm impaction at the fracture site is recommended by many authors (15). Distraction is undesirable, since an uncontrolled shift of the fracture fragments can occur during the period of partial weight bearing, with loss of reduction. In addition, motion at the fracture site may lead to overgrowth of fibrous tissue, limiting the return of vessels across the fracture line into the femoral head fragment.

METHODS OF FIXATION

If the femoral neck fracture were impacted and not subjected to any stresses, it would heal without displacement. The fractured femoral neck, however, is subjected to many forces. While the patient lies in bed, there is an external rotation force on the hip that, coupled with muscular spasms, may displace the fragments. When weight bearing is initiated, a varus stress results. Although the coefficient of friction at the impacted fracture site is moderate and could prevent slippage of the reduction, it is often not sufficient to resist these forces. Thus, various appliances can be placed across the fracture line to hold it reduced by increasing its coefficient of friction (15). Many of these devices incorporate, in addition, a telescoping or sliding mechanism to permit impaction (15).

Since partial resorption with shortening of the femoral neck can occur with healing (especially in the presence of limited motion), it is desirable that the appliance used be so designed as to permit the fracture to remain impacted in spite of the shortening. Thus, a sliding or telescoping feature of the appliance is desirable. Sometimes the shortening is due to collapse of the posterior cortex with angulation. The lateral view should always be checked (10,11).

The Smith-Petersen nail transfixes the fracture and, if shortening of the femoral neck occurs, can slide out through the lateral femoral cortex (Figure 8-5a,b). Knowles pins can also slide out through the lateral femoral cortex (Figure 8-5c). The Ken (8) (Figure 8-6a) and Massie (15) (Figure 8-6b) nails incorporate a telescoping shaft, which can become shorter as the femoral neck shortens (Figure 8-6c). In the Deyerle (7) apparatus (6,18), shown in Figure 8-7a,b, a series of screws are passed through a side plate and across the fracture. If shortening of the neck occurs, these screws can slide through the lateral femoral cortex. Since these screws have screw threads along their entire length, one might expect the screws to bind in the distal fragment; however, they are "over-drilled," that is, the holes in the distal fragment are drilled larger than the diameter of the screw and thus can slide; the holes in the proximal fragment are drilled slightly smaller than the screw so that the screw will bind to it. The compression screw (Figure 8-8a,b) is designed to permit the portion of the appliance in the proximal fragment to be pulled on firmly to impact the fracture, but it also can telescope into the barrel of the distal portion to permit shortening.

Example 8-3. This patient with a mid-left femoral neck fracture demonstrates the placement of a compression screw. Initial films demonstrate anatomic reduction and the placement of K wires to serve as a guide for the screw placement (Figure 8-9a,b). Once an acceptable position has been found with the K wire, a drill is advanced over the wire and a hole drilled for the placement of the screw. The screw is then advanced so that the entire screw thread is in the proximal fragment (Figure 8-9c). If the screw thread is in both the proximal and distal fragments, it can prevent impaction. The barrel of the appliance, attached to the side plate, is then advanced over the shaft of the screw. A tightening device (not shown) is then used to impact the fracture for the final reduction (Figure 8-9d,e). The final films, four months following the fracture (Figure 8-9f), demonstrate healing of the fracture with minimal sclerosis from endosteal (plug) callus. Trabeculae can be identified crossing the fracture line, indicating healing.

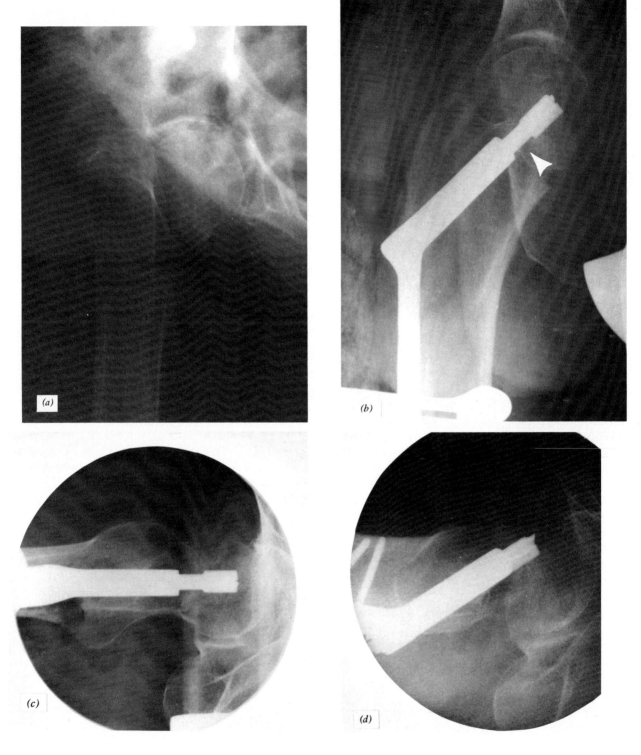

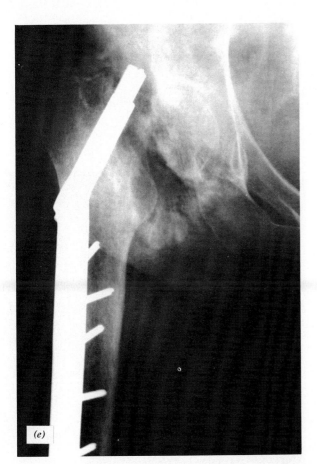
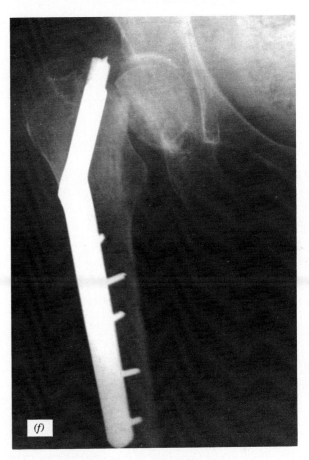

Figure 8-4. Femoral neck fracture treated with a Ken sliding nail, showing rapid loss of reduction. (*a*) The initial film demonstrates the highly osteoporotic bone and the proximal femoral neck fracture. The positions of the lesser and greater trochanters are indicative of marked external rotation. (*b*) Intraoperative films show the placement of the appliance, with distraction along the inferior femoral neck and with moderate valgus of the femoral head. Approximately 1 cm space is left between the fins of the sliding component and the barrel (arrow), permitting up to 1 cm of shortening. No postimpaction films were obtained. (*c*) The lateral intraoperative view demonstrates medial placement of the appliance. On this view, the fins of the appliance anteriorily are close to the fracture line and may not have adequate support to the proximal fragment. The marked comminution of the anterior femoral neck cortex is easily seen in this view. Comminution is common in femoral neck fractures and is one of the predisposing factors for loss of reduction. (*d*) Two weeks later, the lateral view demonstrates that the femoral head has rolled posteriorly and is sliding off the nail. (*e*) Three weeks following surgery, the fins are totally disengaged from the femoral head and the femoral shaft and nail have subluxed superiorly. Extensive ectopic bone formation is present. (*f*) Four years following the fracture, the fracture remains ununited. The patient is nonambulatory.

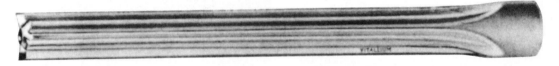

(a)

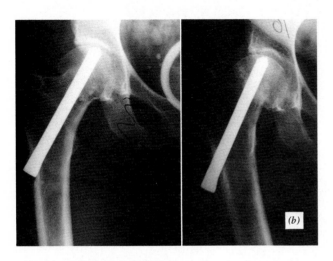

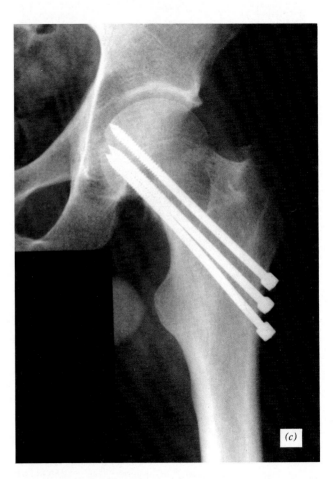

Placement of the Appliance

The placement of the appliance is important. Although a proper reduction is the most important factor, the bone of the femur is not of equal strength in all portions. If the bone structure of an osteoporotic femur from an elderly patient is examined (Figure 8-10), it can be seen that the lateral cortex several centimeters distal to the greater trochanter has a good amount of bone. The trabecular bone is not uniform. It is more marked near the inferior portion of the femoral neck and in the femoral head. Thus, the best bony supports for the appliance are in the lateral cortex, close to the inferior portion of the femoral neck and in the trabecular bone deep within the femoral head.

When the Smith-Petersen nail is used, the inferior portion of the femoral neck provides a second point of fixation for the proximal part of the nail, stabilizing it (10) (Figure 8-11). Placement of the nail near this part of the femoral neck can also reduce the stress on the nail-sideplate junction in an appliance with a sideplate.

Figure 8-5. (*a*) Drawing of Smith-Petersen nail. (Courtesy Howmedica®.) With resorption of the femoral neck or loss of reduction, the nail can slide inferolaterally. (*b*) Smith-Petersen nail sliding through the lateral femoral cortex, with femoral neck resorption. (*c*) Knowles pinning of femoral neck fracture.

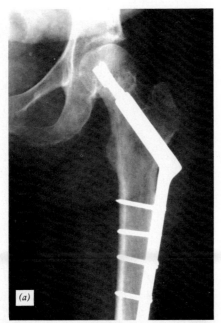

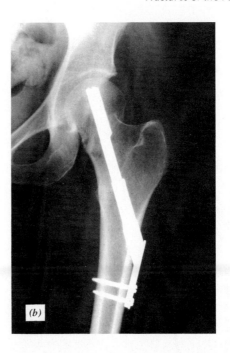

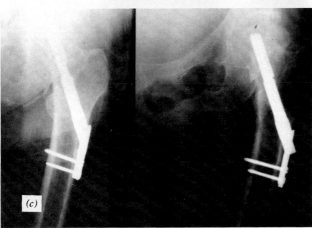

Figure 8-6. (*a*) Ken Nail. (*b*) Massie nail. Both of these nails permit the proximal nail to telescope into the barrel of the distal portion to allow impaction and shortening. The Ken nail (*a*) has a multihole slide plate and a choice of a 135° or 150° nail–side-plate angle. The Massie nail has a two-screw (short) side plate and a 150° barrel–side-plate angle. (*c*) With resorption of the femoral neck, the nail portion of the Massie nail seen in Figure 8-5*b* is progressively telescoping into the barrel. This is probably because of motion at the fracture site, due to lack of adequate impaction at the time of the initial surgery.

RECOGNITION OF THE COMPLICATIONS OF FEMORAL NECK FRACTURE AND ITS SURGERY

Avascular Necrosis

Avascular necrosis is a common complication of femoral neck fractures. Indeed it is interesting that Mary Catto noticed areas of infarcted bone in her nonfractured femoral heads removed at autopsy. In these osteoporotic but otherwise normal femoral heads, the areas of infarcted bone were quite small and usually showed repair fiber bone around them. Transient avascular necrosis is a common if not universal consequence of femoral neck fractures, but it is important to note that it *is* usually transient. Although it might be expected that the avascular bone would not show disuse osteoporosis during the period of immobilization following the femoral neck fracture, this condition usually cannot be recognized with certainty because of the overlying acetabulum. On occasion, a thin rim of bone resorption can be seen just under to the subchondral plate of the femoral articular bone when normal vascularity is present, but such an observation is uncommon; thus, it is useful when present but its absence is of no aid in differentiating normal from absent or decreased vascularity.

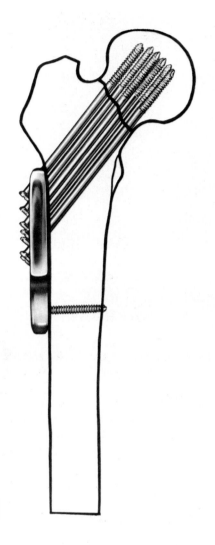

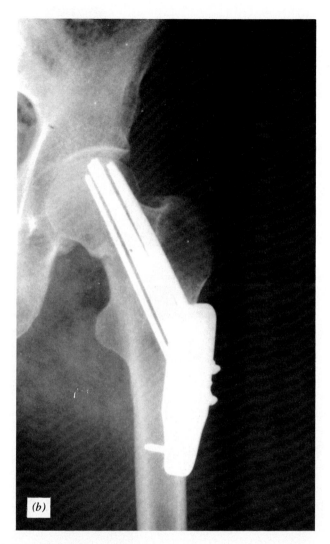

(a)

(b)

Figure 8-7. (*a*) Drawing of Deyerle apparatus. (Courtesy Orthopedic Equipment Company.) (*b*)
The Deyerle apparatus consists of a side plate held to the femoral shaft by a single screw. After
proper reduction of the femoral neck cortices (not achieved in this case), many long screws are
passed through drill holes into the femoral head fragment. When the procedure is properly
performed, the holes are drilled larger than the screws in the distal fragment to permit them to
slide. The screws are individually retightened following operative impaction of the fracture. These
many screws provide a broad surface area, which in turn provides a sharp increase of the coefficient of friction across the fracture. In this case, the inferior femoral neck cortex of the proximal
fragment lies inferior to that of the distal fragment, which would predispose to varus shift with
weight bearing.

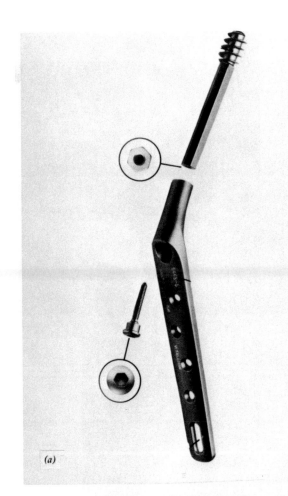

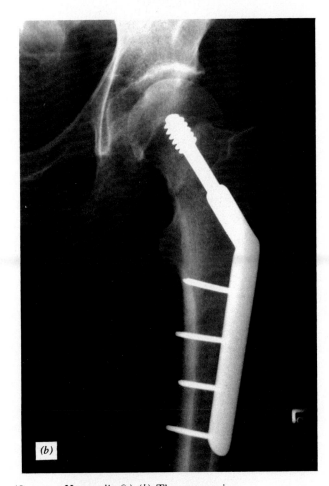

Figure 8-8. (a) Drawing of compression screw. (Courtesy Howmedica®.) (b) The compression screw. The proximal portion has a large screw thread, providing a firm purchase on the proximal fragment. This can be used to pull on the proximal fragment, achieving impaction. The proximal portion can also slide in the barrel of the distal portion to allow shortening. (See Example 8-1.)

Usually, radiographic changes of avascular necrosis cannot be seen until years later, when collapse of the femoral head takes place (Figures 8-12a,b and 8-2e,f). Certainly, one should be alerted to its possible occurrence in patients with a moderate to marked valgus reduction, but even in these cases avascular necrosis may not appear for two to three years following fracture and may not be symptomatic even when it occurs.

Femoral head collapse, when it occurs, may appear either as a thin crescent of lucency beneath the subchondral plate or as more extensive collapse of the femoral head. While increased density in the superior quadrant is often taken as an early sign of avascular necrosis due to other diseases, it is very difficult to apply that finding following placement of a hip nail. On occasion, in osteoporotic bone, the change in the lines of force of weight bearing following femoral nail placement result in moderate thickening (reinforcement) of trabecular bone running

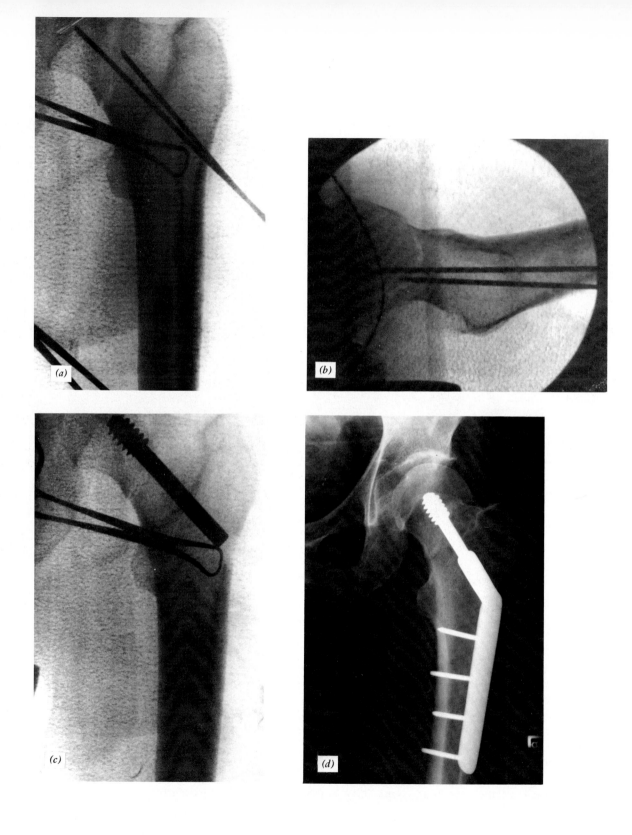

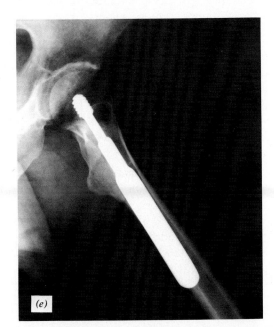 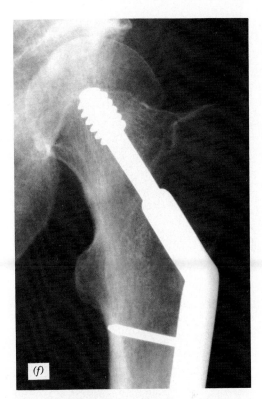

Figure 8-9. Serial radiographs demonstrating placement of a compression screw. Initial frontal and lateral views show anatomic reduction. Two K wires have been placed; the longer wire lies in the midneck and head in each view, a satisfactory position. Following these radiographs, the unsatisfactory K wire is removed and a drill advanced over the properly positioned K wire. A hole is drilled large enough so that the distal, smooth portion of the screw can slide within it. The cortex hole is made large enough for the barrel of the distal component. (a) Frontal view, (b) Lateral view. (c) The screw has now been placed. The screw thread is placed in the femoral head fragment. It is important that the screw thread not extend into the distal fragment, because such overlap would prevent impaction of the fracture. (d,e) The barrel and side plate are then advanced over the smooth portion of the screw component, and the side plate is attached to the femoral shaft. Impaction is then done. The final appearance is shown in these radiographs. (d) Frontal view, (e) Lateral view. (f) Four months following the fracture, trabecula can be identified crossing the fracture line. Slightly increased density at the fracture line reflects the presence of mainly intramedullary callus.

from the weight-bearing surface of bone to the tip of the metal nail (Figure 8-13). This simulates early avascular necrosis, but it is a normal consequence of the change in the pattern of force transmitted through the femur. If the complications of avascular necrosis occur, several salvage procedures and arthroplasties are available and will be discussed in other chapters.

Delayed Union and Nonunion

Delayed union and nonunion of a femoral neck fracture may be easy to recognize if distraction is present; on the other hand, they may be quite difficult to recognize if there is close approximation of the fragments. The best method of demonstrating union is by seeing trabeculae crossing the

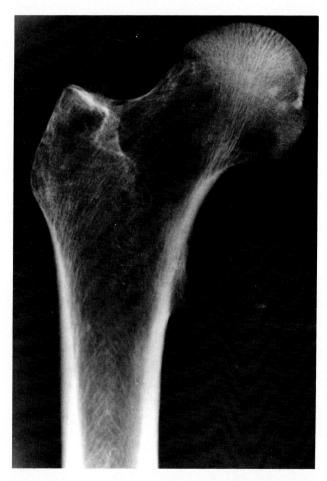

Figure 8-10. Radiograph of a dried osteoporotic proximal femur demonstrating the location of the trabecular bone.

pletely closes off the medullary area of the bone at the fracture site. Its cause is usually motion or intervening muscle or other soft tissue. When the medullary cavity is sealed off from the fracture, it is theoretically impossible for the fracture to unite, unless surgery is done to debride the condensed bone and place the medullary portions of the two fragments into contact.

PENETRATION OF THE FIXATION DEVICE INTO THE ACETABULUM

Penetration of the fixation device into the acetabulum will occur occasionally with all devices used for fixation of femoral neck fractures. It is more common if the articular cortex is penetrated at the time of surgery, even after the nail has been pulled back (3). Although the radiographic appearance of such penetration is frightening, the consequences of this penetration are limited. In one published series (13), Smith-Petersen nails were purposely placed across the joint into the acetabulum to limit motion, with union of the fracture occurring. The patients were not symptomatic as long as weight bearing was limited. Following healing of the fracture and removal of the nail, there was no evidence of degenerative arthritis or other abnormality and no symptoms. While full weight bearing with the nail in place was painful, the pain was thought useful in limiting the patients' activity on the fractured leg. Radiographic change varied, from no evidence of resorption around the nail to resorption around the nail with a new bony shell formation around its tip. Massie (15) indicated some worry that placement of the nail across the joint space might limit the degree of impaction obtainable, thus resulting in lack of impaction and delayed union, but this complication did not occur in Jarry's series (13). Placement of the fixation device across the joint does, however, necessitate a second operation for the removal of the device if full weight bearing is to be resumed (this is not necessary with the usual fixation methods). Many of the patients with femoral neck fractures have only limited ambulation prior to fracture, and thus this potential need for a second operation does not necessarily occur.

fracture line. This can be difficult to see, and on occasion tomography will be necessary to demonstrate the degree of healing. Because of its expense, tomography should be limited to questionable cases.

Delayed union and nonunion have different meanings. A delayed union is still not healed after the usual time for healing has passed. (Massie uses a three-month period). It is usually caused by distraction or motion, and if these factors are corrected, healing will usually take place (15). An established nonunion occurs when condensed bone com-

TREATMENT OF VARUS MALREDUCTION

On occasion, despite initial good reduction, a varus deformity results from slippage of the fragments. When this occurs, it may be treated by nonweight bearing or by reoperation. Surgical approaches are either removal of the appliance with re-reduction and refixation or a peritrochanteric valgus osteotomy to decrease the vertical orientation of the fracture line and thus decrease shearing forces. Both methods appear to be successful in selected cases.

INFECTION

Infection is always a potential complication of any surgery on the hip. The patterns seen are discussed in Chapter 3.

Example 8-4. This 52-year-old man fell down a flight of stairs, sustaining a midfemoral neck fracture. The initial films (Figure 8-14*a*), prior to reduction, suggest that this is a base-of-neck fracture and indicate the difficulty of evaluating the precise level and direction of the fracture line until reduction is achieved. On the postreduction lateral view (Figure 8-14*b*), a portion of the fracture can be seen extending to the region of the lesser trochanter. A Ken nail was placed, and the postplacement films (Figure 8-14*c,d*) demonstrate that the reduction is in moderate valgus, with the calcar portion slightly distracted and with the proximal cortex of the inferior femoral neck lying inferior to the distal cortex. These two factors of malreduction would be predictive of loss of reduction if full weight bearing were allowed. Films at one month (Figure 8-14*c*) demonstrate telescoping of the Ken nail into its barrel to

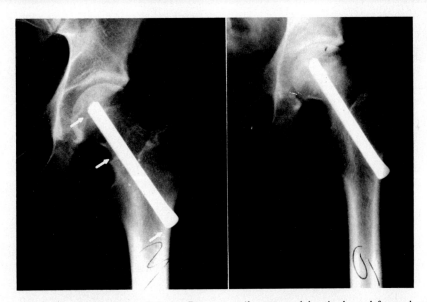

Figure 8-11. A properly inserted Smith-Petersen nail supported by the lateral femoral cortex, the inferior aspect of the femoral neck, and the trabecular bone of the femoral head (arrows). Placing the nail near the inferior femoral neck permits the transfer and diffusion of force from the femoral head to the neck through the nail. If the nail were placed away from the inferior neck, weightbearing might displace the nail with the femoral head fragment inferiorly, resulting in a loss of reduction. The cartilage narrowing that developed in this case represents acute cartilage necrosis (there was no clinical evidence of infection, which must always be excluded in such cases). Acute cartilage necrosis is a common sequella of slippage of the capital femoral epiphysis and is discussed more fully in Chapter 7. It is an unusual sequella of other types of hip injury, with or without surgery.

maximum shortening, with continued separation at the fracture line. At 14 months (Figure 8-14*f*), union was not present (a delayed union). During the year, the patient had pain in the hip and had had several superficial abscesses drained. Thirteen months following surgery, the patient had an increase in severity and duration of pain and was reevaluated. At that time, extensive resorption

around the barrel and sliding portion of the nail was seen. Evidence of inward movement of the side plate was present. The continuing delayed union was also identified. In addition, the development of sclerosis along the fracture line may indicate an early phase in the development of an established nonunion.

As one analyzes the pattern of resorption around the

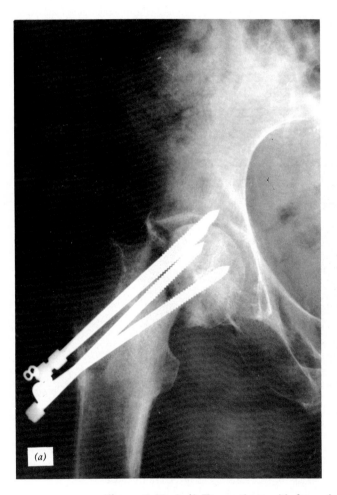 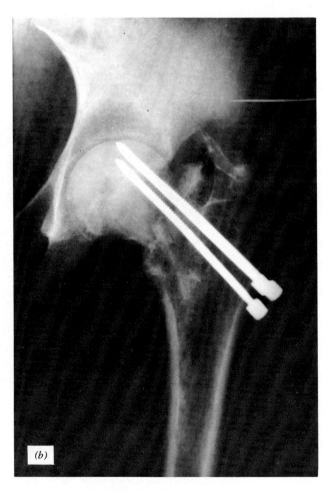

Figure 8-12. (*a,b*) Two patients with femoral neck fractures, treated with Knowles pins, each with loss of reduction, ununited fractures, and changes of avascular necrosis, as shown by the increased density of the femoral heads. In Figure 8-10*a*, the neck is partially resorbed, probably due to movement; one pin has protruded into the acetabulum.

The final film (Figure 8-14*g*), five months following removal of the nail, demonstrates the extent of resorption and of the periosteal reaction present. Union is now present, but changes of secondary degenerative arthritis are seen, with acetabular sclerosis and an acetabular degenerative cyst. At this time, the patient had increasing pain with weight bearing and was being considered as a candidate for a total hip replacement.

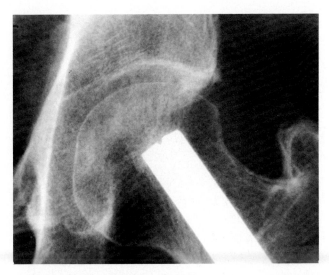

Figure 8-13. The trabeculae superior to proximal tip of the nail are thickened, reflecting the new pattern of stress transfer within the femoral head. this must be differentiated from the changes seen in early avascular necrosis.

proximal portion of the nail, the irregularity and lack of concentric resorption strongly suggest the presence of infective loosening. At the time of surgery for removal of the nail, a deep abscess was found, which grew out staphylococcus epidermitis and a subgroup of Schadler bacillus.

SUMMARY

Femoral neck fractures are common fractures of the elderly but can occur at all ages. The prognosis of any serious illness in these patients is poor, and there is significant mortality from femoral neck fractures, with or without surgery. Accuracy of reduction is probably the most important criterion for a good result. The best reduction is a well-impacted reduction in slight valgus position. Reduction in the lateral view should be near anatomic. Many fixation devices are in use to resist the shear forces across the fractured femoral neck. Complications of avascular necrosis and nonunion can be minimized by proper reduction. Avascular necrosis with femoral head segmental collapse is most common in hips reduced in moderate to marked valgus position.

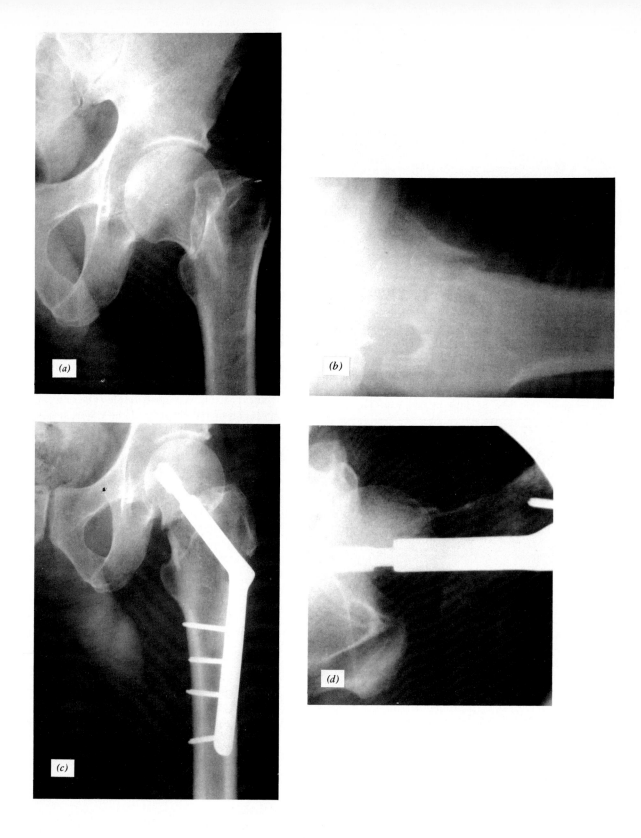

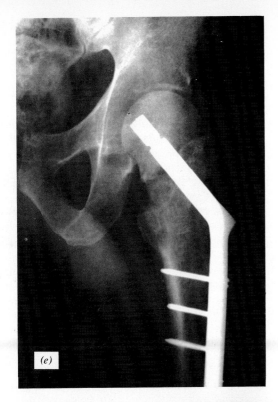

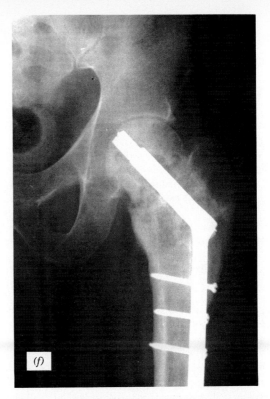

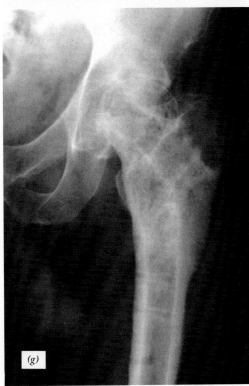

Figure 8-14. Femoral neck fracture with a Ken sliding nail fixation, showing delayed union associated with infection. (*a*) The frontal view demonstrates the base of neck fracture. There is moderate external rotation of the femoral shaft. The ovoid lytic lesion in the region of the greater trochanter represents the fracture site seen en face; it does not represent a lytic metastasis. (*b*) The postreduction lateral view shows a small beak of bone extending from the proximal fragment close to the lesser trochanter. (*c*) Following placement of the Ken sliding nail, the inferior portion of the fracture line is minimally distracted. Radiolucency at the base of the femoral neck medial to the nail results from the displacement of a small bone fragment. (*d*) The lateral view confirms the minimal distraction. (*e*) One month following surgery, the nail has slid into the barrel and is at its shortest length. Minimal distraction is still present. The nail is now holding the fracture distracted and is an impediment to rapid healing. Minimal bone resorption is now present inferior to the barrel of the appliance. This type of bone resorption could have resulted from the appliance repeatedly bending at its attachment to the side plate, bending in response to vertical pressure applied to the femoral head, or from infection surrounding the appliance. (*f*) After 14 months, there is extensive irregular resorption around the barrel and the nail; the joint space is now narrow. These changes are due to infection. The fracture remains ununited. (*g*) Five months following removal of the nail, the changes associated with secondary degenerative arthritis have appeared, with marked cartilage narrowing and a degenerative cyst in the acetabulum.

REFERENCES

1. Barnes R: The Diagnosis of ischemia of the capital fragment in femoral neck fractures. *J. Bone Joint Surg* 44B:1760–1761, 1962.

2. Bentley G: Impacted fractures of the neck of the femur. *J Bone Joint Surg* 50B:551–561, 1968.

3. Brown FT, et al: Transcervical femoral fracture—a review of 195 patients treated by sliding nail plate fixation. *J Bone Joint Surg* 46B:648–663, 1964.

4. Catto M: A histologic study of avascular necrosis of the head of the femur after transcervical fracture. *J Bone Joint Surg* 47B:749–776, 1965.

5. Catto M: The histologic appearances of late segmental collapse of the femoral head after transcervical fracture. *J Bone Joint Surg* 47B:777–791, 1965.

6. Chapman MW, Stehr JH, Eberle CF, et al: Treatment of intracapsular hip fractures by the Deyerle method. *J Bone Joint Surg* 57A:735–742, 1975.

7. Deyerle WM: Multiple pin peripheral fixation in fractures of the neck of the femur: Immediate weight bearing. *Clin Orthop* 39:135–156, 1965.

8. Fielding J Wm, et al: A continuing end-result study of displaced intracapsular fractures of the neck of the femur treated with the Pugh nail. *J Bone Joint Surg* 56A:1464–1472, 1974.

9. Fielding J Wm: Pugh nail fixation of displaced femoral neck fractures. *Clin Orthop* 106:107–116, 1975.

10. Garden RS: Low-angle fixation in fractures of the femoral neck. *J Bone Joint Surg* 43B:647–663, 1961.

11. Garden RS: Stability and union in subcapital fractures of the femur. *J Bone Joint Surg* 46B:630–647, 1964.

12. Garden RS: Mal-reduction and avascular necrosis in subcapital fractures of the femur. *J Bone Joint Surg* 53B:183–197, 1971.

13. Jarry L: Transarticular nailing for fractures of the femoral neck. *J Bone Joint Surg* 46B:674–684, 1964.

14. Massie WK: Functional fixation of femoral neck fractures; telescoping nail technique. *Clin Orthop* 12:230–255, 1958.

15. Massie WK: Fractures of the hip. *J Bone Joint Surg* 46A:658–690, 1964.

16. McElvenny RT: The immediate treatment of intracapsular hip fracture. *Clin Orthop* 10:289–325, 1957.

17. McElvenny RT: The importance of the lateral x-ray film in treating intracapsular fracture of the femur. *Am J Orthop* 4:212–215, 1962.

18. Metz CW, Jr, et al: The displaced intracapsular fracture of the neck of the femur. *J Bone Joint Surg* 52A:113–127, 1970.

19. Meyers MH, Harvey JP Jr, Moore TM: Treatment of displaced subcapital and Transcervical fractures of the femoral neck by muscle-pedicle-bone graft and internal fixation. *J Bone Joint Surg* 55A:257–274, 1973.

20. Meyers MH, Moore TM, Harvey JP Jr: Displaced fracture of femoral neck treated with muscle pedicle graft. *J Bone Joint Surg* 57A:718–720, 1975.

21. Niemann K, Martin H: Fractures about the hip in an institutionalized patient population. *J Bone Joint Surg* 50A:1327–1340, 1968.

22. Smith FB: Effects of rotatory and valgus mal-position on blood supply to femoral head. *J Bone Joint Surg* 41A:800–815, 1959.

9
Femoral Head Replacements

Femoral head replacements are an important adjunct to the management of femoral neck fractures, especially in elderly patients. While they have traditionally been used also for the treatment of arthritis of the hip, this application has been largely supplanted by the total hip replacement.

ing, with extensive bone resorption around the metal strut. Loosening is not always symptomatic. Although this prosthesis is no longer used, it is still occasionally seen. The patient shown in Figure 9-1c was satisfied with his hip for 20 years following surgery, until the plastic femoral head finally fragmented.

THE JUDET PROSTHESIS

The earliest widely used femoral head prostheses were the Judet and related stem prostheses. (Figure 9-1a,b,c). Each of these consisted of a plastic femoral head with a metal strut (stem) anchoring it to the proximal femur. The strut was passed through the femoral neck to exit in or just distal to the distal portion of the greater trochanter. The plastic femoral head component is radiolucent, and thus only the metal strut is visible on radiographs. Variations of the prosthesis include several designs with a metallic femoral head and stem (Figure 9-2). The Judet prosthesis has been supplanted by the Moore and Thompson prostheses and their variants because of its tendency for early failure by dislocation, subluxation, loosening, or infection. In Salvati's review (17), the Judet prosthesis had a 25% failure rate in the first five years, with a 15% incidence of subluxation or dislocation. It is common for even the successful Judet prostheses to show evidence of loosen-

THE AUSTIN-MOORE PROSTHESIS

The Austin-Moore prosthesis (Figure 9-3), developed in 1939, is a metallic prosthesis made either of Vitallium or stainless steel. It consists of a femoral neck and head. The head (available in several sizes) attaches to a stem of various lengths and widths. The stem is most commonly fenestrated. Recent redesign has optionally eliminated the fenestrations. The prosthesis may be seated in the medullary bone of the femoral canal or in methylmethacrylate (Figure 9-4a,b).

Size

Selection of the correct size is important in obtaining good results. The femoral head should fit snugly in the acetabulum and should approximately equal the size of the replaced femoral head (with its articular cartilage). This is best evaluated at the time of surgery by a suction fit. The accuracy of the fit is more difficult to judge on radiographs, but concentricity of the prosthetic head and acetabulum is usually present. Occasionally, despite

This chapter is based on materials originally printed in the *Radiology Clinics of North America,* vol 8, pp 45–56, 1975. Portions reprinted with permission.

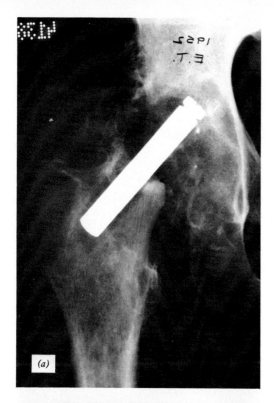

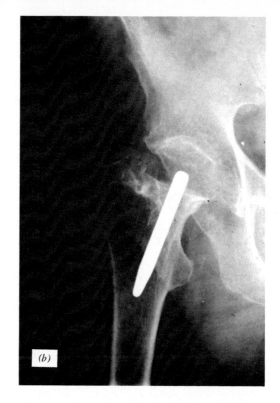

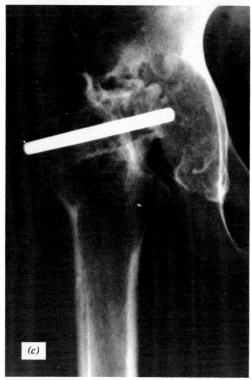

Figure 9-1. Three different modifications of the Judet prosthesis, each with a metal stem and a plastic femoral head (radiolucent). The stem of each of these prostheses is loose and has a wide zone of bone resorption around it. (*a,b*) The stem is placed in an intramedullary site. (*c*) The lateral femoral cortex is penetrated by the stem for added support. The prosthesis was in place for 20 years.

proper placement, the roentgenogram will demonstrate a lack of concentricity because of normal or degenerative variation in the thickness of acetabular cartilage. Because of this, only marked discrepancy in the size of the acetabulum and prosthetic femoral head can be interpreted as indicating incorrect size. A very small femoral head predisposes to progressive cartilage narrowing and sclerosis of the acetabulum, which is often painful. A large femoral head may result in the patient experiencing a sticking or jelling sensation during hip motion. If the head is much too large, it may cause constant subluxation and recurrent dislocation.

Placement of the prosthesis so that the femoral neck is of the proper length is also important and is determined in part by the surgeon's choice of the site of the femoral neck osteotomy and the degree of anteversion selected. The correct length can be estimated before or during surgery by roentgenography. One method is to take a roentgenogram of the hip with a pelvimetry ruler placed next to the hip at the same distance from the film as from the hip. Alternatively, this measurement can be determined with sufficient accuracy by assuming a 20% magnification factor on films taken at a distance of 40 inches (9). The proper neck length can also be estimated by comparison with the opposite hip if the degree of rotation is equal. A short femoral neck may decrease the tension in the muscles around the hip, which may result in weakness of abduction and predispose the hip to dislocation. A long femoral neck may result in painful muscle spasms and a sticking sensation (7,9).

Position

Position of the stem is important in avoiding excessive varus angulation, which would predispose the prosthesis to loosening; neutral to slight valgus position is preferred. The femoral neck should be placed in neutral or slight anteversion. Most important, the position should be firmly maintained by bony contact and the flange of the prosthesis (at the base of the femoral neck portion) should be in contact with femoral cortical bone on both frontal and lateral views. Incomplete contact may lead to loosening, possibly with settling of the prosthesis deeper into the femur (9). This would have the same consequence as the presence of an initially short femoral neck. Intraoperative roentgenograms are desirable to assure accurate initial placement. The flange should rest on approximately ⅝ in. of bone of the femoral neck medially to achieve proper fit in the greater trochanteric region.

Example 9-1. This 78-year-old woman fell during a visit to a neighbor's house. Physical examination revealed a shortened and externally rotated right lower extremity. Radiographs disclosed a midfemoral neck fracture and Paget's disease of the pelvis, including the acetabulum (Figure 9-5a). Asymmetric narrowing of the superomedial

joint cartilage is present. A long-stemmed Austin-Moore prosthesis was inserted (Figure 9-5b). Although the femoral head prosthesis is asymmetric within the acetabulum and might be thought to be too small, this is solely a reflection of the degenerative narrowing of the articular cartilage of the acetabulum. The patient was placed on partial weight bearing 10 days following surgery and was without hip complaints three months later when seen for an unrelated illness.

THOMPSON PROSTHESIS

The F.R. Thompson prosthesis (Figure 9-6) was developed in 1951 and demonstrates several structural differences from the Austin Moore prosthesis. The Thompson prosthesis has a longer prosthetic femoral neck and is designed to sit at the base of the femoral neck along the intertrochanteric line. The Thompson prosthesis is therefore preferred for low neck fractures. The Thompson's stem is not fenestrated. Proper positioning and size selection are otherwise essentially the same as for the Austin Moore prosthesis (20). The Thompson prosthesis, however, is easier to remove than the Austin Moore prosthesis, even if fixed in methacrylate. Similar prostheses can be designed to be replaced easily by the femoral portion of a total hip replacement, should this be desirable later. (Figure 9-7b,c). Stabilizing the Thompson prosthesis in methacrylate appears to decrease the incidence of complications (8,21).

Example 9-2. This elderly woman fell and was found to have a femoral neck fracture. On the initial film, increased density was present along the medial edge of the fracture line (Figure 9-7a). This occasional finding of focal sclerosis may be seen prior to the development of the fracture or at the time of the acute fracture and suggests that certain femoral neck fractures represent the completion of stress fractures. The prosthesis used is a variant of the Thompson type, designed for easy total hip replacement (Figure 9-7b). A comparison of its appearance to that of the femoral component of a Charnley-Miller prosthesis (Figure 9-7c) clearly shows the similarity of the stem, flange, and neck. Should this patient need a total hip re-

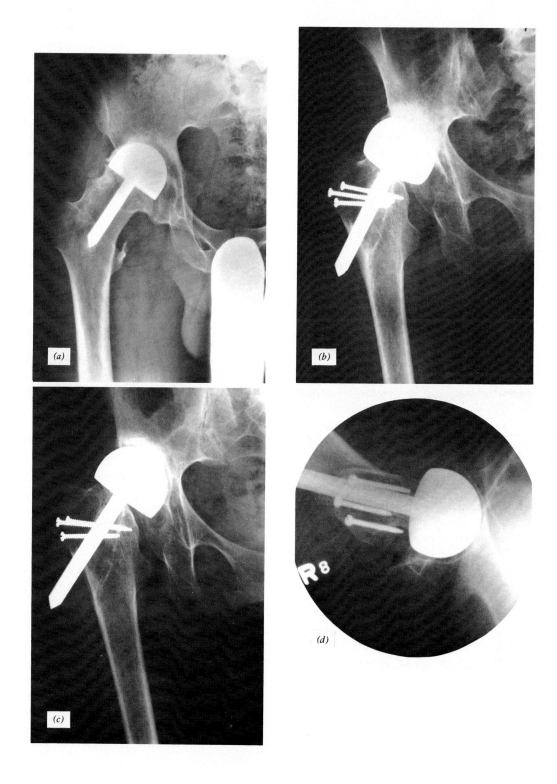

148

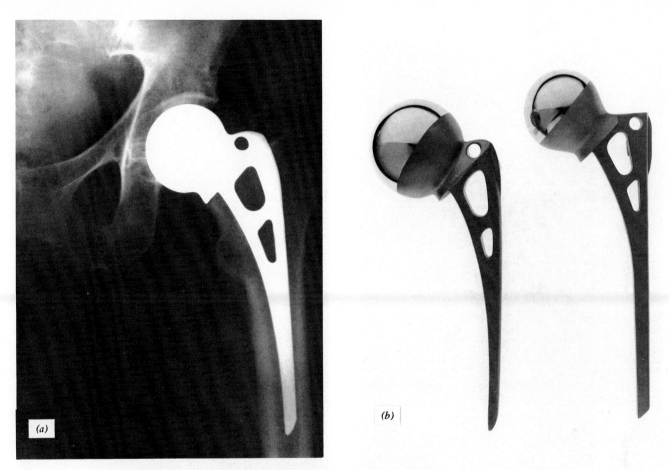

Figure 9-3. The Austin-Moore prosthesis. Identifying characteristics of this prosthesis include the fenestrations in the stem, the hole at the base of the lateral portion of the neck to aid in removal, and the relatively short neck. Properly positioned, the flange of the prosthesis should rest on approximately ⅝ in. of medial femoral neck. The head should be approximately the size of the replaced femoral head and its articular cartilage.

Figure 9-2. Modifications of the Judet prosthesis, with metallic femoral heads. (*a*) The stem is placed in the medullary canal. The sclerosis at the tip of the prosthesis probably reflects a focal reinforcement of trabeculae to better distribute the transmitted force. The prosthetic femoral head articulates with an eroded and superiorly placed acetabulum, as do all of the Judet-type prostheses shown. While preoperative films are not available in these cases, this view suggests a tendency for the prosthesis to erode the acetabulum superiorly. A modified Judet stem prosthesis with varus shift, increasing over a three-year period. Widening of the zone of radiolucency around the stem has increased. The prosthesis articulates with a superiorly placed pseudoacetabulum. (*b*) Earliest film, (*c*) 3 year follow-up view. (*d*) The lateral view shows that the screws are not part of the prosthesis. They were probably used to reattach the greater trochanter during surgery. A temporary intraoperative osteotomy through the greater trochanter during surgery can simplify surgery on the hip and is discussed more fully in the chapter on total hip replacements.

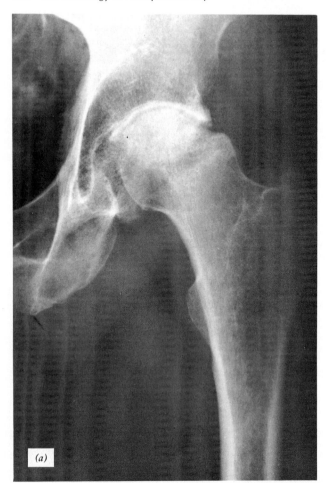

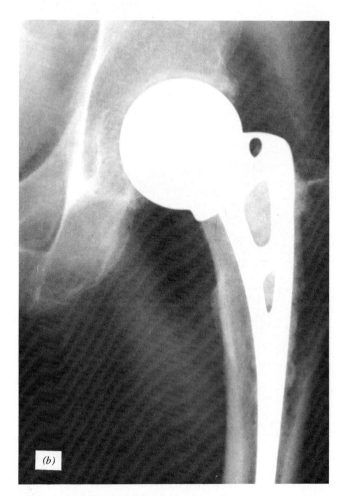

Figure 9-4. Austin-Moore prosthesis in methylmethacrylate. (*a*) Preoperative view shows sclerosis and collaspe of the superior quadrant of the femoral head characteristic of avascular necrosis. (*b*) The Austin-Moore prosthesis has been placed in radiopaque methylmethacrylate. The Moore prosthesis is not usually placed in methacrylate, because the methacrylate in the fenestrations would make it very difficult to remove the prosthesis, should it be necessary.

placement in the future, this femoral component can easily be replaced by the total hip replacement femoral component. The prosthesis is seated in minimally radiopaque methylmethacrylate.

NORMAL FINDINGS

Size, appearance, and positioning have already been discussed. Several changes in the bone of the femoral shaft and the acetabulum can be seen following femoral head and neck replacement; these changes should not be confused with abnormality.

Periostitis

Following surgery, it is possible to see a small amount of periosteal new bone along the lateral aspect of the femur, particularly if the prosthesis was inserted during a second operation on the hip. After several months, this periosteal new bone will show progressive maturation and stabilization. Occasionally, a minimal amount of additional periosteal new bone can be seen developing adjacent to the tip of the stem of the prosthesis years later, in the absence of symptoms (20).

Increased Bone Density

Increased bone density with a cotton-wool-like appearance may develop over many months in the medullary cavity adjacent to the tip of the prosthesis (Figure 9-8*a,b*). Occasionally this density resembles cortical bone and blends with the lateral or medial cortex. Similar sclerosis can occur with a loose prosthesis and is thought to partially support it (Figure 9-9). Increased density also occurs along the calcar femoris adjacent to the medial aspect of the flanges of the prosthesis (14,20). A minor degree of increased density in the acetabulum is frequently seen. Although a greater degree of acetabular sclerosis is usually

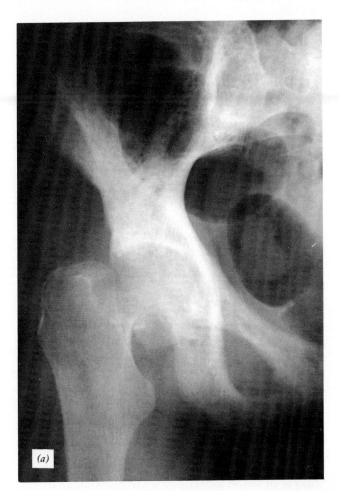

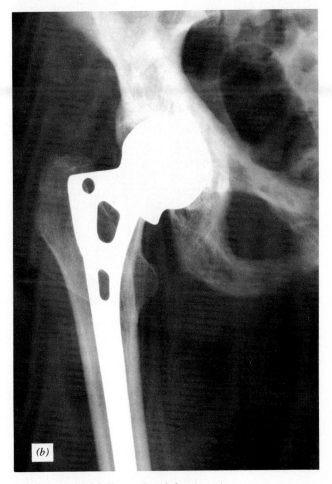

Figure 9-5. Example 9-1. Use of the Austin-Moore prosthesis. (*a*) Midfemoral neck fracture. At least ⅝ in. of the medial femoral neck is attached to the distal fragment. The acetabulum cartilage is of normal thickness. Paget's disease is present in the pelvis. (*b*) A long-stemmed Austin-Moore prosthesis has been inserted. The cartilage is narrowed medially, probably due to the arthrosis associated with Paget's disease.

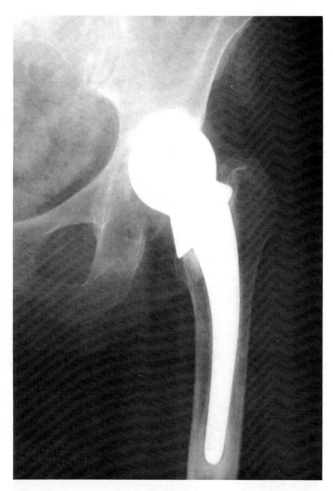

Figure 9-6. The Thompson prosthesis. Identifying characteristics include the absence of fenestrations and the longer femoral neck, which permits the placement of the prosthesis at the base of the femoral neck. The curved proximal portion and straight distal portion of the stem help to distinguish it from similar prosthesis.

painless, pain sometimes will occur. Moderate sclerosis seems to be more common following reaming of the acetabulum or in the presence of preexisting degenerative arthritis of the hip (14,20).

Thickening of the cortex of the femur just distal to the tip of the stem of the prosthesis is common in the more active patient.

Resorption of the Medial Femoral Neck

Following placement of the Austin-Moore prosthesis, it is common to see a small amount of resorption of the remaining portion of the femoral neck. Associated settling of the prosthesis may or may not occur. Occasionally, 5 to 10 mm of calcar can be resorbed over many months in the absence of symptoms. More marked resorption seems to occur in particularly firmly seated protheses and presumably represents disuse atrophy, as shown in Figure 9-10 (6,20).

Zone of Radiolucency Around Prosthesis

Approximately one-third of all patients will demonstrate a thin zone of radiolucency around the stem of the prosthesis, with a thin band of dense bone surrounding the radiolucency (Figure 9-11). The bands of radiolucency and sclerosis usually measure less than 1 mm each. When this radiolucency is seen, the prosthesis is usually asymptomatic, but occasionally, it will be painful and loose. When the zone of radiolucency exceeds 2 mm, the incidence of loosening is higher. It is important to be certain, however, that the prosthesis was not placed in radiolucent methylmethacrylate, since that gives a wide zone of radiolucency around the prosthesis (6,20).

Acetabular Protrusion

This sequela of femoral head replacement may be symptomatic or asymptomatic. It is common in cases of rheumatoid arthritis and Paget's disease (Figure 9-12a,b). Acetabular protrusion is also common if the acetabulum has been reamed (4) (e.g., for treatment of degenerative arthritis) and is also seen with unevenly seated prostheses (9). The same sequela would be expected in osteomalacia. (1,2,3,4,6).

Sinking of the Prosthesis into the Femoral Shaft

This is usually a sign of loosening, but occasionally the prosthesis shifts to a position of firmer impaction and remains well seated.

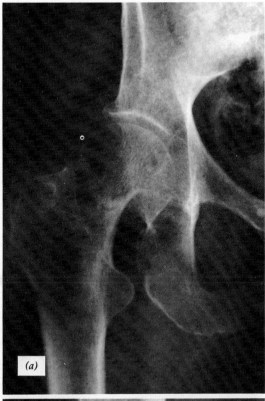

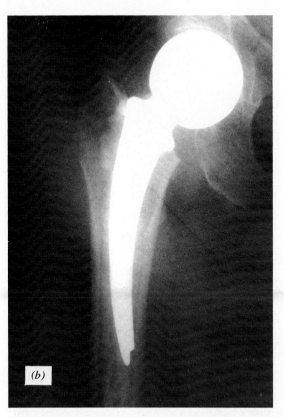

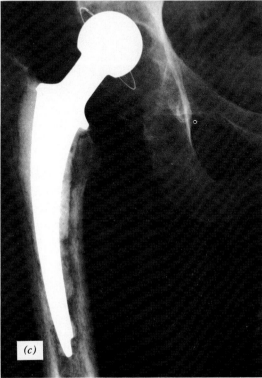

Figure 9-7. Example 9-2. The Muller femoral head prosthesis used for femoral neck fracture. (*a*) Midfemoral neck fracture with varus deformity. (*b*) The Muller prosthesis has been placed in slightly radiopaque methacrylate. The curve of the stem is designed for easy removal and replacement with the femoral component of a total hip prosthesis. (*c*) A Muller total hip prosthesis with the same stem as the Muller femoral head prosthesis.

COMPLICATIONS

Fracture

Fracture at the time of insertion is an anticipated, fairly common, complication of treatment when the bone is osteoporotic (2). The fractures can occur during reaming of the medullary canal, at the time of the impaction of the prosthesis into the intertrochanteric portion of the femur, or, during surgery, on reduction of the dislocated hip. The intertrochanteric fractures can be very subtle and careful scrutiny is necessary to detect them prior to displacement, which may occur on the initiation of weight bearing.

153

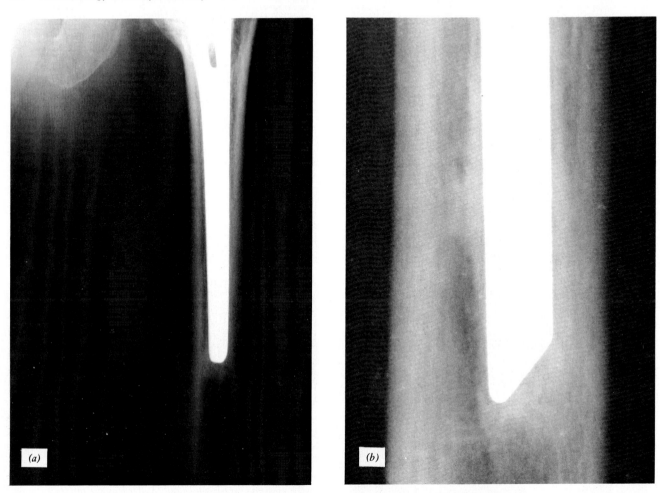

Figure 9-8. (a,b) Two patients with firmly seated Moore prostheses. Sclerosis at the tip of these prostheses reflects a reactive bone hypertrophy in response to stress.

Example 9-3. This 86-year-old woman with a healed sub- and intertrochanteric fracture fell at home and developed hip pain. She was seen at a local hospital, given analgesics, and either left of her own will or was sent home. Because of increasing pain she was brought to another hospital where a right midfemoral neck fracture was identified. The healed subtrochanteric and lesser trochanteric fracture can be seen with several circlage (encircling) wires in (Figure 9-13a). Ectopic bone formation is present superolateral to the hip joint. A midfemoral neck fracture is present with superior displacement of the distal fragment. Although the lateral view is of poor quality, the discrepancy of the angle between the femoral neck and the position of the acetabulum implies a great amount of posterior femoral neck comminution (Figure 9-13b). This fracture was treated with an Austin-Moore prosthesis. Because of the deformity from the prior fracture a straight stem prosthesis was chosen. At the time of insertion of the Moore prosthesis, a fracture through the osteoporotic greater trochanter occurred. A long-stem Moore prosthesis was used to help transfer force distally (Figure 9-13c). Limited ambulation was started one week postoperatively,

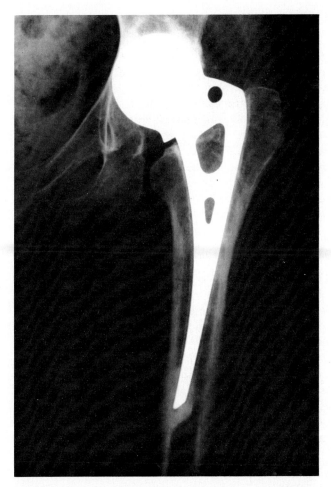

Figure 9-9. Loose Austin-Moore prosthesis with sclerosis at tip. Extensive sclerosis near the tip of the prosthesis reflects the transfer of force distally. This occurs when there is insufficient support at the medial femoral neck. A high degree of sclerosis often means that the prosthesis is or was loose. On occasion, loose prostheses settle to a new position of firm fixation. In this patient there has also been resorption of the femoral neck and of the acetabular cartilage. Sclerosis of the acetabular rim is due to degenerative arthrosis.

and the patient was ambulatory with a four-legged walker three weeks postoperatively. Seven months postoperative, the greater trochanter fracture had healed and the patient was ambulating well at home (Figure 9-13*d,e*).

Traumatic fractures, months to years later, can occur

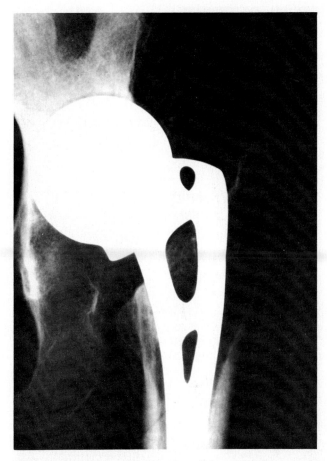

Figure 9-10. Progressive resorption of the medial femoral neck demonstrated on serial films. This is a normal finding. At surgery, this prosthesis was firmly seated. There was no evidence of infection. Sclerosis of the acetabulum was due to degenerative arthrosis. The prosthesis was painful because of secondary degenerative arthrosis. (Reprinted by permission, Radiologic Clinics of North America, April 75.)

either through the bone surrounding the stem of the prosthesis or just distal to it (15). Such fractures heal normally.

Limp

A limp can result from pain (discussed later) or from muscle weakness. Occasionally, the muscle weakness is related to a short femoral neck, resulting in weak abductors (abductor lurch). Proper femoral neck length can be esti-

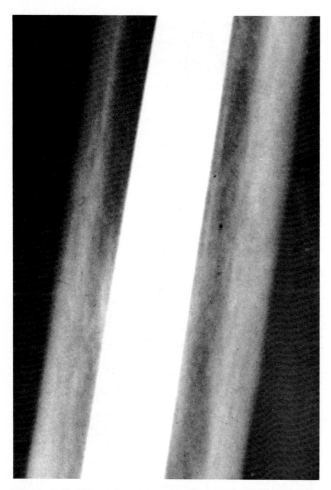

Figure 9-11. Normal reaction of bone to the stem of an Austin-Moore prosthesis. A thin zone of radiolucency is separated from the medullary trabecular bone by a thin band of condensed bone. Asymptomatic patient. No evidence of loosening on follow-up. (Reprinted by permission, Radiologic Clinics of North America.)

mated by comparing the operated and nonoperated sides. Occasionally, a large prosthetic femoral head will cause sticking and a limp.

Dislocation

Dislocations are seen in 2 to 8% of femoral head prostheses. These dislocations can occur in the early postoperative period or years later (5,8,19).

Cartilage Necrosis

Cartilage necrosis is usually painful when the patient walks, but may be asymptomatic. Cartilage necrosis commonly occurs following femoral head replacement for avascular necrosis and in patients with evidence of preoperative cartilage narrowing. It is often progressive in these patients following femoral head replacement, as can be seen in Figure 9-14 (20). If cartilage narrowing is seen in a patient with a previously radiographically normal joint space and normal-appearing cartilage at the time of surgery (and in the absence of avascular necrosis of the femoral head preoperatively), infection should be suspected (see Figure 9-18).

Degenerative Arthritis

Degenerative arthritis is a common cause of postoperative pain following femoral head replacement. The usual cause is preoperative degenerative arthritis that remains symptomatic following surgery; this is not surprising, since femoral head replacement treats only one side of the joint (9,10). Degenerative arthritis of the joint may develop following surgery in a previously normal joint, though this is less likely in the relatively inactive older patient. Avascular necrosis of the femoral head appears to predispose to degenerative arthritis following prosthetic replacement (Figure 9-14).

Sinking of the prosthesis and acetabular protrusion may be symptomatic or asymptomatic; they have been discussed previously.

Loosening

Loosening is an important, frequent complication of femoral head replacements. The frequency of loosening increases the longer the prosthesis is in place. Loosening may be mildly uncomfortable (not requiring treatment) or severely painful, requiring further surgery. A loose prosthesis may be infected but may demonstrate no specific changes due to infection.

Loosening can be detected by observation of a wide or widening zone of radiolucency around the stem of the prosthesis (Figure 9-15a,b,c,d). A 1 mm zone of radiolucency is usually normal; wider zones of radiolucency are suspect (1,2,6,9,11). (However, one must remember that the prosthesis may be placed in radiolucent methylmethacrylate, resulting in a wide band of radiolucency around the prosthesis.) Progressive widening over serial films is diagnostic. Occasionally a 3–4 mm zone of radiolucency is seen, limited to the intertrochanteric region in the absence of symptoms, which presumably is a normal variant.

Occasionally the zone of radiolucency becomes dumbbell shaped, representing toggling around a center point. Sink-

ing of the prosthesis may be associated with loosening or occur as an isolated finding, as seen in Figure 9-16a,b (6).

Loosening can be demonstrated by comparing the distance of the flange of the prosthesis from the calcar femoris or lesser trochanter on films taken before and at the end of 15 minutes of 10 lb of skin traction on the leg (to relax muscle pull) (6,9,11). A brief pull may be insufficient to overcome muscle spasm, particularly with a painful prosthesis (9). Arthrography can also be used to demonstrate loosening and may show tracking of contrast

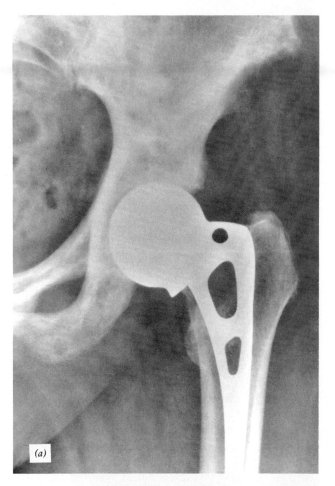 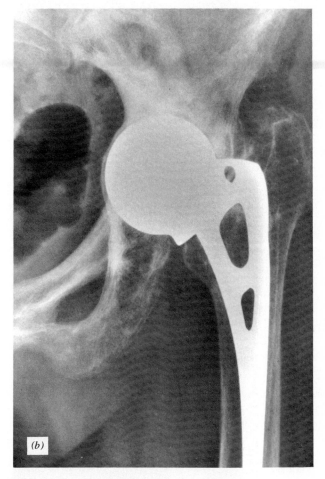

Figure 9-12. Acetabular protrusion. (a,b) Progressive acetabular protrusion is seen on sequential taken films five years apart. Paget's disease is present in the pelvis. (Reprinted by permission, Radiologic Clinics of North America.)

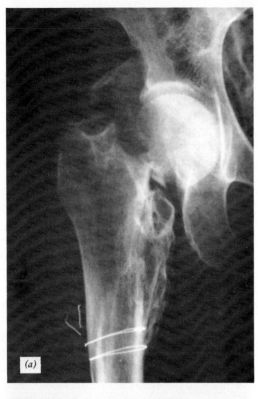

(a)

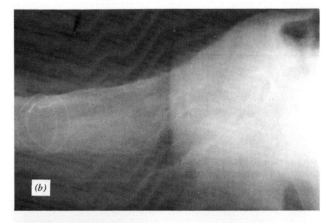

(b)

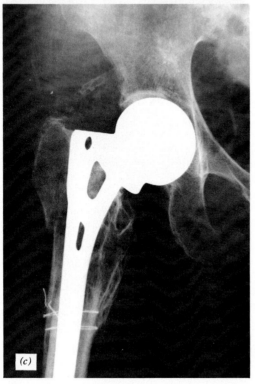

(c)

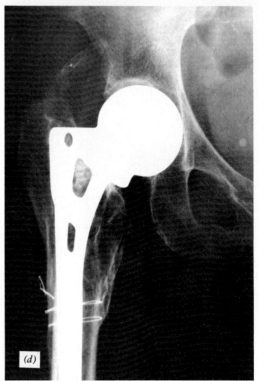

(d)

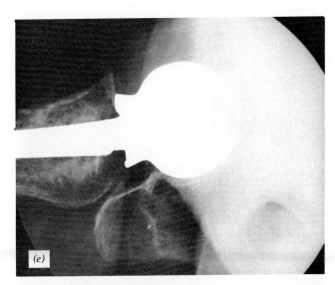

Figure 9-13. Example 9-3. Fracture on insertion of Austin-Moore prosthesis. (*a*) An acute femoral neck fracture is present. A healed medial and subtrochanteric fracture is present. Two circlage wires are present. (*b*) The lateral view shows the posterior rotation of the femoral head usually associated with marked posterior comminution of the femoral neck. (*c*) A fracture through the greater trochanter occurred intraoperatively. Because of this, a long-stem Moore prosthesis was used. Seven months following surgery, the greater trochanter fracture has healed. The prosthesis is in firm contact with the femoral bone on both frontal (*d*) and lateral (*e*) views.

around the prosthesis (16). Tracking of contrast material around a limited portion of the prosthesis is of uncertain significance.

Example 9-4. This 65-year-old woman developed bilateral avascular necrosis of the femoral heads following steroid therapy of thrombocytopenic purpura. Because of severe pain, bilateral Austin Moore prostheses were placed.

Left Hip
Preoperatively, the left hip radiograph demonstrates marked flattening of the femoral head with osteophytes and degenerative cysts in the acetabulum (Figure 9-17a). The changes are due to healed avascular necrosis with secondary degenerative arthrosis.

The next film (Figure 9-17*b*) was taken approximately three months postoperative. At that time, the size of the femoral head prosthesis was correct and was concentric with the acetabulum. Minimal thinning of the acetabular cartilage is visible superiorly and a few osteophytes are adjacent to the lateral acetabular rim. The length of the remnant of femoral neck is approximately the desired 5/8 inch. The prosthesis lies adjacent to trabecular bone.

Seven months later (Figure 9-17*c*) the superior acetabular cartilage is narrower and minimal sclerosis may be developing in the acetabular roof. The remnant of the femoral neck is now shorter. Because the flange of the prosthesis is still adjacent to the calcar remnant, the prosthesis has settled deeper into the femoral shaft. A thin zone of demarcation is visible around the prosthesis, with minimal radiolucency surrounded by a thin sclerotic band. While the settling indicates a degree of loosening, it is possible for the settling to lead to a tight impaction of the prosthesis within the femoral canal. The zone of demarcation around the prosthesis is a normal finding.

One year later (Figure 9-17*d*) there has been additional loss of articular cartilage, with no other change or additional settling. At this time the patient is asymptomatic regarding her hips.

Five years post operative (Figure 9-17*e*), the patient is seen with slowly increasing hip and knee pain. Because of increasing pain she now walks with two Canadian crutches. The radiograph demonstrates additional sclerosis of the acetabulum, a degenerative finding, which may be associated with pain. The calcar femoralis is now almost totally resorbed and the prosthesis has sunk deeper into the shaft. Surrounding the prosthesis is a wide zone of radiolucency, demarcated from the adjacent medullary bone by a thin band of sclerosis. There has been progressive resorption of the bone within the fenestrations in the stem of the prosthesis. These are all signs of loosening of the prosthesis.

Right Hip
Preoperatively, the right hip radiograph (Figure 9-17*f*) demonstrates focal sclerosis and lucency within the femoral head, with marked osteophyte proliferation at the base of the femoral head. Many degenerative cysts are present in the acetabulum. There is asymmetric cartilage narrowing.

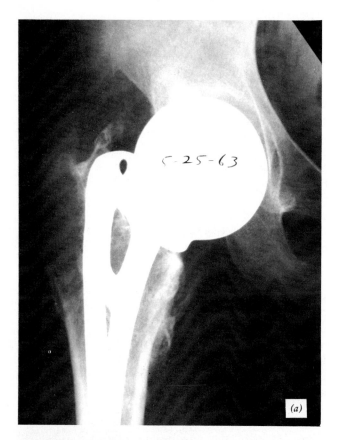

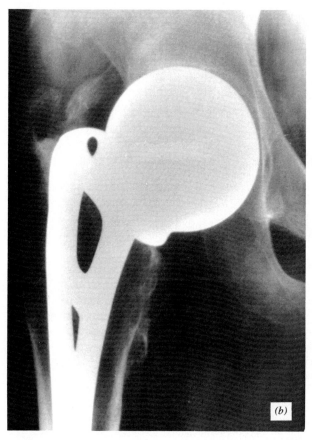

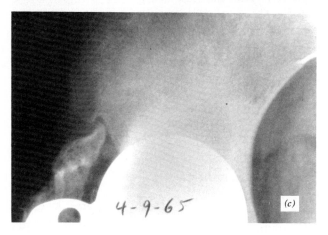

Figure 9-14. Cartilage necrosis leading to degenerative arthrosis. (*a*) Austin-Moore prosthesis used as treatment for avascular necrosis of the femoral head. Postoperative view discloses normal cartilage thickness, properly seated Austin-Moore prosthesis, and minimal ectopic bone. (*b*) Five months later, the articular cartilage is moderately narrowed. (*c*) Two years later, the articular cartilage is destroyed and there is sclerosis of the acetabular bone. At this time the prosthesis is also loose (same patient as in Figure 9-15). At surgery degenerative arthrosis, loosening, but no evidence of infection were found. (Reprinted by permission, Radiologic Clinics of North America.)

Changes are due to avascular necrosis, with secondary degenerative arthrosis of the hip.

Nine months following surgery, the radiograph (Figure 9-17*g*) demonstrates irregularity of the acetabular roof. This irregularity is a normal finding in the healing phase

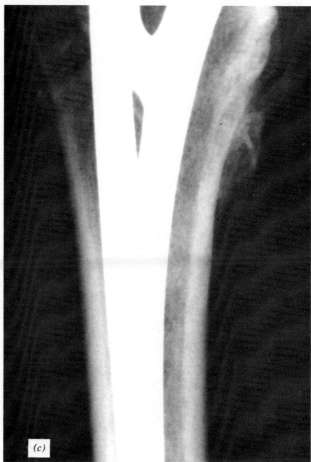

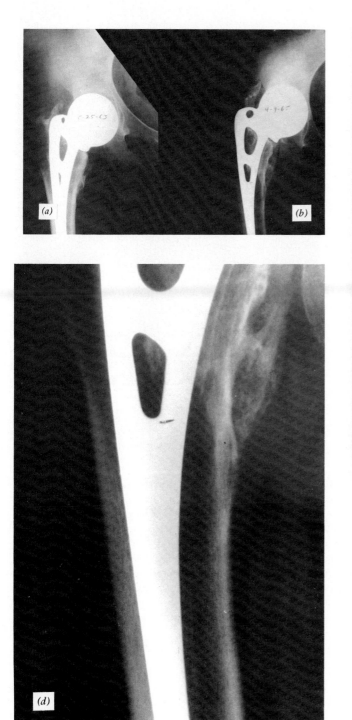

Figure 9-15. Loose Austin-Moore prosthesis. (Same patient as in Figure 9-14. (*a,b*) Films two years apart demonstrate the development of a thick zone of lucency around the stem of the Austin-Moore prosthesis. Resorption of the bone within the fenestration has also developed. (*c,d*) Close-up views of (*a*) and (*b*) reveal the wide band of radiolucency that has developed. (Reprinted by permission, Radiologic Clinics of North America.)

following reaming of the acetabulum for correction of the deformity resulting from degenerative arthrosis of the hip. If reaming has been done, this irregularity should not be considered a manifestation of infection. The femoral neck remnant appears short; this is partially a projectional artifact due to obliquity. Note that the flange appears round.

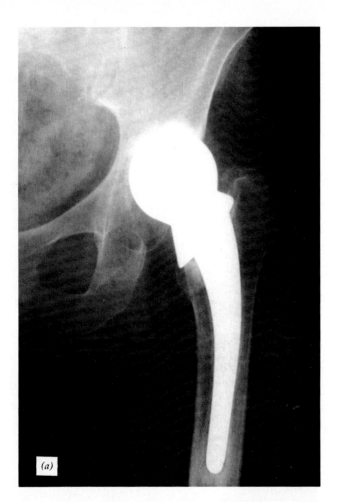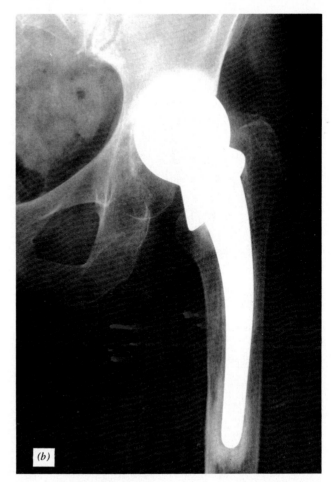

Figure 9-16. Settling of Thompson prosthesis—probable loose prosthesis. (*a*) Four years following insertion of Thompson prosthesis for hip pain, the prosthesis appears well seated with only a thin zone of radiolucency around it. The sclerosis at the tip of the stem of the prosthesis is within normal limits. There is moderate acetabular sclerosis. At this time the patient had mild thigh and hip pain, but was able to walk around the house and to walk two blocks using one cane. (*b*) Sixteen months later, the prosthesis has settled into the femoral shaft. This is detectable by comparing the position of the flange (or skirt) of the prosthesis to the lesser trochanter. An increase in the thickness of the zone of radiolucency is also present. No change in hip symptomatology was present. The loose prosthesis may have minimal or no pain associated with it. In this minimally symptomatic patient, there was no clinical justification to do anything for the probable loosening of the prosthesis.

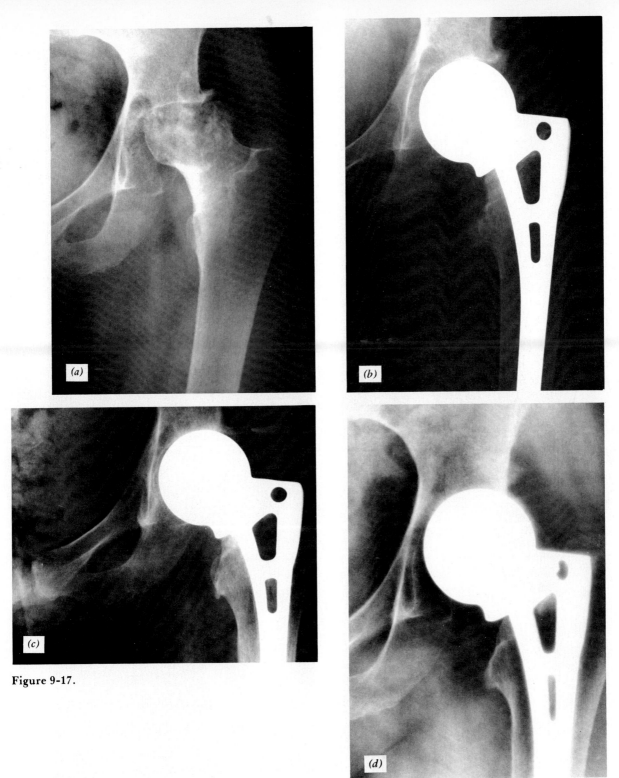

Figure 9-17.

(*Legend on page 165*)

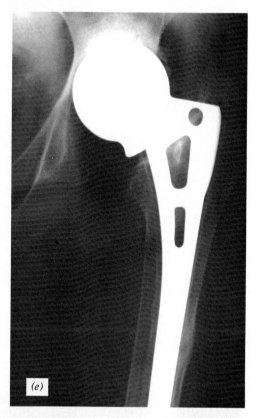

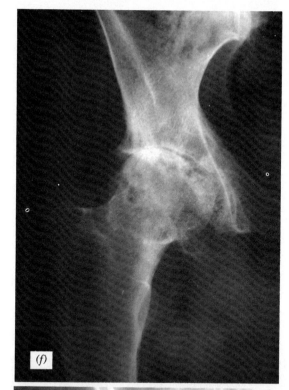

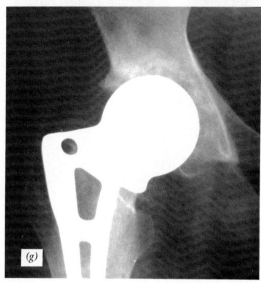

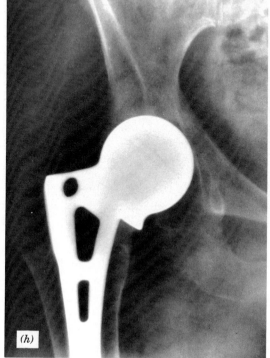

Figure 9-17. (*Continued*)

(*Legend on next page*)

164

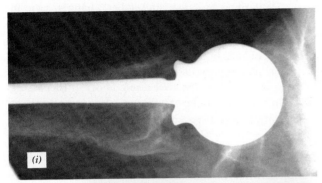

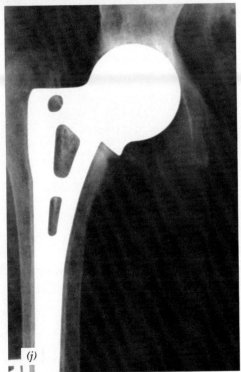

Figure 9-17. Example 9-4. Austin-Moore prosthesis used for treatment of bilaterial avascular necrosis of the femoral heads following steroid use for thrombocytopenic purpura. (*a* to *e*) Left hip. (*f* to *j*) Right hip. (*a*) Deformity of the femoral head and narrowing of the articular cartilage are due to avascular necrosis. (*b*) Three months following surgery, the Austin-Moore prosthesis is well seated on approximately ⅝ in. of medial femoral neck. Minimal narrowing of the acetabular cartilage is present. (*c*) Ten months following surgery there has been minimal resorption of the medial femoral neck with a small amount of sinking of the prosthesis into the femoral shaft. The prosthesis is now demarcated by a thin band of sclerosis and a thin zone of radiolucency from the medullary bone. (*d*) Twenty-two months following surgery, the hip is asymptomatic. The sinking of the prosthesis has ceased. (The film is blurred because of poor screen contact on the original.) (*e*) Five years following surgery, the prosthesis is loose, and degenerative arthrosis has developed. The prosthesis has sunk further into the femoral shaft; there is a wide zone of radiolucency surrounding the stem of the prosthesis; sclerosis of the acetabulum is present. (*f*) Preoperatively, the right hip shows the changes brought on by avascular necrosis and by moderate degenerative arthrosis. (*g*) Nine months following surgery, the acetabular roof shows irregular radiolucencies. This is a normal finding following reaming of the acetabulum during placement of the prosthesis; if the acetabulum has been reamed, this does not indicate infection. (*h*) Twenty-two months following surgery, the acetabular roof has largely reformed. There is now a normal demarcation between the medullary femoral bone and the prosthesis with a thin zone of radiolucency and sclerosis. (Blurring of film due to poor screen contact on the original.) (*i*) Lateral view demonstrating the shape of the flange. (*j*) Five years following surgery, the prosthesis is loose. It has settled into the femoral shaft, and the zone of radiolucency around it has widened. A minimal joint space has developed in the acetabulum, probably due to the development of fibrocartilage.

When viewed from its true side, the flange is nearly straight (Figure 9-17*h*). The lateral view of this prosthesis, in the early postoperative period (Figure 9-17*i*) shows the contour of the flange and suggests why it would appear rounded if seen obliquely.

One year later (Figure 9-17*h*), the neck fragment appears longer (due to the better positioning), but is still slightly shorter than the ideal ⅝ inch. The acetabular roof

has largely reformed and is smooth, with only minimal sclerosis. Demarcation of the prosthesis from the trabecular bone has now occurred, with a thin band of sclerosis appearing slightly separated from the prosthesis.

Five years following surgery (Figure 9-17*j*), settling of the prosthesis into the femoral shaft has occurred, with resorption of the femoral neck fragment. A zone of radiolucency of intermediate thickness surrounds the prosthesis, demarcated from the trabecular bone by a thin band of sclerosis, and the bone in the fenestrations has partially resorbed. These are signs of loosening. The sclerosis of the acetabular roof has increased minimally, a degenerative change sometimes associated with pain. A minimal joint space has developed following reaming of the acetabulum. Histologically, this space is often filled by fibrocartilage.

When last seen, the patient was being considered for bilateral total hip replacements.

Infection

These patients usually have constant pain. Radiographic changes include joint-space narrowing, permeative and destructive lesions of bone, and other changes seen in classical osteomyelitis and septic arthritis (Figure 9-18a,b). Extensive heterotopic bone formation is a common late sequela. It is important to remember, however, that cartilage narrowing and resorption of the calcar can occur in the absence of infection (as discussed above). Increasing density of the acetabular bone can also occur with or without infection and is a nonspecific finding (6,18,20).

Example 9-5. This 78-year-old woman fell, sustaining a femoral neck fracture. This was treated with an Austin-Moore prosthesis. Results were satisfactory for three months, but then pain developed in the upper one-third of

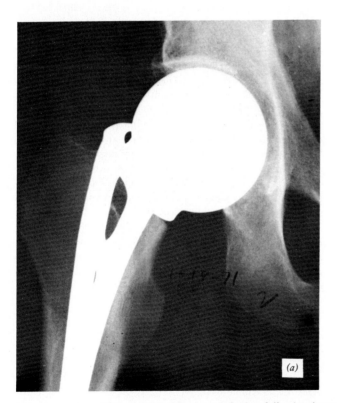
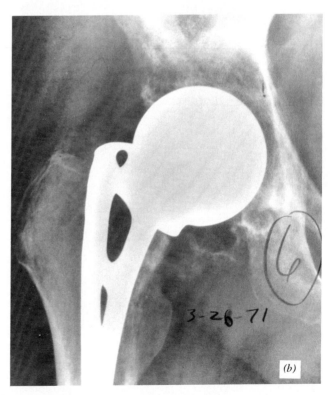

Figure 9-18. Hip joint infection following insertion of an Austin-Moore prosthesis. (*a*) Normal appearance of Austin-Moore prosthesis inserted as treatment for a pathologic fracture of the femoral neck in this 53-year-old man with lymphoma. (*b*) Nine weeks later, while the patient was receiving chemotherapy for lymphoma, this roentgenogram was taken because of recurrent hip pain. Permeative radiolucencies in the superior acetabular rim are present. Joint aspiration and culture documented a pseudomonas infection, which responded to appropriate antibiotics. (Reprinted with permission, Radiologic Clinics of North America.)

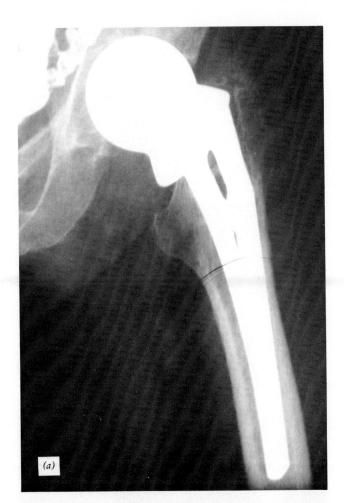

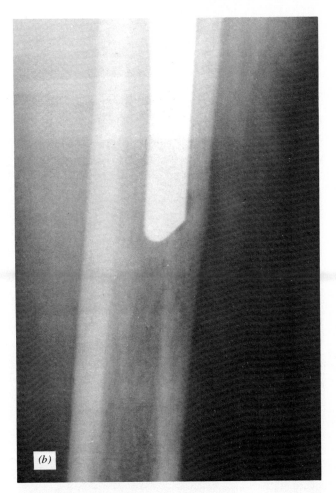

Figure 9-19. Infected Austin-Moore prosthesis, one year following surgery. (*a*) A wide zone of radiolucency lies between the prosthesis and the greater trochanter. The remainder of the prosthesis is in close contact with the medullary bone. This zone of radiolucency cannot be explained as the result of mechanical stress because of the lack of resorption elsewhere; rather, it suggests infection. (*b*) Slight focal resorption of the cortex near the tip of the prosthesis associated with a small amount of adjacent periosteal new bone reflects a focal accumulation of granulation tissue and osteomyelitis.

the anterior thigh. This pain increased over the next nine months, by which time severe pain was present with any movement of the hip. Radiographs obtained one year following surgery demonstrated changes suggestive of infection, but not of loosening (Figure 9-19*a,b*). Hip aspiration was positive twice for infection with staphyloccus epidermidis. Surgical debridement was carried out and a total

hip replacement was inserted. Extensive granulation tissue was present at surgery. The prosthesis was firmly seated.

Heterotopic Bone Formation

A minor amount of heterotopic bone formation is a common complication of femoral head replacement surgery.

Associated with occasional mild pain, it does not seem to affect motion adversely in the majority of patients in whom it occurs (6,13).

MISCELLANY

Breakage of Prosthesis

An older man with severe rheumatoid arthritis was treated with an Austin-Moore prosthesis for severe hip arthritis.

Sudden right hip pain developed, associated with breakage of the prosthesis (Figure 9-20a,b).

Moore Replacing Jewett Appliance

The screws from the Jewett appliance were left in place when the Moore prosthesis was placed (Figure 9-21). If the metals are dissimilar, there is danger of electrolysis with breakage of the prosthesis. If the metals are the same, this is an acceptable approach.

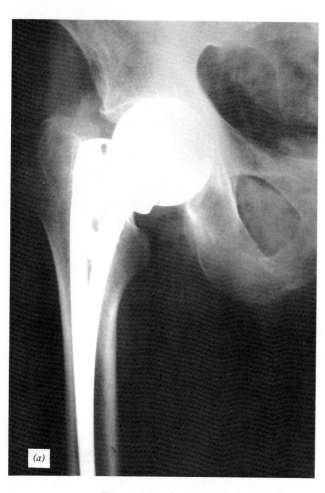
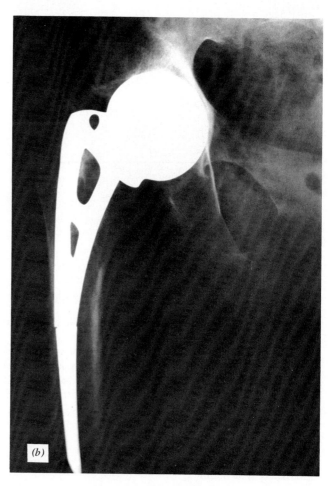

Figure 9-20. Breakage of the stem of an Austin-Moore prosthesis. (*a*) Austin-Moore prosthesis. Extensive cartilage narrowing due to underlying rheumatoid arthritis. (*b*) The stem of the prosthesis is broken. At surgery, the proximal portion was loose and extensive granulation tissue was present. The distal portion was more firmly seated.

Moore Prosthesis Placed in Cup Arthroplasty

Each of two patients had combined Austin-Moore and cup arthroplasties (see also Chapter 14). This technique was used in an early attempt at a total hip replacement. The procedure is no longer used (Figure 9-22*a,b*).

SUMMARY

The Austin-Moore and Thompson prostheses play an important role in the treatment of patients with femoral neck fractures (5,8,12). The results obtainable with the use of these prostheses rival those obtained for internal fixation of femoral neck fractures. In the early postoperative period, intraoperative fractures in 4.5% of the patients (2), early infection in 8% (17), and dislocation in 1 to 3% (2,9) are the major local complications. Long-term results demonstrate increasing frequency of complications, particularly loosening of the prosthesis, but, for the mainly elderly and sedentary population who sustain femoral neck fractures, these prostheses permit a majority of their recipients to resume ambulation quickly.

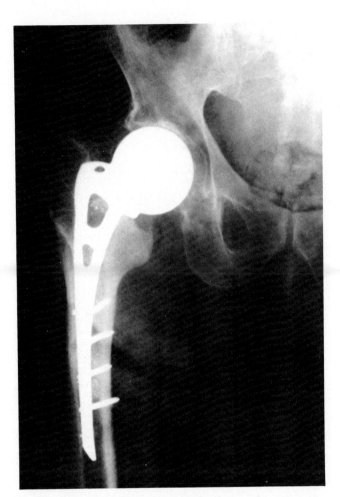

Figure 9-21. Austin-Moore prosthesis following removal of a Jewett appliance. The screws from the Jewett appliance are still present.

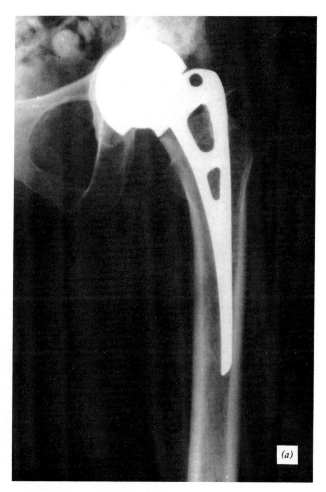
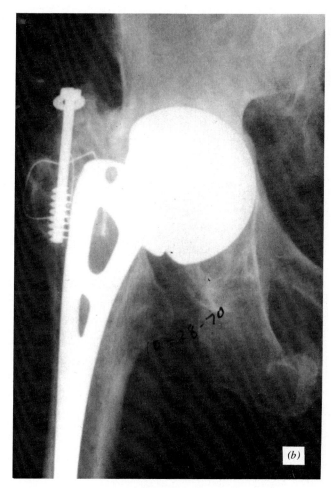

Figure 9-22. (*a,b*) Austin-Moore prosthesis placed in cup arthroplasty. Two different patients.

REFERENCES

1. Anderson G, Nielsen JM: Results after arthroplasty of the hip with Moore's prosthesis. *Acta Orthop Scand* 43:397–410, 1972.

2. Anderson LP, Hamsa WR, Waring TL: Femoral head prostheses: A review. *J Bone Joint Surg* 46A:1049–1065, 1964.

3. Apley AG, Millner WF, Porter DS: A follow-up study of Moore's arthroplasty in the treatment of osteoarthritis of the hip. *J Bone Joint Surg* 51B:638–647, 1969.

4. Barr J, et al: Arthroplasty of the hip. *J Bone Joint Surg* 46A:249–266, 1964.

5. Chan RN-W, Bath, Hoskinson J: Thompson prosthesis for fractured neck of femur. A comparison of surgical approaches. *J Bone Joint Surg* 57B:437–443, 1975.

6. Coventry M: Salvage of the painful hip prosthesis. *J Bone Joint Surg* 46A:200–212, 1964.

7. Crenshaw AH: *Campbell's Operative Orthopedics.* St. Louis, C. V. Mosby Co., 1963, pp 663–667.

8. D'Arcy J, Devas M: Treatment of fractures of the femoral neck by replacement with the Thompson prosthesis. *J Bone Joint S* 58B:279–286, 1976.

9. Deyerle Wm M: Complications of hip prosthesis. *Clin Orthop* 53:61–79, 1967.

10. Eftekhar H: The cemented endoprosthesis. Lecture presented at Current Status of Joint Replacement, Miami, FLA, Dec 15, 1973.

11. Evarts CM: Endoprosthesis as the primary treatment of femoral neck fractures. *Clin Orthop* 92:69–76, 1973.

12. Goodwin RA: The Austin-Moore prosthesis in fresh femoral neck fractures. A review of 611 postoperative cases. *Am J Orthop Surg* 10:40–43, 1968.

13. Hamblen DL, Harris WH, Rottger J: Myositis ossificans as a complication of hip arthroplasty, abstracted. *J Bone Joint Surg* 53B:764, 1971.

14. Hinchey JJ, Day P: Primary prosthetic replacement in fresh femoral neck fractures. *J Bone Joint Surg* 46A:223–240, 1964.

15. Parrish T, Jones J: Fracture of the femur following prosthetic arthroplasty of the hip. *J Bone Joint Surg* 46A:241–248, 1964.

16. Razzano CD, Nelson CL, Wilde AH: Arthrography of the adult hip. *Clin Orthop* 99:86–94, 1974.

17. Salvati E, Wilson P: Long-term results of femoral head replacement. *J Bone Joint Surg* 55A:516–524, 1973.

18. Sarmiento A: Austin-Moore prosthesis in the arthritic hip. *Clin Orthop* 82:14–23, 1972.

19. Smith DM, Oliver CH, Ryder CT, Stinchfield FE: Complications of Austin-Moore arthroplasty. Their incidence and relationship to potential predisposing factors. *J Bone Joint Surg* 57:31–33, 1975.

20. Thompson FR: 2½ Years experience with the vitallium intramedullary hip prosthesis. *J Bone Joint Surg* 36A:489–500, 1954.

21. Wrighton JD, Woodyard JE: Prosthetic replacement for subcapital fractures of the femur: A comparative survey. *Injury* 2:287, 1971.

10
Intertrochanteric Fractures

Intertrochanteric fractures are common fractures, usually occurring in the elderly patient and usually involving osteoporotic bone. They may be stable or unstable, with the stability most closely related to the degree of comminution of the medial femoral cortex (5,8,13,17,19). Systemic complications of pneumonia and pulmonary emboli are common.

The unstable fracture presents the orthopedist with a complex problem. Anatomic reduction with internal fixation will decrease pain and simplify care in bed, but prolonged nonweight bearing will be necessary. Alternately, several techniques utilizing purposeful nonanatomic alignment may provide sufficient stability to permit early ambulation. Careful analysis of the fracture is needed to evaluate the appropriateness of these alternate methods. Metal by itself is usually insufficient to support an unstable fracture. The realigned fractures are held stable by a complex interdependence of bone and metal. Until the 1950s, most intertrochanteric fractures were treated without open surgery or appliances. Traction followed by external support with a spica cast yielded good results, with only rare cases of nonunion and with moderately good hip function returning after fracture healing. Many of the fractures shifted into varus malalignment, but this did not significantly interfere with eventual function. The more comminuted fractures required prolonged bed rest, and pneumonia and pulmonary emboli resulted in many deaths. Excellent nursing care was needed to prevent bed sores. Stable fractures generally did well (8,16).

Example 10-1. This 77-year-old man with severe cardiac and respiratory disease fell several weeks prior to his routine appointment. He rested for several weeks because of severe right hip pain. At his next visit, radiographs demonstrated an impacted, partially healed, stable high intertrochanteric fracture (Figure 10-1*a,b*). Because of minimal symptomatology and severe pulmonary disease, he was treated with restricted weight bearing. He did well, showing only minimal symptoms. Progressive varus shift of the fracture occurred (Figure 10-1*c*).

THE USE OF HIP NAILS

During the 1950s, the use of hip nails in intertrochanteric fractures became standard. The hip nail greatly simplified nursing care, decreased the duration of hospitalization, and often permitted the patient to be out of bed within a week or two (usually with limited or no weight bearing on the fractured hip). With the patient upright, systemic complications decreased in frequency, but local complications of fracture displacement and problems with the appliances became relatively common (9). This chapter will focus on these local complications.

TYPES OF APPLIANCES

The comminuted intertrochanteric fracture is quite difficult to hold reduced. The variety of internal fixation

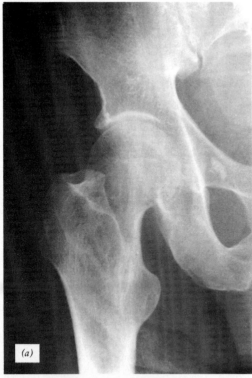

(a)

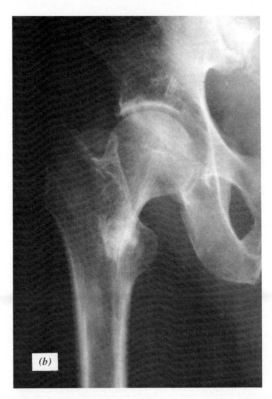

(b)

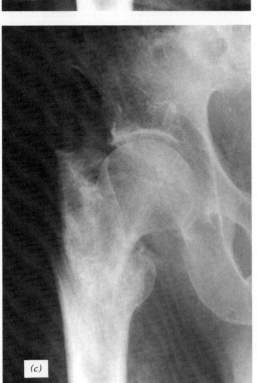

(c)

Figure 10-1. Example 10-1. A 77-year-old man with an impacted intertrochanteric fracture of the right femur; no surgical therapy. (a) A prefracture view for comparison, two years prior to injury. (b) An impacted intertrochanteric fracture is present. The sclerosis represents callus. The patient came in for therapy several weeks after his injury. (c) Four weeks later, the fracture has shifted into varus. This position remained stable. Partial healing is present.

devices suggests that none completely solves the problem of holding the fracture in a stable position. When dealing with the problems inherent in these fractures, it is informative to consider the variety of approaches used to achieve a stable reduction. The methods used to achieve a firm hold on the proximal and distal fragments vary with the different appliances. The methods for preventing or counteracting shear forces along the fracture line vary. Some prostheses are rigid to help counteract the shear along the fracture line, but this rigidity may permit the nail to penetrate through to the acetabulum if reduction is lost. Other prostheses are flexible, so that if the reduction is lost they will bend, allowing deformity but protecting the joint. Some appliances permit progressive impaction; others are designed to limit the telescoping of fractures to prevent the penetration of the nail into the acetabulum.

Following the success of the Smith-Petersen nail for the treatment of fractures of the femoral neck, attempts were made to modify that nail for use in the intertrochanteric fracture. While the fixation in the proximal fragment seemed sufficient, the lateral portion of the nail often rested in or near the fracture line and was unstable. Because of this situation, new devices were designed to provide a better attachment to the distal fragment. The first of these devices was a side plate bolted to the Smith-Petersen nail and held by screws to the distal fragment (Figure 10-2a,b). This method is still used. The side plates may have a fixed or variable angle for the nail attachment.

Welding of the side plate to the Smith-Petersen nail was the next advance. This appliance is now forged as a single piece. The Jewett nail (Figure 10-3a,b) is the most common of this basic type of appliance. Modified over the years since its development, it now is available with nails in several lengths, with several nail-side-plate angles, and with several lengths of side plate. The Holt nail (11,12,14), shown in Figure 10-4a,b, is a similar type of nail, but is designed for maximal strength. It has a round, unfinned nail, and the side plate is bolted to the femoral shaft. The proximal end of the nail is flat, providing a broad support surface.

Three other types of appliances are also frequently used. The compression screw (7,10) (Figure 10-5), used for femoral neck fractures, is also suited for the treatment of intertrochanteric fractures. It is composed of three main pieces: a proximal component with a broad screw thread is placed within a barrel that is attached to a side plate and can telescope within the barrel. The third piece is a tightening screw, a compression device, inserted through the lateral portion of the barrel and into the proximal component. When turned, this pulls the larger pieces together, impacting and compressing the fracture.

The Zickel nail (Figure 10-6) combines an intrafemoral rod with a variant of the Smith-Petersen nail. The in-

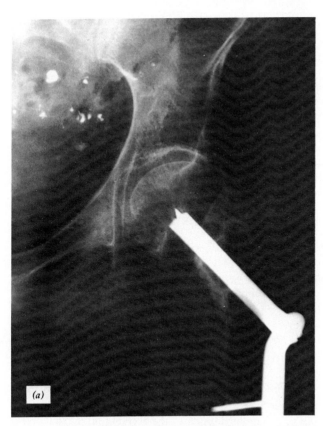

(a)

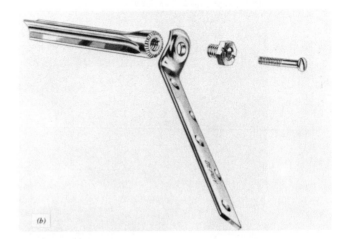

(b)

Figure 10-2. (a) A Smith-Petersen nail bolted to a side plate, which in turn is held to the femoral shaft by screws. (b) Drawing of a Smith-Petersen nail with side plate. (Courtesy DePuy.)

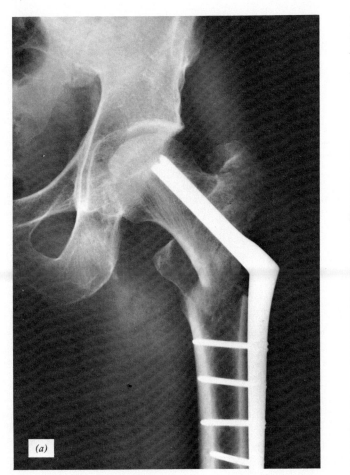

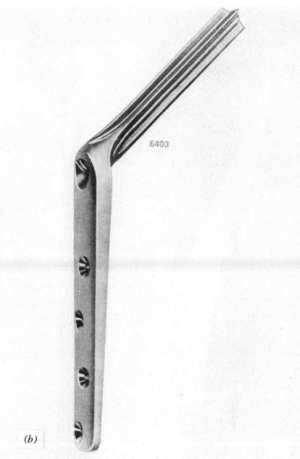

Figure 10-3. (a) A Jewett appliance. (b) A drawing of a Jewett appliance. (Courtesy Howmedica®.)

tramedullary rod serves as the distal attachment and is also usually anchored to the proximal fragment near the greater trochanter, providing a second site of attachment for the proximal fragment.

The Enders nail (Figure 10-7a,b) is also an intramedullary appliance. It consists of three long rods, which are inserted into the medial femoral condyle and passed proximally through the femoral shaft across the fracture site. Because the rods are inserted near the knee, the operative exposure necessary for placement is much simpler than for the other devices (4).

Prosthetic Replacement of the Comminuted Intertrochanteric Fracture

Experimental work has been reported in which a femoral head and neck replacement prosthesis is fixed in methylmethacrylate to replace the proximal end of the fractured upper end of the femur (20,21). This bypasses many of the problems inherent in nail fixation of these fractures. Additional follow-up is needed before the proper place of this procedure in the orthopedist's armamentarium is known.

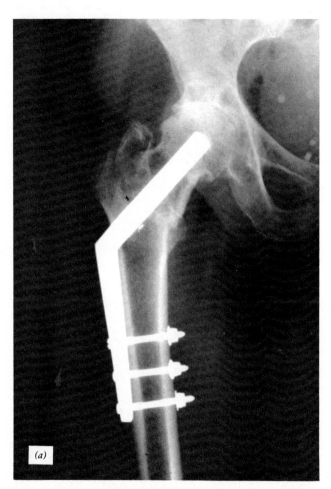

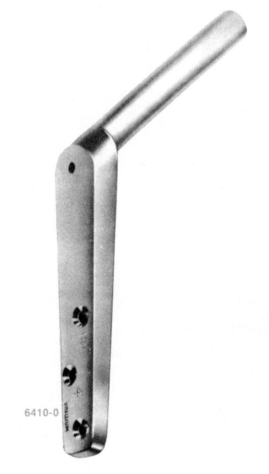

6410-0

Figure 10-4. (*a*) A Holt nail held to the femoral shaft with a Barr bolt. (*b*) Drawing of Holt nail and Barr bolt. (Courtesy Howmedica®.)

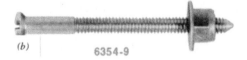

(*b*)   6354-9

FIXATION OF THE APPLIANCE TO THE DISTAL AND PROXIMAL FRAGMENTS

The success of an appliance reflects its ability to hold the fracture reduced. An important part of this ability is the need to hold to the proximal and distal fragments without slippage, fixation to the distal fragment is usually easier than to the proximal fragment.

Fixation to the Distal Appliance

Fixation of the appliance to the distal fragment may require the use of an intramedullary rod or a side plate. The Zickel nail (Figure 10-6) and the Enders nail (Figure 10-7a,b) use intramedullary femoral rods to stabilize the distal fragment. The intramedullary rod of the Zickel nail should closely approximate the size of the narrowest portion of the femoral canal for maximal support.

Most appliances use a side plate held to the femoral shaft by screws. Because the trabecular bone in the upper portion of the femoral shaft is sparse, the screws are usually placed through the lateral femoral cortex and screwed into the medial cortex. Failure to place the screws into both cortices weakens the hold of the screws and may permit them to pull out. Holes are drilled for the placement of the screws. Drill bits may break and be left within the bone (Figure 10-13c).

The side plate of the Holt nail (Figure 10-4a,b) is bolted to the femoral shaft. These bolts are less likely to pull out

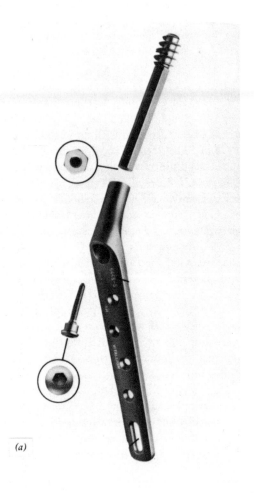

(a)

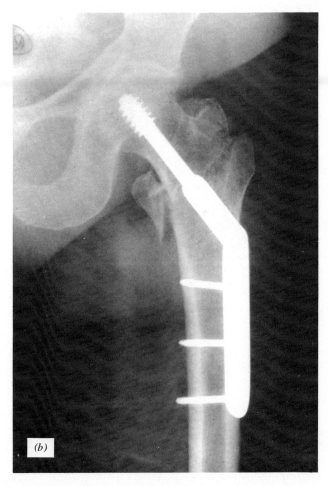

(b)

Figure 10-5. (a) The compression screw. (b) Drawing of a compression screw. (Courtesy Howmedica®.)

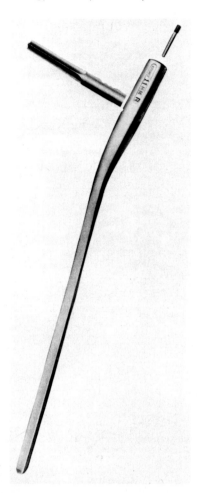

Figure 10-6. Zickel appliance. (Drawing courtesy of Howmedica®.)

of the bone than screws, but because the bolts consist of two separate pieces, they are slightly more difficult to fasten.

Fixation to the Proximal Fragment

It is often difficult to achieve a firm hold on the proximal fragment. the nail is held within the proximal fragment by trabecular bone. The amount of trabecular bone varies with the degree of osteoporosis and varies at different sites within the proximal fragment, reflecting the lines of stress.

A nail placement that is satisfactory in a young patient may cut through the osteoporotic bone of the elderly. One must relate position to osteoporosis in evaluating the degree of fixation (2). In osteoporotic bone, the best trabecular bone lies within the femoral head, and many authors believe that the tip of the nail should be placed there (2,9,12,17,22); if the nail is placed too far into the femoral head, and should further impaction take place, the nail may penetrate into the joint space or acetabulum, requiring reoperation (3,17,18). In osteoporotic bone, the trabeculae close to the medial femoral neck are denser than those in the superolateral portion of the neck, and placement of the nail inferiorly in the neck and into the femoral head is preferred by some authors (2,3,9,14,18).

Example 10-2. This 62-year-old male pedestrian was hit by a car and sustained a comminuted intertrochanteric fracture. Reduction and internal fixation with a compression screw left him with an unstable reduction (Figure 10-8a,b). The factors contributing to the instability included a failure of proper fixation in the proximal fragment and failure of anatomic reduction of the medial femoral cortex. The placement of the screw in the proximal fragment would have been adequate except for the presence of moderate osteoporosis. The tip of the screw, although lying slightly within the femoral head, missed most of the thick vertical trabeculae of the femoral head. Laterally, because of the associated fracture of the greater trochanter, support was also limited. Added to this was the instability resulting from failure of anatomic contact of the medial, anterior, and posterior cortices. The minimal displacement medially of the distal fragment was sufficient to limit the cortex to cortex transfer of force, leading to instability. This remains an unstable fracture.

The patient was treated with partial weight bearing. Two weeks following surgery (Figure 10-8c), radiolucency was noted around the inferior portion of the screw, indicating minimal cutting through of the screw. Because of the slippage of the fragments, the patient was placed nonweight bearing.

Seven months following surgery (Figure 10-8d), further cutting through of the screw could be seen. The fracture fragments shifted into varus and the shaft shifted medially. The fracture was only partially healed, a delayed union.

When last seen two years following the fracture, the hip was asymptomatic. Because of shortening of the leg, a shoe lift was advised.

This initially unstable fracture might have been held better if the initial cortical reduction had been anatomic. Better fixation within the proximal fragment could have resulted from placing the screw further into the trabecular bone of the femoral head, either by using a longer screw or by placing it lower within the proximal fragment. This later position would have caused the screw to intersect the denser trabeculae.

Early recognition of the shift of the fragments permitted the patient to be placed on nonweight bearing, limiting the degree of loss of reduction. Careful follow-up of all intertrochanteric fractures is required so that if loss of reduction is occurring, its early detection can lead, as in this case, to a good final result by the institution of nonweight bearing.

ACHIEVING A STABLE REDUCTION

Metal alone will not hold the fracture fragments in position. Fractures are held by a dynamic interrelation of bone and metal, where each must hold the other in position. Even a limited shift of the fragments can delay union; greater displacement may impair future hip function.

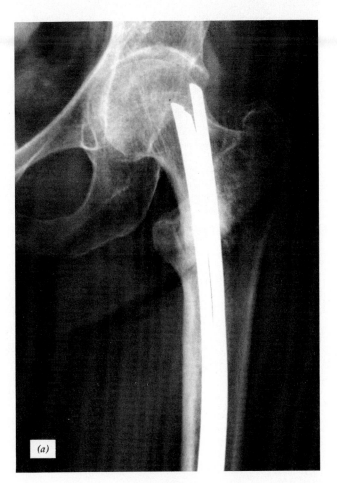
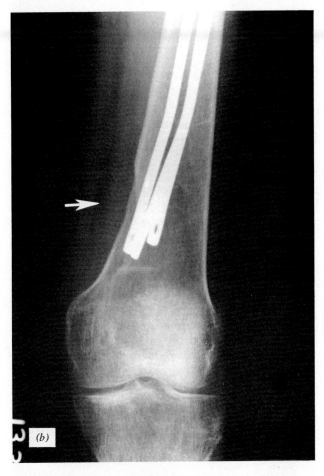

Figure 10-7. (*a,b*) Enders nails. (*b*) The cortical defect (arrow) is the site of insertion.

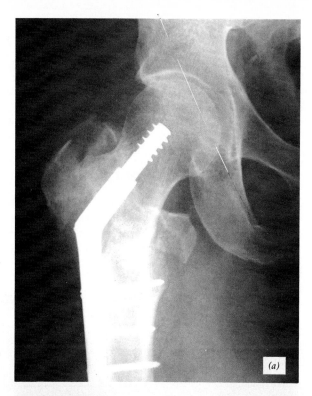

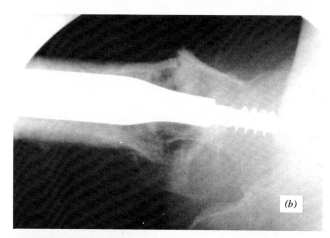

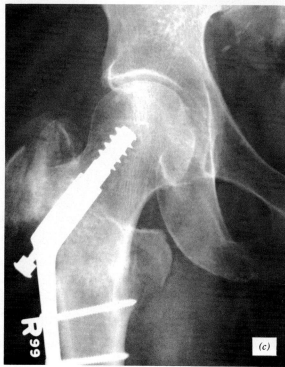

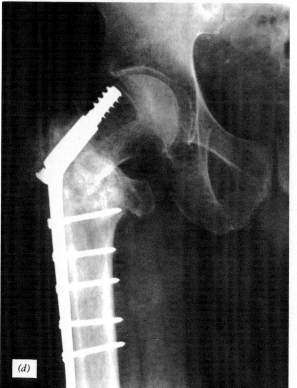

To evaluate the reduction, consideration must be given to the forces acting at the fracture site to increase or decrease stability. The position seen on the initial postfracture films usually reflects the direction of instability, but a more detailed analysis is often necessary.

INCREASING STABILITY BY PURPOSEFUL NONANATOMIC ALIGNMENT

Stability may be achieved by anatomic reduction of the medial femoral cortex (if its comminution is limited) or by purposeful nonanatomic alignment. Two methods of nonanatomic alignment can be used. The first is by medial displacement of the distal fragment with impaction of the proximal fragment into it (Figure 10-9). This method gives cortical support to the femoral neck medially and to the fractured cortex laterally (1,2,5,10,13).

The second method is by valgus repositioning, often with a high-angle nail (Figure 10-10). This valgus shift decreases shear forces along the fracture line and increases impaction. Valgus angulation with the use of a high-angle nail, however, may lead to penetration of the nail into the acetabulum if the fracture is unstable and telescopes.

FORCES ACTING ON THE FEMORAL FRACTURE SITE

Five main forces act on the proximal femur to displace or prevent displacement of the fracture fragments: shear along the fracture line; impacting forces; forces shifting the distal fragment medially; varus angulation forces; and external rotation forces. Each must be considered in evaluating the stability or instability of a fracture, its reduction, and its fixation. If a stable reduction can be achieved, early ambulation with partial or full weight bearing may be possible, but the fracture must be followed carefully. If significant shifting of the fragments is observed, weight bearing should cease and the patient should be maintained nonweight bearing until the fracture has healed.

SHEAR FORCES

Shear force causing displacement along the fracture line results mainly from weight bearing (20) and is related to the degree of vertical inclination of the fracture line or lines (19). Muscular activity adds to the shear. This force is most commonly counteracted by careful apposition of the fracture surfaces, with impaction of the many small interdigitations of bone, which then provide a high coefficient of friction. The placing of an appliance or appliances across the fracture line also increases the coefficient of friction. Appliances differ in their degree of resistance to shear forces. This resistance to shear depends mainly on the amount and strength of trabecular bone with which the appliance is in contact, and, to a lesser extent, on the appliance's intrinsic strength. The ability of the appliance to permit impaction (to be discussed shortly) also affects the fracture's resistance to shear.

The amount of trabecular bone with which the appliance is in contact depends on three things: the degree of osteoporosis; the site of placement of the appliance within the bone; and the geometry of the appliance. Trabecular bone is nonuniform in its distribution within the femur (Figure 10-11). In osteoporotic bone, only the trabecular bone within the femoral head may be present in sufficient quantity to anchor the appliance. In more normal dense bone, any portion of the proximal fragment may be sufficiently strong. When there is insufficient support of the

Figure 10-8. Example 10-2. Compression screw cutting through the proximal fragment. (*a,b*) Initial reduction with lack of contact of medial, anterior, and posterior cortices. (*c*) Two weeks following surgery radiolucency appears inferior to the screw; it is caused by a slight cutting through of the appliance. Telescoping of the screw into the barrel has occurred. The tightening screw is now visible. (*d*) Seven months following surgery, further cutting through has occurred. The triangular radiolucency in the superior femoral neck represents bone resorption in the path of the nail's migration. The fragments have shifted into varus.

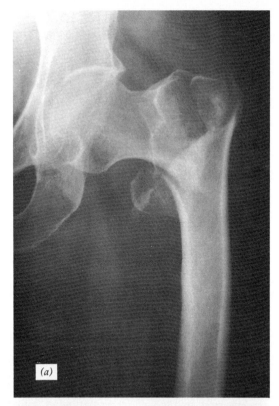

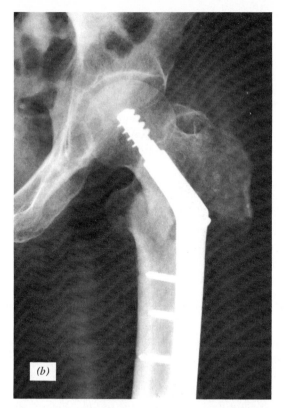

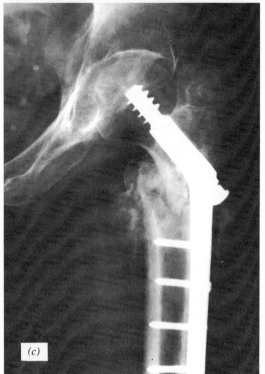

Figure 10-9. Unstable intertrochanteric fracture treated by medial displacement and impaction. (*a*) Comminuted intertrochanteric fracture with comminution of the medial femoral cortex. (*b*) Position postreduction, with medial displacement of the femoral shaft and impaction of the proximal fragment into the distal fragment. Fixation with a compression screw. (*c*) Four months later there is partial healing with moderate callus. A small medial shift of the femoral shaft has occurred. The compression screw has guided the direction of impaction.

nail, it will usually cut through the proximal fragment, with loss of reduction.

The intrinsic strength of the appliance also affects the resistance to shear (20). If the appliance does not cut through the trabecular bone, the nail should hold, bend, or break, depending on its strength (Figure 10-12*a,b,c,d*). Over the years, the available types of nails have been redesigned to make them stronger. Early Jewett nails were more flexible than current models. The Holt nail has exceptional intrinsic strength. Whether it is preferable for the nail to bend or to cut through is unclear. Clearly it is most desirable for the nail and the reduction to hold.

Example 10-3. This 59-year-old man tripped, falling down several steps and landing on his left side. A long, spiral, comminuted intertrochanteric and subtrochanteric fracture occurred (Figure 10-13a,b). The vertical inclination of this fracture increases the shear forces along the fracture line. Apart from this, the fracture is well suited to resist most of the major forces acting on proximal femoral fractures. The medial cortex is not comminuted, providing stability against varus deformity. The inferomedial extension of the proximal fragment should prevent medial displacement of the distal fragment. The bone density is moderately good, particularly in the inferior femoral neck and femoral head.

The large posterior comminution fragment adds a degree of instability, as does the extension of the fracture into the subtrochanteric region. With adequate fixation, a good result can be expected.

The patient was treated with a 10-hole (long side plate), 135°, 3-inch-long Jewett nail (Figure 10-13c). The long side plate is important in stabilizing the subtrochanteric portion of the fracture. The 3-inch nail extended not quite to the femoral head neck junction, perhaps a little short. Most importantly, the fracture was left distracted. Because of the marked shear resulting from the vertical orientation of the fracture line and because of the lack of impaction, shift along the fracture line would be expected.

At 15 days, the patient was walking with a walker; at six weeks he walked with protective weight bearing. At three months (Figure 10-13d), further impaction of the fracture was noted, with bending of the upper two screws and minimal cutting through of the nail in the femoral neck. The patient was placed nonweight bearing for one month, at which time callus was thought sufficient to prevent further fragment shift, and partial weight bearing was permitted. At six months, the fracture was healed and full weight bearing was allowed. No further displacement of the fracture occurred.

Use of a longer nail and firm impaction might have prevented the minimal displacement. Careful follow-up with cessation of weight bearing on identification of fragment shift was proper, through perhaps overcautious,

since the position achieved by the fragment shift was more stable than the initial one.

IMPACTING FORCE

Force applied perpendicular to the fracture line leads to impaction of the fragments (20). This force results from a combination of muscle pull and weight bearing, and it counteracts the shear force along the fracture line by increasing the coefficient of friction along this line. The impaction force is related to the angle of the fracture line and the degree of weight bearing or muscle pull. Metal appliances guide the direction of impaction and permit intraoperative impaction by blows on the distal fragment: only the compression screw actively impacts the fracture. Since impaction (shortening) may progress following surgery, the appliance should be placed to permit additional impaction. If it does not allow such impaction, the appliance may hold the fragments distracted, decreasing the resistance to shearing force and delaying union. Normally dense, nonosteoporotic bone may prevent or limit impaction and hold the fracture distracted (1).

Sliding nails permit progressive impaction (7). The sharp tips of the fins of a Jewett appliance usually permit the appliance to cut deeper into the femoral head as impaction progresses. The Deyerle screws (Figure 10-14) also permit progressive impaction by sliding through the lateral side plate (6). The Holt nail, with its broad, flat end, can hold the fragments distracted if the bone beyond its tip has not been sufficiently drilled. High-angle nails, by their more vertical orientation, tend to guide the force of weight bearing more directly into an impacting force. Purposeful valgus reduction, by decreasing the vertical inclination of the fracture line, tends to convert shear forces into impacting forces.

Penetration Into the Acetabulum

If the reduction is not sufficiently stable to prevent progressive impaction, a fixed nail, like the Jewett, may eventually penetrate through the femoral head, requiring additional surgery. The broad, flat end of the Holt nail tends to prevent this penetration. The sliding nail and

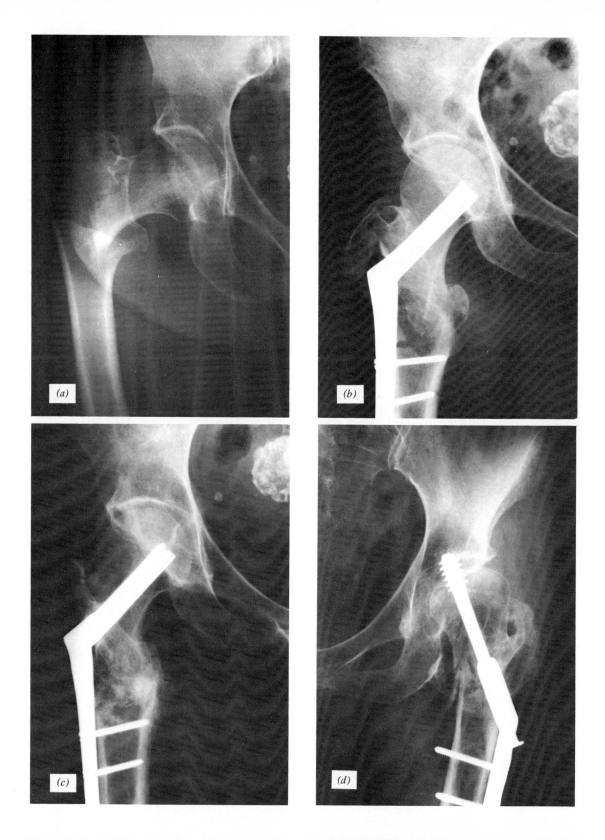

184

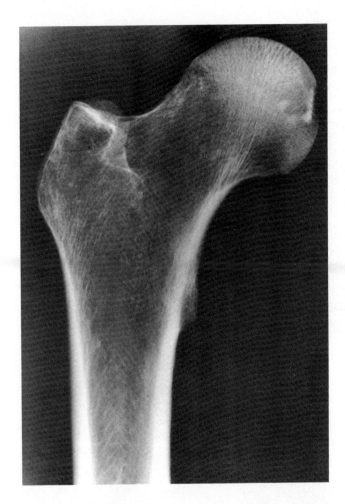

Figure 10-11. Radiograph of a dried femur specimen demonstrating the nonuniform trabecular pattern in moderate osteoporosis. The vertical trabeculae in the femoral head are usually the sites of greatest strength in the proximal fragment in an intertrochanteric fracture.

Deyerle appliance usually will not penetrate through the articular surface.

Prevention of penetration by the nail depends most on the stability of the reduction. A reduction that prevents progressive shortening can be achieved by cortex-to-cortex apposition. Anatomic reduction is best, if it can be prevented from slipping (9). If anatomic reduction is unstable because of comminution (19)—mainly of the medial femoral cortex—medial displacement of the femoral shaft with impaction of the proximal into the distal shaft fragment can give a firm cortex-to-cortex support (1,2,5,10,13,19) (Figure 10-9), as can a valgus osteotomy shaped to give cortex-to-cortex support (Figure 10-10).

If impaction is not sufficient, fracture displacement may occur and delayed union is common.

Example 10-4. This elderly woman fell onto her right hip and sustained a high intertrochanteric fracture (Figure 10-15a). Only minimal comminution is present, and, despite the moderate osteoporosis, a stable reduction should be possible. The 40° oblique inclination of the fracture should decrease shear across the fracture; it should also prevent medial displacement of the femoral shaft. The medial cortex is not comminuted and anatomic reduction should prevent varus shift.

During surgery, an iatrogenic lateral cortical fracture occurred, and for this reason vigorous impaction was avoided. The fracture was left minimally distracted.

The patient was kept nonweight bearing, although the distraction was noted. At 3½ months (Figure 10-15b), the patient was started on partial weight bearing to permit gentle impaction of the fracture.

At one year (Figure 10-15c), the fracture was considered partially healed (a delayed union), and protected weight bearing was continued.

Figure 10-10. Unstable intertrochanteric fracture treated by valgus repositioning. (a) Comminuted intertrochanteric fracture in a 43-year-old woman. (b) Initial reduction with valgus realignment. A Jewett nail is used to hold the reduction. (c) 14 months later the fractue is healed and reduction is maintained. (d) Acetabular protrusion of a compression screw.

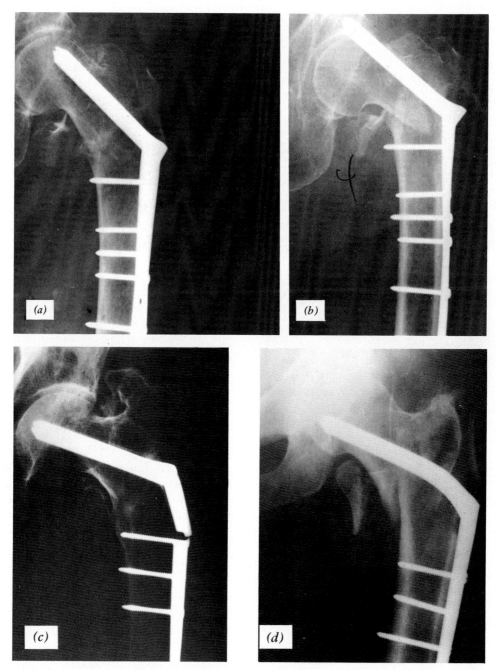

Figure 10-12. Three patterns of appliance failure in unstable intertrochanteric fractures. (*a,b*) Cutting through a Jewett nail, with varus shift of the fragments. (*c*) Breakage of a Jewett nail, showing varus shift. (*d*) Bending of a Jewett nail, with varus shift.

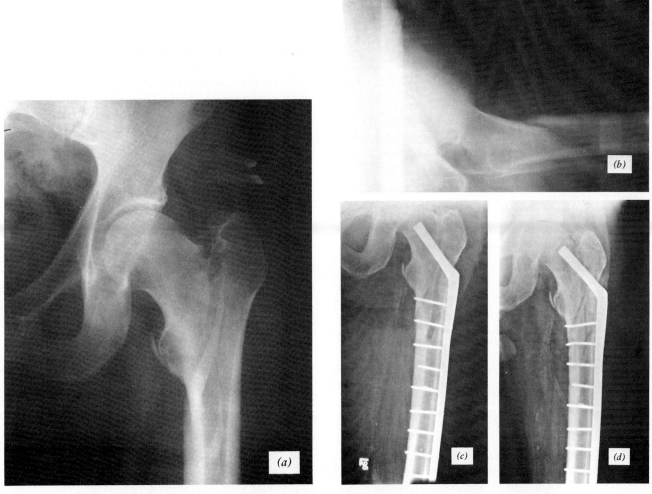

Figure 10-13. Example 12-3. Shear along vertical fracture with bending of screws. (*a,b*) Comminuted inter- and subtrochanteric fracture, showing a near vertical fracture line. (*c*) After reduction with a long side plate Jewett nail. The fracture is minimally distracted. (*d*) The fracture fragments have shifted slightly because of movement along the fracture line, impaction of the fracture, and bending of the two top screws. A small portion of a drill bit appears near the fifth screw.)

MEDIAL DISPLACEMENT FORCES ON THE FEMORAL SHAFT FRAGMENT

The hip adductors (and the iliopsoas muscle, if attached to the distal fragment) tend to pull the femoral shaft medially and into adduction deformity (1). The inclination and contour of the fracture line best determine the potential for medial shift (1). Cortical bone support extending superiorly from the lateral portion of the distal fragment provides good protection against medial shift (Figure 10-15a). A transverse fracture provides little support (Figure 10-16). A fracture obliquely inclined superomedially

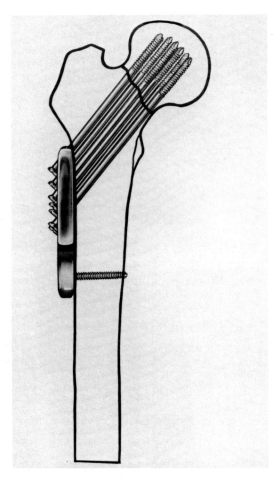

Figure 10-14. Drawing of the Deyerle apparatus, which can be used for femoral neck or intertrochanteric fracture. (Courtesy Orthopedic Equipment Company, Inc.)

increases the instability (Figure 10-17a)(1,8). Large interdigitations of the proximal and distal fragments tend to prevent medial displacement (1). Shift of the distal fragment medially may permit the nail to penetrate through the proximal fragment and may predispose to varus angulation (to be discussed shortly).

Example 10-5. This 42-year-old blind woman fell down a flight of stairs, sustaining a comminuted sub- and intertrochanteric fracture of the femur (Figure 10-17a). The in-

ward and upward slope of the fracture line markedly increases its instability and may permit medial migration of the distal fragment. The medial cortex is not comminuted; anatomic reduction would probably prevent varus angulation, but medial migration will be difficult to avoid.

A Jewett nail with a long side plate was used to hold an anatomic reduction (Figure 10-17b). The large lateral comminution fragment was secured with a screw and a circlage wire. Cancellous bone graft was added. Reduction was felt to be adequate, but nonweight bearing for six months to one year was contemplated.

Analysis of the reduction demonstrates an anatomic reduction. The nail has been placed low within the femoral neck and into the good trabecular bone of the femoral head. A 135° nail was used; it enters the lateral cortex of the proximal fragment. The side plate and nail therefore interconnect the two lateral cortices in a configuration which should prevent medial shift.

Four months following surgery (Figure 10-17c) minimal medial shift has occurred. The nail has moved closer to the medial femoral neck. The inferolateral proximal fragment cortex, which was helping to prevent medial shift, has fractured and is displaced medially (arrow).

At nine months (Figure 10-17d), the medial displacement is more marked. The nail is cutting through the cortex of the medial femoral neck and there is a greater shift of the lateral cortical fragment, which once prevented medial migration. At this point the patient had marked hip pain with hip motion. A delayed union was felt to be present.

After the fracture healed, the nail was removed (Figure 10-17e), and treatment was instituted for a moderate flexion contracture of the hip.

Methods for preventing medial displacement of the distal fragment include purposeful nonanatomic alignment, where the medial cortex of the proximal fragment is placed medially to the medial cortex of the distal fragment (locking this position with cortical bone to prevent medial displacement), combined with placement of the nail close to the medial cortical fracture to fix it in a medial-lateral position (18). Appliances that transfix the cortex of both proximal and distal fragments will also prevent medial displacement. The Zickel appliance, with its rod extending

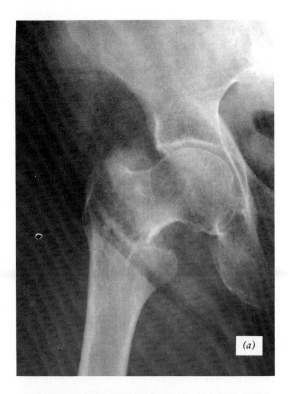

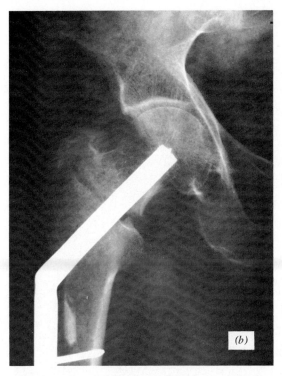

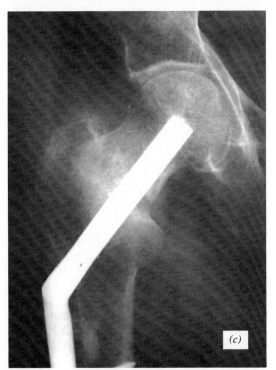

Figure 10-15. Example 10-4. Stable intertrochanteric fracture with distraction and delayed union. (*a*) A high intertrochanteric fracture. The medial femur is not comminuted. There is moderate roation of the shaft. (*b*) At 3½ months, distraction of the main fragments is present. (*c*) One year after fracture, it is incompletely healed. Medial distraction is still present.

proximally through the cortex of the greater trochanter, accomplishes this fixation, as does the use of a buttress plate. A buttress plate is a separate plate attached to the superior two screws of Jewett appliance, which extends proximally and can be screwed into the lateral cortex of the proximal fragment, locking its medial-lateral position (1).

Loss of reduction by medial displacement is also prevented by purposeful medial displacement of the femoral shaft with fragment impaction, as demonstrated previously.

Placement of the nail low in the neck near the fracture line may also stabilize it (1), but failed to do so in the example shown.

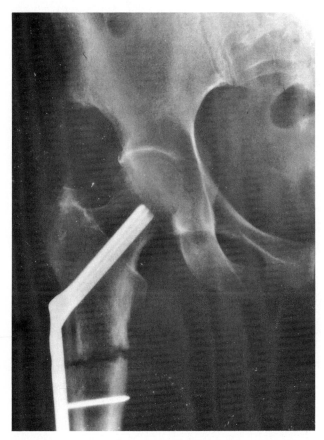

Figure 10-16. A transverse subtrochanteric fracture. Medial-lateral instability is present. The long side plate of the Jewett appliance should prevent displacement.

VARUS ANGULATION FORCES AT THE FRACTURE SITE

Weight bearing tends to shift the intertrochanteric fracture fragments into varus position. This displacement is accentuated by the pull of the adductors and of the gluteus maximus. Varus malposition results in a short limb and may result in a limp. It is usually not of serious consequence, except that fragment shift can delay the time at which weight bearing can begin, delaying union. Varus malposition may also cause a nail to cut through the proximal fragment, which may then require reoperation.

This same type of malposition may result from or be associated with movement along the fracture line (related to shear forces) or may be associated with loss of reduction from medial displacement of the femoral shaft.

The medial femoral cortex, when anatomically aligned, is the site of major transfer of the force of weight bearing from the proximal to the distal fragment. If it is not anatomically reduced, varus shift can occur, since trabecular bone cannot resist this force. Placement of the medial cortex of the proximal fragment lateral to the medial cortex of the distal fragment often leads to varus shift. The reverse placement, with the medial cortex of the proximal fragment medial to the medial cortex of the distal fragment is thought by some to increase stability (18). Although this placement does help prevent medial shift of the distal fragment, one biomechanical study suggests that varus shift will still occur (20).

Anatomic reduction or purposeful medial displacement of the distal fragment with impaction remain the best ways of preventing varus shift (1,2,5,10,13).

Example 10-6. This 50-year-old man fell while intoxicated, landing on his left hip. A four-piece intertrochanteric fracture with varus shift was found. (Figure 10-18a). A small, but important, comminution fragment of the medial femoral cortex was seen (it is more visible postoperatively). This fracture line should prevent medial displacement of the distal fragment. Bone density is good within the femoral head and neck.

Intraoperative views (Figure 10-18b,c) demonstrate anatomic reduction, but a gap is present in the medial femoral cortex. A Jewett nail has been placed, running in the midneck on the anterior view and in the posterior neck on the lateral view. Minimal distraction is present. The proximal portion of the lateral cortex of the distal fragment is now fractured, decreasing medial-lateral stability.

The first postoperative view (Figure 10-18e) demonstrated minimal varus shift and minimal medial displacement of the distal fragment. This position was unstable and progressive varus shift would have been anticipated if weightbearing were permitted. The nail extended into the femoral head to an area of moderately good trabecular bone. Because of the instability of the fracture, the patient was treated with non-weight bearing for four months.

Despite this, progressive shift of the fragments was seen (Figure 10-18*f*). This progressive varus shift was associated with a delay in fracture healing. At eight months the fracture was still incompletely healed and clinically was considered a delayed union. Full weight bearing was permitted at 12 months. At the end of two years the hip continued to be painful whenever the patient got up from a sitting position. Clinically, this is thought to represent osteoarthritis.

Example 10-7. This 76-year-old woman sustained a comminuted intertrochanteric fracture (Figure 10-19*a,b*). The fracture was treated by medial displacement of the shaft and Jewett nail fixation (Figure 10-19*c*). The tip of the nail lies in the distal portion of the femoral head. Moderate osteoporosis is present. The realignment has placed the medial cortex of the proximal fragment in the midportion of the femoral shaft. While the medial neck cortex appears to be in contact with the medial cortex of the distal fragment, review of the acute fracture films discloses that this area is comminuted, and firm cortex-to-cortex support is not present.

Three weeks following surgery (Figure 10-19*d*), the nail is cutting through the femoral neck and the fragments have shifted into varus malalignment.

The medial displacement osteotomy, as described by Harrington (10), required contact between the medial cortices of the proximal and distal fragments to prevent varus shift (2,10). The final film demonstrates that the fragments have shifted into the recommended position, where they stayed, suggesting that it is a position of greater stability.

EXTERNAL ROTATION STRESS

When lying supine in bed, the major force active across the fracture site is that of external rotation (5,18). External rotation stress also occurs during ambulation. This external rotation stress may be sufficient to disrupt an otherwise stable reduction. Most important in preventing this disruption is anatomic reduction of the posterior cortex, which is best evaluated in the lateral view.

Unequal rotation of the proximal and distal fragments will leave a gap visible on the anterior view as a radiolucent defect in the greater trochanteric region (15). This gap should not be confused with a comminution fragment. Its presence postnailing suggests hidden instability of the fracture (15). If the instability is recognized, the addition of external support to prevent external rotation in bed may prevent the loss of reduction. Occasionally, unequal rotation of the proximal and distal fragments intraoperatively will permit the nail to be misdirected posteriorly, missing or partially missing the proximal fragment (15).

Example 10-8. This 81-year-old woman fell onto her hip, sustaining a comminuted intertrochanteric fracture of the femur. On the initial view (Figure 10-20*a,b*), a radiolucent area is present in the trochanteric region. This is due to differences in rotation of the proximal and distal fragments and does not represent a lytic metastasis or displaced comminution fragment.

During surgery, the patient developed several severe hypotensive episodes, and therefore surgery may have been abbreviated. The intraoperative Polaroid® films (Figure 10-20*c,d*) demonstrates superficially adequate reduction on the frontal view. If one looks carefully at the trochanters, however, a difference in rotation of the proximal and distal fragments can be detected: the lesser trochanter indicates minimal external rotation and the greater trochanter indicates either moderate internal or external rotation. The lateral view (Figure 10-20*d*) is underexposed. If the probable position of the femoral head and neck from the position of the acetabulum is reconstructed, it seems that the nail is positioned outside of the proximal fragment.

On the predischarge films (Figure 10-20*e,f*) four days following surgery, the Jewett nail is seen in a different position than on the intraoperative views (suggesting a shift). A gap is present in the bone of the greater trochanter, indicating incomplete reduction of the anterior or posterior cortex. Although the nail appears to be largely within the femoral neck on the frontal and lateral views, it is important to remember that the femoral neck is a cylinder, not a cube, and that two right-angle views will occasionally demonstrate an appliance within the bone, when oblique views would show it to be outside.

Two weeks later, the nail was noted to have "cut out" of the femoral neck. The patient was slowly ambulated,

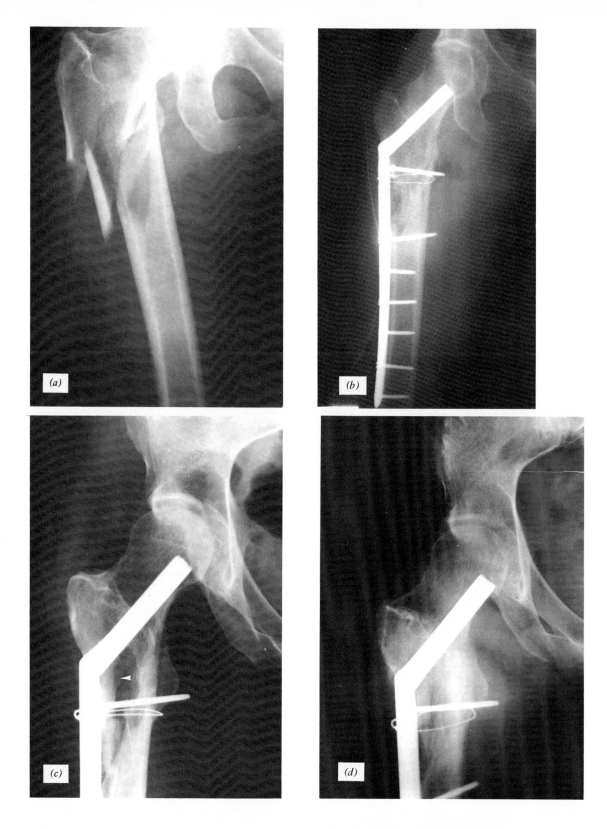

192

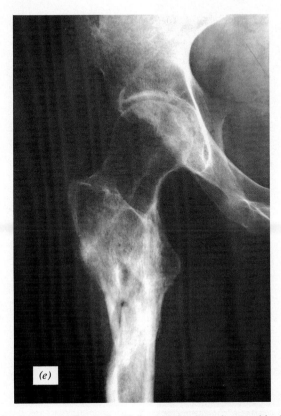

(e)

Figure 10-17. Example 10-5. A comminuted, unstable inter-trochanteric fracture, with medial shift of the distal fragment following reduction and fixation. (*a*) The inward and upward angulation of the major fracture line is accompanied by medial and proximal displacement of the distal fragment. (*b*) After reduction using a Jewett appliance with a long side plate. Reduction is anatomic. (*c*) A slight medial shift of the distal fragment is present. The nail has cut medially and inferiorly towards the cortex of the femoral neck. A small projection of bone of the distal lateral cortex of the proximal fragment (arrow) has fractured and is slightly displaced medially. (*d*) Six months after fracture, the nail has cut through the neck inferiorly. The medial shift of the femoral shaft is more readily identifiable. (*e*) One year following fracture, the fracture has healed. The nail has been removed.

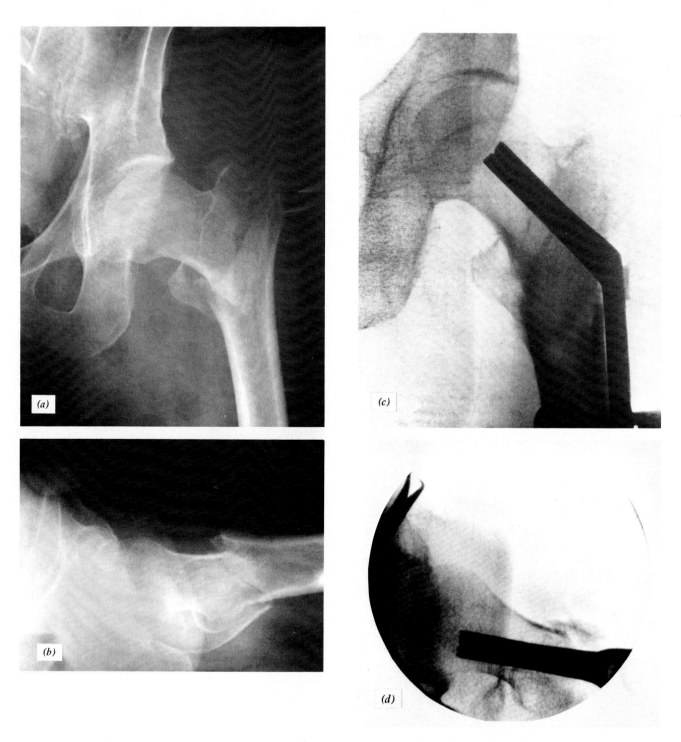

194

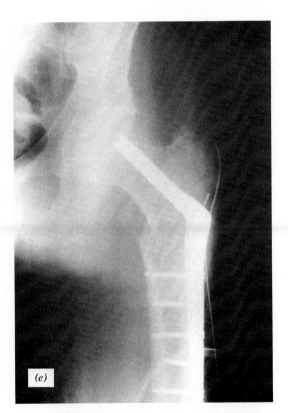

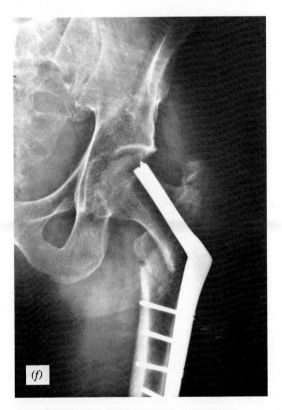

Figure 10-18. Example 10-6. Unstable intertrochanteric fracture with progressive varus deformity. (*a*) This initial view shows the minimally comminuted intertrochanteric fracture. Minimal comminution of the medial femoral cortex is present. (*b*) The initial lateral view demonstrates different rotations of the fragments. The proximal fragment is mildly rotated externally, as shown by the location of the greater trochanter. The distal fragment is markedly rotated externally, as demonstrated by the thickness and curvature of the anterior femoral cortex. This cortex corresponds well to the shape and thickness of the medial femoral cortex. (*c,d*) AP and lateral intraoperative Polaroid view demonstrating anatomic reduction with minimal distraction. (*e*) Later during the day surgery took place, the fracture fragments shifted. It can be seen that the distal fragment has shifted medially. Cortical support is no longer present medially. (*f*) During the next month progressive varus shift occurred. Subsequent follow-up showed that further shift did not occur.

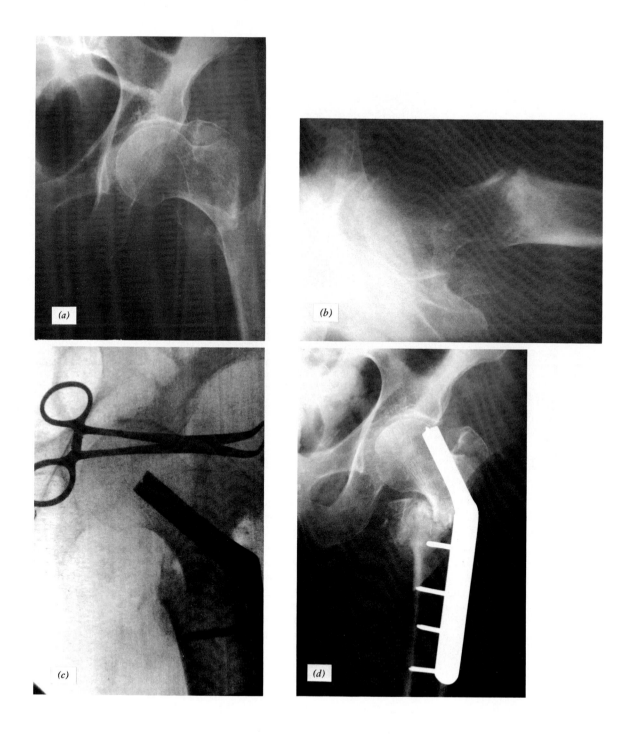

Figure 10-19. Example 10-7. Unstable intertrochanteric fracture treated by medial displacement but with insufficient cortical contact, showing varus shift. (*a*) Initial view demonstrates varus angulation and a comminuted medial femoral cortex. A moderate posterior greater trochanter comminution fragment is present. (*b*) The lateral view demonstrates moderate external rotation of the distal fragment, as shown by the contour of the anterior surface of the distal fragment. This is the contour of the anteromedial femoral cortex. (*c*) Intraoperative view showing final operative position. The distal fragment has been displaced medially and the medial cortices appear almost in contact. (In Figure 19*a*, the medial cortex, which here appears intact, is comminuted.) (*d*) Three weeks following surgery, the nail is cutting through and varus angulation has occurred due to the lack of support from the comminuted medial cortex of the distal fragment.

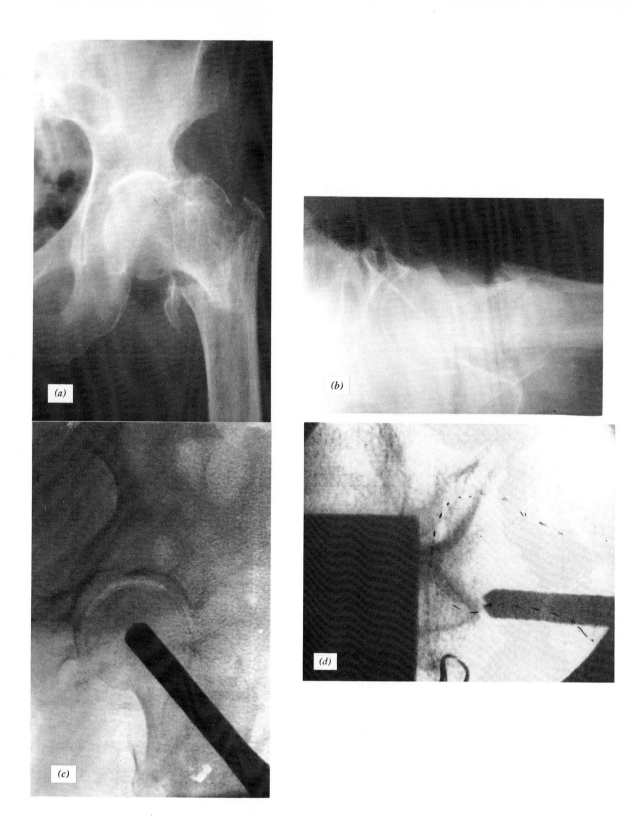

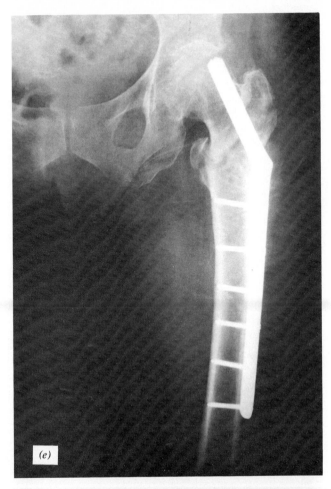

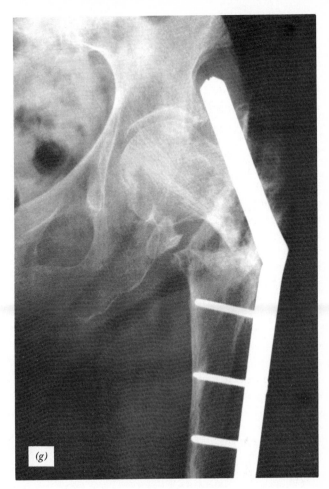

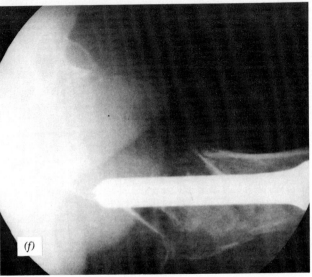

Figure 10-20. Example 10-8. Malreduction and incomplete correction of rotation, with placement of the nail posterior to the proximal fragment. (a) Initial view with a slightly comminuted intertrochanteric fracture. The femoral shaft is moderately rotated externally. (b) The lateral view demonstrates the external rotation of the femoral shaft. Landmarks of the acetabulum can be identified. (c) Intraoperative Polaroid view. Only the proximal fragment is easily seen, and the position of the nail appears good within it. Careful observation of the trochanters shows differential rotation of the fragments. (d) Intraoperative lateral Polaroid view. Underexposed view with probable position of the femoral head reconstructed by acetabular landmarks. The nail is probably posterior to the femoral head and neck. (e) Four days following surgery, the nail has shifted in relation to the proximal fragment. (f) The lateral view four days following surgery demonstrates moderate anterior angulation of the distal fragment. The nail projects partially from the femoral neck. (g) Seven months postsurgery, the nail lies above the femoral neck and articulates with the ilium.

199

and nine months following surgery was able to ambulate with a walker with only minimal symptoms. No further surgery was advised. On the final film (Figure 10-20*g*), the nail can be seen to articulate with the ilium. There is delayed union of the fracture.

Several important points are illustrated by this example. Intraoperative life-threatening complications can occur, such as severe hypotension, cardiac arhythmia, and seizures, any of which may lead the surgeon to abbreviate the operation. Thus, while the radiologist should evaluate the radiographs critically, he should not be judgmental.

Adequate radiographs are essential for proper orthopedic management, and it is the responsibility of the radiologist to be certain that the orthopedist has adequate radiographs.

As mentioned before, the femoral neck is a cylinder, not a cube, and an appliance may be positioned outside of it, even if it appears to be within it on two views. If the appliance is close to the edge of a cylindrical bone on two views, oblique views should be obtained.

Even the most disastrous-appearing radiographs may be compatible with acceptable function of the patient. This patient who had limited mobility preoperatively, is satisfied with the results of surgery and does not desire or require additional surgery.

SUMMARY

Intertrochanteric fractures, when comminuted, are complex fractures requiring careful evaluation and follow-up. The five stresses—shear force; impacting force; medial displacement forces on the distal fragment; varus stress; and external rotation stress—should be evaluated in each fracture pre- and postreduction, and the available alternatives in therapy should be considered for each patient.

REFERENCES

1. Anderson LD: Fractures, in Cremshaw AH (ed): *Campbell's Operative Orthopedics,* St. Louis, CV Mosley, 1971, pp 572–586.
2. AuFranc OE, et al: Fractures of the hip: head, neck and trochanter, in Cave EF, et al (eds): *Trauma Management.* Chicago, Yearbook Publishers, 1974, pp 619–680.
3. Cleveland M, et al: A ten-year analysis of intertrochanteric fractures of the femur. *J Bone Joint Surg* 41A:1399–1408, 1959.
4. Collado HF et al: Condylocephalic nail fixation for trochanteric fractures of the femur. *Orthop Clin North Amer* 5:4:669–678, 1974.
5. Deyerle Wm M: Surgical impaction over a plate and multiple pins for intertrochanteric fracture. *Orthop Clin North Amer* 5:3:615–628, 1974.
6. Dimon J, Hughston J: Unstable intertrochanteric fractures of the hip. *J Bone Joint Surg* 49A:440–450, 1967.
7. Ecker ML, Joyce JJ III, Kohl EJ: The treatment of trochanteric hip fractures using a compression screw. *J Bone Joint Surg* 57A:23–26, 1975.
8. Evans EM: The treatment of trochanteric fractures of the femur. *J Bone Joint Surg* 31B:190–203, 1949.
9. Evans EM: Trochanteric fractures. *J Bone Joint Surg* 33B:192–204, 1951.
10. Harrington K, Johnston JO: The management of comminuted unstable intertrochanteric fractures. *J Bone Joint Surg* 55A:1367–1376, 1973.
11. Holt EP Jr: Hip fractures in the trochanteric region: Treatment with a strong nail and early weight bearing. *J Bone Joint Surg* 45A:687–705, 1963.
12. Holt EP Jr: Rigid Fixation by use of the Holt nail. *Orthop Clin North Amer* 5:3:601–613, 1974.
13. Hughston JC: Intertrochanteric fractures of the femur (hip). *Orthop Clin North Amer* 5:3:585–600, 1974.
14. Johnson LL, Lottes JO, Arnat J: The utilization of the Holt nail for proximal femoral fractures. *J Bone Joint Surg* 50B:67–78, 1968.
15. May JMB, Chacha PB: Displacements of trochanteric fracture and their influence on reduction. *J Bone Joint Surg* 50B:318–323, 1968.
16. Murray RC, Frew JFM: Trochanteric fractures of the femur. *J Bone Joint Surg* 31B:204–219, 1949.
17. Sarmiento A: Intertrochanteric fractures of the femur. *J Bone Joint Surg* 45A:706–722, 1962.
18. Sarmiento A: Avoidance of complications of internal fixation of intertrochanteric fractures: Experience with 250 consecutive cases. *Clin Orthop* 53:47–59, 1967.
19. Sarmiento A, Williams E: The unstable intertrochanteric fracture: Treatment with valgus osteotomy and I-beam nail-plate. *J Bone Joint Surg* 52A:1309–1318, 1970.
20. Sonstegard DA, et al: A biomechanical evaluation of implant, reduction, and prosthesis in the treatment of intertrochanteric hip fractures. *Orthop Clin North Amer* 5:3:551–570, 1974.
21. Tronzo RG: The use of an endoprostheses for severely comminuted trochanteric fractures. *Orthop Clin North Amer* 5:4:679–681, 1974.
22. Tronzo RG: Special considerations in management. *Orthop Clin North Amer* 5:3:571–583, 1974.

11
Fracture Through Metastases: A Brief Note

Fracture through metastases is a common cause of increased morbidity in the patient with metastatic cancer. Despite the almost inevitable fatal outcome, these patients have a mean survival of 5 to 15 months (2,7), with some living for many years. Procedures to diminish pain and improve function are therefore important. With proper choice of methods, as many as 94% of the patients ambulatory prior to fracture can regain the ability to walk (2), and marked decrease in pain can occur (1,2). The prognosis is improved and healing following surgery is more rapid when the potential fracture can be treated by surgery and irradiation prior to actual bony disruption. Improved prognosis and healing are possible because the healing of a complete fracture involves callus with its cartilage, while the healing of a lytic metastasis without fracture occurs without the development of cartilage. The change from cartilage to bone is more radiosensitive than the direct replacement of bone (2).

Because the metastasis has destroyed bone stock, it may not be possible to achieve a stable reduction. Appliances may bend or break when subjected to the full force of weight bearing. To cope with this problem, several different approaches have evolved.

The best approach is to treat the metastasis before it has fractured through; in this way the remaining bony stock will give added stability. Treatment can include radiotherapy, chemotherapy, and internal fixation. If the metastatic disease involves only a small area of bone, standard nails may be sufficient (4). Special nails and plates are used more often because of the usually extensive degree of bone lysis. These devices may be supplemented by methylmethacrylate to fill the space left by the bone lysis. Prosthetic replacement may also be used when it is possible to replace the region of weakened bone by the prosthesis. The same methods are used following fracture, but greater morbidity usually results.

Example 11-1. This 60-year-old woman, with limited metastases from carcinoma of the breast, returned five years after her initial diagnosis with a right femoral ache. Two months following her initial pain, the subtrochanteric portion of the femur fractured. This condition was treated with a blade plate having a long side plate and with radiotherapy. Because of initial malalignment, reoperation was necessary.

Two years following this surgery, the patient was ambulatory (Figure 11-1a).

Eight months later, the plate and femur had fractured (Figure 11-1b). Refixation was attempted unsuccessfully, because of the extension of lysis into the femoral neck (Figure 11-1c). Since that time the patient has been nonambulatory.

Radiotherapy, along with the two initial operations, had given this patient three years of ambulation.

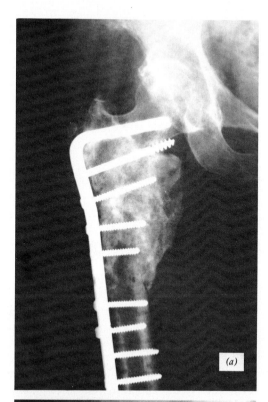

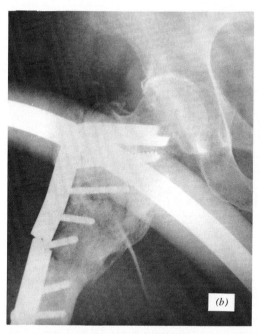

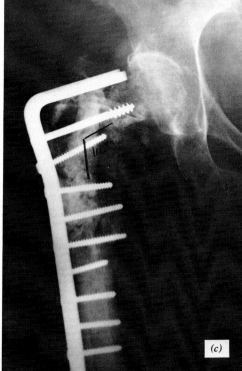

Figure 11-1. Breakage of plate and refracture of the femur. Lytic and blastic metastases of breast carcinoma. (*a*) Two years following blade-plate fixation and irradiation, the patient is ambulatory. Moderate lysis is present, distal to the fourth screw. (*b*) Nearly three years following the initial fracture, the plate and the femur have refractured. (*c*) Re-reduction and fixation with a new blade plate supported in part by radiopaque methylmethacrylate have failed because of the extension of bone lysis into the femoral neck, with fracture of the femoral neck.

The Zickel Nail

Subtrochanteric fractures are a common site of fracture through metastases. They are often difficult to stabilize, and refracture is common. One method of stabilizing such a fracture is that developed by Dr. Zickel; the device is a special nail, which seems to provide sufficient support to the bone to prevent a loss of reduction and a major shift of the fragments. The appliance consists of a long intramedullary rod, providing support through almost the entire length of the femur. The rod is attached to a nail, which fits in the femoral neck and head to prevent rotation of the proximal fragment (Figure 11-2). This appliance is quite helpful in these problem cases (3,5,7). Dr. Zickel

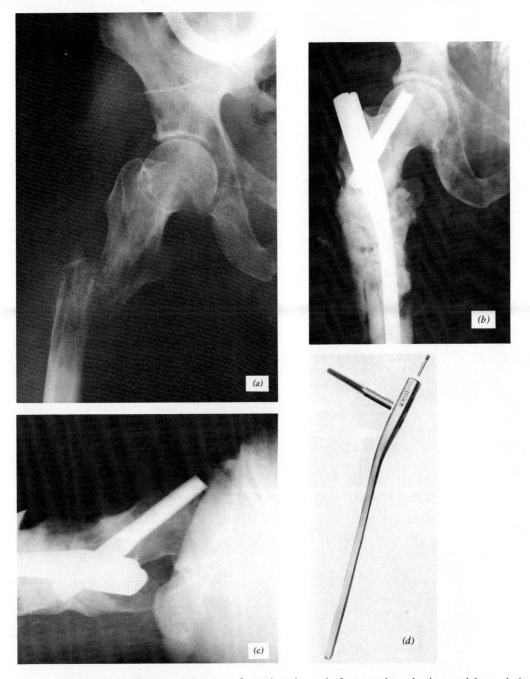

Figure 11-2. Zickel nail fixation of a subtrochanteric fracture through abnormal bone: lytic metastasis from carcinoma of the colon. (*a*) The fracture and extensive bone lysis of the proximal femoral shaft are coincident with many smaller lytic metastases of the bony pelvis. A colostomy appliance is present over the lower abdomen. (*b,c*) The abnormal bone of the femoral shaft has been resected and replaced by radiopaque methylmethacrylate. The Zickel appliance is in place. (*d*) The Zickel appliance. (Courtesy Howmedica®.)

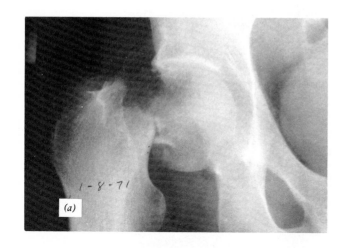

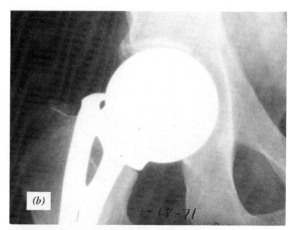

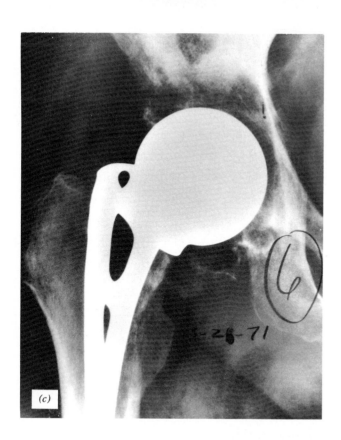

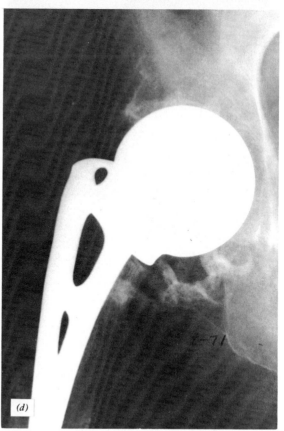

204

prefers to use his appliance without methacrylate; however, in the example shown, methylmethacrylate is used to replace the diseased bone.

The Use of Methylmethacrylate to Replace Diseased Bone

Most appliances do not have sufficient strength to support the weight of the body, and they will bend or break if used when there is insufficient bone for a stable reduction. In these situations, methylmethacrylate can be used to replace the diseased bone, thus providing sufficient support for the internal fixation device. Large quantities of methylmethacrylate can be used in this fashion. Although the duration of success of methacrylate used in this fixation is uncertain, it does seem to exceed the usual life expectancy of these patients (Figure 11-2) (6).

Replacement of the Diseased Bone by a Prosthesis

If the diseased bone is in a limited area, a prosthetic replacement of that area can be quite successful. For example, if the femoral head or neck are involved, an Austin-Moore or Thompson prosthesis can be used to replace it. If the Moore prosthesis is chosen, a variation of it with a long intramedullary stem is often used to distribute forces over an extensive area of the femur. When the acetabulum is involved, a total hip replacement can be used (2,4).

Example 11-2. This 49-year-old man with lymphosarcoma developed sudden right hip pain. A radiograph revealed a pathologic fracture of the right femoral neck (Figure 11-3a). A bone survey disclosed no other lytic lesions. Because of the location of the fracture, the patient's femoral head and neck were replaced by an Austin-Moore prosthesis (Figure 11-3b). Radiation therapy of the proximal femur was then given. Six months following surgery, the patient developed increasing pain in the hip. Radiographs at that time (Figure 11-3c) disclosed a permeative lesion in the right acetabular roof compatible with either tumor or infection. Hip joint aspiration revealed klebsiella. The patient responded to antibiotic therapy, and the infection cleared. Three months later, the bone of the acetabulum had returned towards normal (Figure 11-3d).

SUMMARY

One-sixth of all fractures through skeletal metastases are in the proximal portion of the femur (4). While metastatic disease to bone usually indicates an eventual fatal outcome, the mean survival is 9 to 15 months.

If the patient can regain the ability to walk, and, using appropriate techniques, as many as 94% can, the quality of life is much improved (2). Careful analysis of the extent of metastatic disease is important in choosing the best procedure for each patient. Treatment is often easier and healing is faster if the metastasis is recognized and treated in its prefracture or impending fracture stage.

REFERENCES

1. Douglass H, Shukla SK, Mindell E: Treatment of pathologic fractures of long bones excluding those due to breast cancer. *J Bone Joint Surg* 58A:1055–1060, 1976.

Figure 11-3. Lymphosarcoma metastatic to the femoral neck, with a pathologic fracture treated by replacement with an Austin-Moore prosthesis. Complicated by joint-space infection. (a) The initial view demonstrates the femoral neck fracture associated with the lysis of bone in the femoral neck. (b) Normal postoperative appearance of the Austin-Moore prothesis. (c) Extensive permeative destruction of the superior acetabular bone due to klebsiella infection. Minimal heterotopic bone is present inferior to the head of the prosthesis. Joint-space narrowing is present. (d) The bone of the acetabulum has partially reossified three months after antibiotic therapy of the infection. (Reprinted with permission, *Radiologic Clinics of North America*, 8:45–56, 1975.)

12
Intertrochanteric Osteotomies for Degenerative Joint Disease

Intertrochanteric osteotomies for degenerative joint disease are often successful in relieving symptoms of the pain of degenerative arthrosis of the hip for 2 to 10 years. Because the osteotomies take 3 to 12 months to heal, total hip replacements are now preferred, and it is unlikely that many new intertrochanteric osteotomies for degenerative arthrosis will be seen except in young patients (9). However, many patients who have had these osteotomies done in the past continue to return for follow-up and are satisfied with their results; thus it is important to know the radiological features of these procedures.

A simple transverse osteotomy of the proximal femur will often relieve the pain of hip arthrosis for one to two years, even if the fragments are not displaced (3). This symptomatic relief is probably related both to the immobilization of the extremity for 3 to 12 months and to the hyperemia resulting from the osteotomy. Transverse osteotomy coupled with appropriate displacement of the fragments, however, can result in long-lasting pain relief, which may last ten or more years. A simple transverse osteotomy usually does not reverse the radiographic changes of degenerative arthrosis (3), whereas osteotomy with appropriate displacement of fragments often does. (1) The choice of an appropriate position is therefore of major importance.

Example 12-1. This 72-year-old man's hip problems date to age 21, at which time he sustained a severe injury to his left hip while playing ice hockey. Although he was aware of decreased motion in the hip for many years, the hip remained relatively pain free until age 58. Over the next five years the pain progressively increased, and at age 63 became sufficiently severe so that he sought medical advice. A radiograph at the time (Figure 12-1a) demonstrated severe degenerative arthrosis with joint narrowing, sclerosis, degenerative cyst formation, and osteophyte formation. The femoral head was laterally shifted and osteophytes partially filled in the acetabulum. A tomogram (Figure 12-1b) demonstrates the severity of the cyst formation.

A McMurray medial displacement osteotomy with varus angulation was recommended and performed (Figure 12-1c). A straight spline was used to hold the fragments. The osteotomy healed (Figure 12-1d), and a repeat tomogram one year later demonstrated partial healing of the degenerative cysts (Figure 12-1e). Radiographs two years following surgery (Figure 12-1f) demonstrated further healing of the degenerative cysts.

Seven years following the surgery, the pain began to recur and within a year was severe enough to lead the patient to desire reoperation. Radiographs at that time

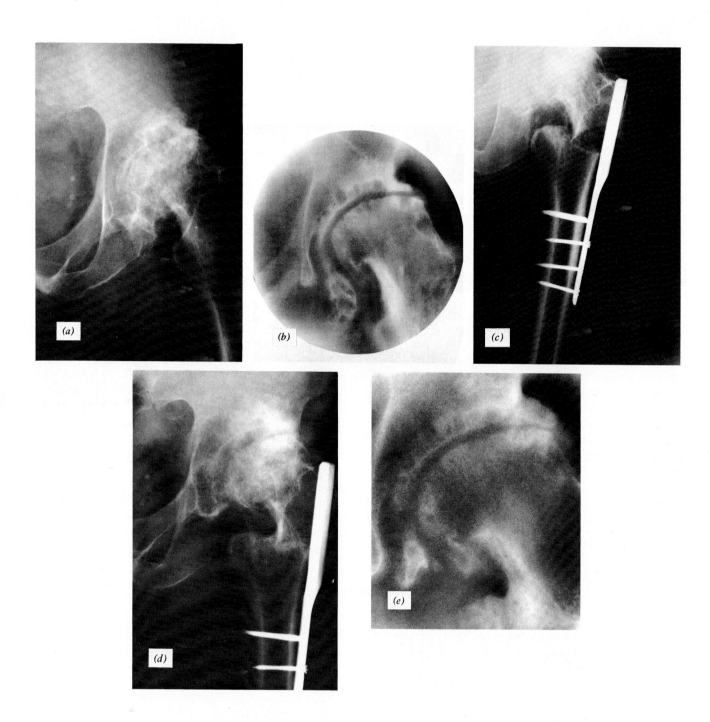

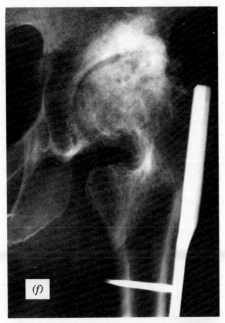

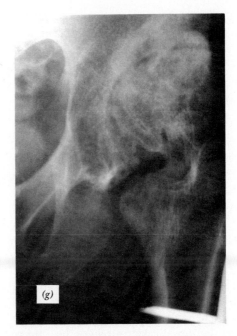

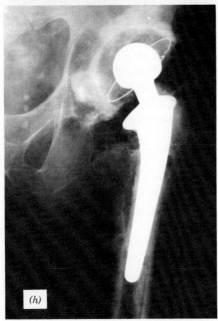

Figure 12-1. Example 12-1. McMurray osteotomy for severe degenerative arthrosis of the hip. (*a*) Patient age 63. Preoperative view. Changes of severe degenerative arthrosis can be seen, along with joint-space narrowing, degenerative cysts, and osteophytes. The medial acetabulum is filled in with osteophytes, and the femoral head is shifted laterally. (*b*) Preoperative view, tomogram, demonstrates the severity of degenerative cyst formation. (*c*) Early postoperative view, McMurray and varus osteotomy. This is an opening wedge osteotomy; the lateral portion of the osteotomy line is distracted. Minor dense areas within this space between the fragments probably represent chips of bone graft. (*d*) Following healing of the osteotomy (one year after surgery), the joint space appears wider, and partial healing of the degenerative cysts has taken place. (*e*) Tomography confirms this partial healing. A thin line of acetabular roof bone now separates most of the cysts from the joint space, a sign of healing. (*f*) Two years following surgery, the acetabular degenerative cysts have healed. (*g*) Seven years following surgery, the pain and the degenerative cysts have recurred. (*h*) A Charnley-Muller straight-stem total hip prosthesis was used as treatment for the recurrent degenerative arthrosis.

(Figure 12-1*g*) disclosed a recurrence of the acetabular degenerative cysts. A Charnley-Muller straight stem total hip prosthesis was used (Figure 12-1*h*).

POSITIONING OF FRAGMENTS

The choice of position is influenced by several factors: deformity by itself often accentuates the pain of the arthrosis, and, therefore, correction of deformity is a prime goal. In degenerative arthrosis, the damage to cartilage is often asymmetrical; an attempt is made to reposition the femoral head so that the thickest cartilage is in the weight-bearing position. Muscle imbalance and increased muscular tension across the hip are though to be partial etiologies both for the development of degenerative arthrosis and its pain; repositioning attempts to change the relative lever arms and therefore the relative strengths of the abductor and adductor muscles of the hip (11,12).

The success of the hanging hip operation, in which the muscles around the hip are divided to relieve the pain of degenerative arthrosis, supports the importance of muscle pull as a factor in the pain of degenerative arthrosis (13).

To achieve these varied results, a careful preoperative clinical and radiological evaluation is usually carried out. Films are obtained of the hip in internal and external rotation and in maximum adduction and abduction. From these films and the clinical examination, the desired position can be derived (3,7). This position can be achieved at the time of surgery by a combination of varus or valgus realignment and internal and external rotational realignment (4,5). These realignments may be combined with medial displacement of the distal femoral shaft fragment. If the choice of position has been appropriate, pain relief will usually persist for a period of 2 to 10-years, and the radiographic changes of degenerative arthrosis will diminish; it is thought that proper selection of the type of realignment will increase the likelihood of prolonged pain relief.

THE VARUS OSTEOTOMY

The prototype of the varus osteotomy is the work of Pauwels, who did a closing-wedge osteotomy on the medial side of the proximal femur by removing a wedge-shaped piece of bone. The varus osteotomy is thought to be effective because it raises the position of the greater trochanter in relation to the hip joint, thus reducing the tension on the hip from the gluteus medius. The osteotomy also lengthens the lever arm of the gluteus medius, permitting this muscle to apply a greater rotational and stabilizing force across the hip. The varus osteotomy is usually coupled with division or partial division of the adductor muscles tendons.

The varus osteotomy is best in the subluxing hip, especially the subluxing hip with coxa valga and a shallow acetabulum. Moderate motion at the hip should still be present, and ample abduction should be present to allow the femoral head to be seated well within the acetabulum (11). This osteotomy can be used in the child with a subluxing hip prior to the development of degenerative arthrosis or in the adult after pain has developed.

Patients who can benefit from the varus osteotomy may demonstrate an antalgic limp, they may manifest abduction deformity, and they will often have pain on adduction. If abduction is limited, the osteotomy will increase adduction deformity with increasing pain (3). The varus osteotomy can be combined with a rotational osteotomy and with displacement of the shaft medially. If the tension of the iliopsoas is great, and the medial shaft displacement does not diminish it, the iliopsoas tendon can be divided. When divided, the tendon will usually heal with a greater length, thus helping to relieve pressure across the hip joint.

THE VALGUS OSTEOTOMY

The valgus osteotomy is thought to be the best procedure in patients with adduction deformity, particularly if abduction is painful. Because it shifts the femoral head into adduction, the valgus osteotomy is limited to patients in whom it is possible to adduct the hip further. On occasion, the presurgical radiograph will disclose a large osteophyte on the superolateral lip of the femoral head (3,11) (Figure 12-2*c*). Valgus repositioning helps in the relief of pain in such patients.

THE MEDIAL DISPLACEMENT OSTEOTOMY (MCMURRAY OSTEOTOMY)

Medial displacement of the femoral shaft decreases the tension in the iliopsoas muscle, often leading to a decrease in the pain of degenerative arthrosis of the hip. Lessening of this muscle tension can also lead to regression of the radiographic changes of degenerative arthrosis (11).

The medial displacement osteotomy was popularized by McMurray in several articles and by his personal teaching (8). Intertrochanteric osteotomies with medial displacement of the distal fragment are usually called McMurray osteotomies for that reason. McMurray's actual operation has been modified by most surgeons to improve its results. Originally, McMurray's operation involved a steeply oblique (angled medially and cranially) osteotomy, with the aim that some of the force of weight bearing would be transferred from the pelvis directly to the upper end of the femur. He combined medial displacement with rotation of the femoral head so that a less damaged portion of articular cartilage could assume the weight bearing. Initially he treated his patients in plaster without internal fixation.

As others used his operation, certain modifications were introduced and these are now commonly incorporated into the so-called McMurray osteotomy. Instead of being steeply oblique, the osteotomy is now usually transverse. Metallic appliances are now used to hold the position of the fragments. Both straight splines (Figure 12-2b) and angled plates (Figure 12-2d) may be used. The straight spline has the advantage that it permits progressive impaction, which is often limited by the angle of the blade plate (3,11). Olsson (10) reports the angled compression plate gives better results than the straight spline in his series of 82 hips. With the use of the transverse osteotomy and internal fixation, the incidence of nonunion and loss of desired position is lowered.

Example 12-2. This middle-aged man developed progressive pain in his left hip. A radiograph (Figure 12-2a) disclosed a lateral femoral head degenerative cyst. A McMurray medial displacement osteotomy (Figure 12-2b) was performed with good relief of symptoms for the next six years. Toward the end of this period a mild adduction deformity developed. An adduction radiograph (Figure 12-2c) revealed a large, laterally placed osteophyte on the lateral femoral head. In adduction, the osteophyte did not impinge on the acetabulum, and a repeat osteotomy was performed to shift the femoral head into valgus (Figure 12-2d). Good pain relief was achieved. Four years following the reoperation (Figure 12-2e), the patient's pain recurred, and he was then considered for a total hip replacement.

EXPECTED RADIOLOGIC CHANGES FOLLOWING OSTEOTOMY

Following osteotomy, the thickness of the articular cartilage is usually increased. This should not be surprising, since one of the major aims of the operation is to shift thicker cartilage to the weight-bearing surface. Many early articles interpreted this increased thickness of articular cartilage as a result of regeneration of cartilage. Only recently have several authors (2,14) correctly pointed out that the appearance of thicker articular cartilage is due simply to the shift of more normal cartilage to the position of weight bearing. Since the change is positional, it would be expected that the cartilage could appear thicker and thinner on serial films because of changes in the position of the hip and not because of the presence of new disease in the hip (14). Thinning of the cartilage following surgery should not be interpreted as indicative of infection unless other clinical and radiological signs are present.

Osteophytes and degenerative cysts often resolve following osteotomy (see Example 12-1). This is probably the result of the hypervascular response, the repositioning of thicker and more normal articular cartilage, and perhaps from the postoperative immobilization. When pain does recur following intertrochanteric osteotomy, the osteophytes, degenerative cysts, and other changes of degenerative arthritis usually recur as well.

COMPLICATIONS OF INTERTROCHANTERIC OSTEOTOMY FOR DEGENERATIVE ARTHROSIS

Prior to the use of internal fixation, it was common to see a shifting of fragments back towards the preoperative posi-

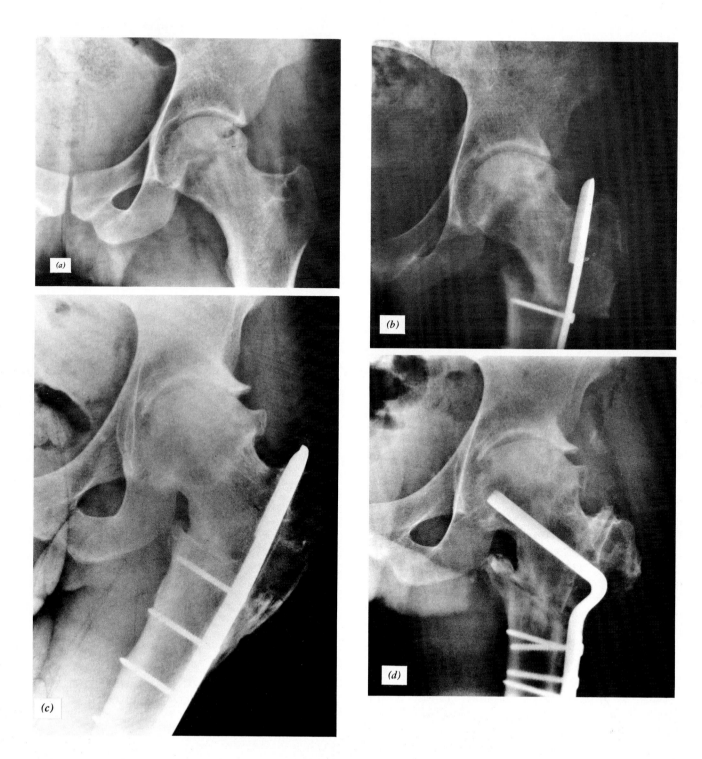

214

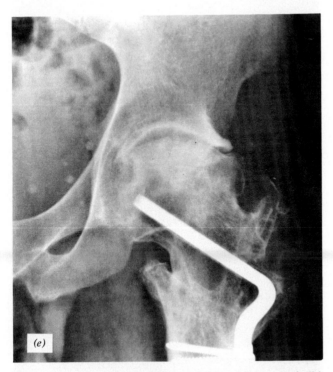

(e)

Figure 12-2. Example 12-2. Degenerative arthritis treated with a McMurray osteotomy. Retreated using a valgus osteotomy, six years later for recurrent pain. (*a*) Presurgical view. A moderate-sized degenerative cyst is present in the superolateral portion of the femoral head. (*b*) Appearance following a McMurray medial displacement osteotomy. The fragments are held with a straight spline. (*c*) Six years following surgery, adduction view demonstrates the large lateral femoral head osteophyte. This would impinge on the acetabulum in abduction, limiting motion and causing pain. (*d*) Following valgus osteotomy, the position is held with an angled blade-plate. With the shaft in neutral position, the osteophyte on the femoral head is now away from the acetabulum, permitting some abduction. (*e*) Four years following reoperation, the lateral femoral head osteophyte has grown and again limits abduction. Because of recurrent pain, the patient is now being considered for a total hip replacement.

An interesting pattern can be seen with delayed union of intertrochanteric osteotomies. One can see a slight shift into varus position, resulting in distraction of the lateral femoral cortex. Callus fills in the medial portion of the osteotomy line, with a delay in healing occurring laterally (15). In one series, approximately 20% of the cases involved had failed to unite totally at one year, and 10% were not completely united at two years. The longer the delay in union, the greater the chance of varus malalignment. Delay in union is the major cause of continued pain postosteotomy (15). On occasion, tomography may be helpful in evaluating the extent of union. Several factors have been related to the presence of delayed union and nonunion: these include medial displacement of the distal fragment by greater than 50%; distraction at the osteotomy site (which may be more common when angled internal devices are used); and marked obliquity of the osteotomy as in the original McMurray technique (6,16). When internal fixation devices are used in patients with delayed union or nonunion, resorption around the proximal portion of the fixation plate is often seen (16).

CONVERSION TO TOTAL HIP REPLACEMENT

A specific problem may arise when an attempt is made to revise an intertrochanteric osteotomy to a total hip replacement. When valgus reposition or medial displacement has occurred during the osteotomy, the curved, normal stem of the femoral component of the total hip replacement appliance may not fit or may fit only with difficulty into the reshaped femoral shaft. As a result, the stem of the femoral component may be forced through the medial cortex of the femur (Figure 12-3*a,b,c,d*). This problem can be avoided if a special straight stem femoral prosthesis is used (Figure 12-1*h*).

SUMMARY

Although the intertrochanteric osteotomy has now probably been largely supplanted by the total hip replacement, there are still many patients with successful osteotomies who are benefiting from the pain relief which the

tion. This condition is less common with metallic internal fixation. Progressive varus deformity is, however, seen on occasion and is more common in patients with delayed union or nonunion. Delayed union and nonunion occur in 3 to 13% of osteotomies (6,15). Infection occurs occasionally.

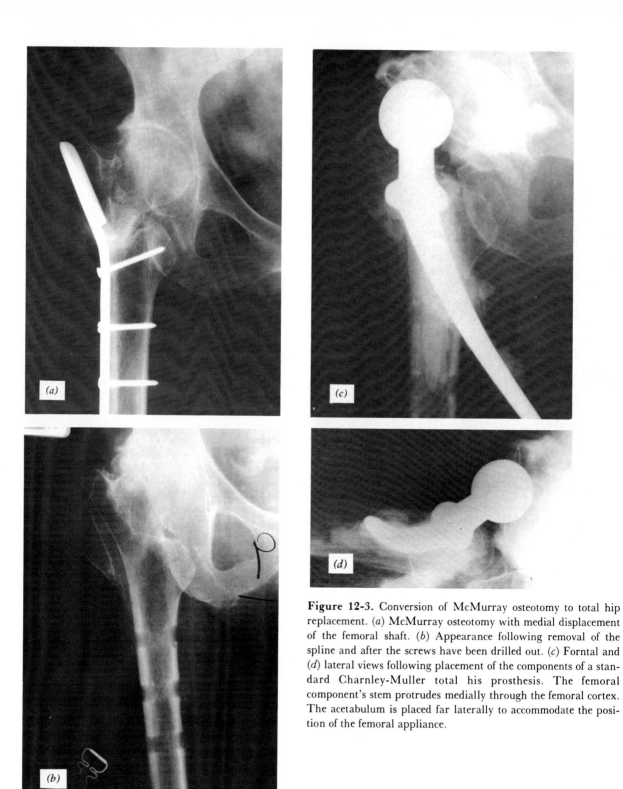

Figure 12-3. Conversion of McMurray osteotomy to total hip replacement. (*a*) McMurray osteotomy with medial displacement of the femoral shaft. (*b*) Appearance following removal of the spline and after the screws have been drilled out. (*c*) Forntal and (*d*) lateral views following placement of the components of a standard Charnley-Muller total his prosthesis. The femoral component's stem protrudes medially through the femoral cortex. The acetabulum is placed far laterally to accommodate the position of the femoral appliance.

procedure can give. The major complications are delayed union and the difficulties that may be encountered in the conversion of an intertrochanteric osteotomy to a total hip replacement.

REFERENCES

1. Adam A, Spence AJ: Intertrochanteric osteotomy for osteoarthritis of the hip. *J Bone Joint Surg* 40B:219–226, 1958.

2. Arden GP: Variations in joint space of the hip as shown radiographically. *J Bone Joint Surg* 39B:750–751, 1957.

3. Blount WP: Osteotomy in the treatment of osteoarthritis of the hip. *J Bone Joint Surg* 46A:1297–1325, 1964.

4. Ferguson AB Jr: High intertrochanteric osteotomy for osteoarthritis of the hip. *J Bone Joint Surg* 46A:1159–1175, 1964.

5. Ferguson AB Jr: The pathologic changes in degenerative arthritis of the hip and treatment by rotational osteotomy. *J Bone Joint Surg* 46A:1337–1352, 1964.

6. Green JP: Union of Intertrochanteric Osteotomies. *J Bone Joint Surg* 49B:488–494, 1967.

7. Knodt H: Osteoarthritis of the hip joint. *J Bone Joint Surg* 46A:1326–1336, 1964.

8. McMurray TP: Osteoarthritis of the hip joint. *J Bone Joint Surg* 21:1–11, 1939.

9. Mendes DG: Intertrochanteric osteotomy for degenerative hip disease. *Clin Orthop* 106:60–74, 1975.

10. Olsson SS, Goldie IF, Irstam LKH: Intertrochanteric osteotomy for osteoarthritis of the hip. *J Bone Joint Surg* 57B:466–470, 1975.

11. Ottolenghi CE, Frigerio E: Intertrochanteric osteotomies in osteoarthritis of the hip. *J Bone Joint Surg* 44A:558–596, 1962.

12. Ottolenghi CE, et al: Effects of intertrochanteric osteotomy in the hip joint. *Clin Orthop* 39:157–170, 1965.

13. Radin EC, Maquet P, Parker H: Rationale and indications for the "hanging hip" procedure. *Clin Orthop* 112:221–230, 1975.

14. Robins RHC, Piggot J: McMurray osteotomy with a note on the regeneration of articular cartilage. *J Bone Joint Surg* 42B:480–488, 1960.

15. Rosborough D, Stiles PJ: Nonunion after intertrochanteric osteotomy with internal fixation for osteoarthritis of the hip. *J Bone Joint Surg* 49B:462–474, 1967.

16. Scott PJ: Nonunion of oblique displacement intertrochanteric osteotomy for osteoarthritis of the hip. *J Bone Joint Surg* 49B:475–487, 1967.

13
The Cup Mold Arthroplasty

Cup mold arthroplasty of the hip is a good, but not perfect, method for restoring mobility to the hip. It is a type of interposition arthroplasty in which the femoral head and acetabular surfaces are reshaped to restore their congruence and in which an inert material is interposed between the surfaces to permit motion during healing. The interposition arthroplasty using fascia has wide application in many joints in the body, but, in the weight-bearing joints, fascia is often too fragile for success. Dr. Smith-Petersen (6), in a fascinating review, summarizes the development of an indestructable, interposable mold. Glass, then Celluloid, then Pyrex, then Bakelite, and finally Vitallium metal were used to provide the mold for the new hip joint. Figure 13-1*a,b* shows the result of the use of a Pyrex cup mold in the late 1930s. Although the Pyrex cup mold eventually broke (Figure 13-1*b*) and had to be removed, the patient was left with a mobile hip, because in the intervening 18 months cartilage had formed on both femoral head and acetabular surfaces. The current molds are made of metal and are of various shapes and sizes. In the original procedure the mold was always removed, but with Vitallium metal this was found to be unnecessary, and the molds are now left in place.

When it works, the cup mold arthroplasty provides a strong, mobile, stabile, but occasionally mildly to moderately painful hip. The importance of the procedure is that, although it does not totally relieve pain, the patient

This chapter is based in part on material originally printed in the *Radiologic Clinics of North America*, 8:45–56, 1975, and portions are reprinted with permission.

need not favor his or her hip. It is ideally suited for the laborer who must carry heavy loads or the athlete who places strenuous demands on his or her hip.

The success of the cup mold arthroplasty depends only partially on the surgical procedure. Of major importance is postoperative nursing and rehabilitation. Following surgery, the patient must work his hip despite the presence of pain, since motion of the hip is essential for the formation of cartilage surfaces on the articular bone and for the prevention of adhesions. Six months of intensive rehabilitation is often required. Because of the extensive rehabilitation necessary (six months of total disability and one year of additional partial disability), this procedure is suitable only for well-motivated patients (2).

Example 13-1. At the age of 9 months, this 43-year-old woman experienced a dislocated left hip, which was treated by closed manipulation. At the age of 18 months, surgical reduction of the left hip was attempted with only partial success. At age 7 years, a left shelf arthroplasty was performed. About age 30, bilateral hip pain developed (more severe in the left hip than in the right), and at age 39 bilateral cup arthroplasties were performed. At the present, four years following this surgery, the patient has a mild muscle ache in her right hip and is aware of limitation of motion of both hips. She is fairly active, swims, takes care of her house and her four children, but occasionally uses a cane. The radiograph (Figure 13-2) demonstrates the bilateral metallic cup molds; they are quite large (decreasing the chance for progressive protrusio

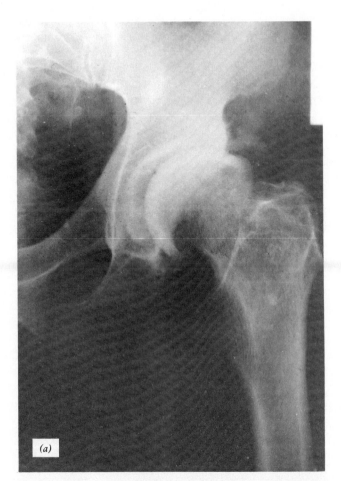 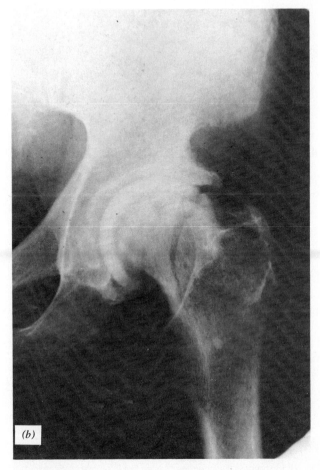

Figure 13-1. Cup mold arthroplasty with Pyrex cup, dating from about 1939. (*a*) The Pyrex cup mold in place. A good joint space is present. (*b*) The Pyrex cup has broken through its base. The cup was removed and the patient was left with a satisfactory hip.

acetabuli). The right cup is medially placed, with mild protrusio acetabuli present. The greater trochanter (attached with wires) has been shifted distally to improve the length and therefore strength of the gluteus muscles. The left cup has been placed under the overhanging shelf of bone from the previous shelf procedure.

Example 13-2. This 73-year-old woman had a Moore femoral head replacement of the right hip performed at age 62 for unknown cause. This became painful and was replaced by a shaft cup arthroplasty. (Although it is

preferable to place the cup mold on the femoral head, in cases where it has been removed, as in this patient with a previous Austin Moore arthroplasty, the cup can be placed on the shaped greater trochanter or on the femoral shaft). This shaft cup arthroplasty was complicated by a joint infection, which was drained in 1971. Since that time the patient has had persistent pain. After discussing the available options, the patient decided not to have surgery at this time.

The radiographs (Figure 13-3*a,b*) show the special shaft arthroplasty cup which has a neck portion. A joint space is

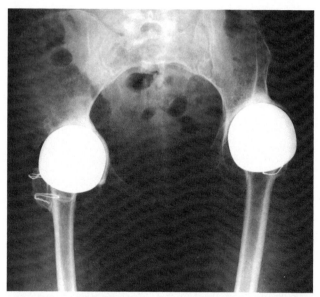

Figure 13-2. Example 1. Bilateral cup mold arthroplasty for sequella of bilateral congenital displacement of the hips. The left cup articulates with the shelf from a prior shelf arthroplasty.

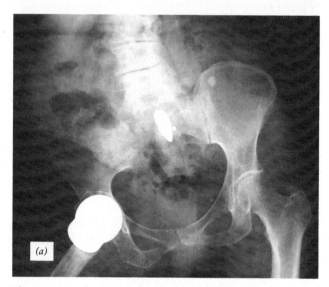

Figure 13-3. Example 13-2. Shaft cup mold arthroplasty. (*a*) The cup mold is placed on the femoral shaft. There is moderate pelvic tilt and severe degenerative disc disease of the lower lumbar spine. (*b*) The abduction view demonstrates motion of the cup within the acetabulum and motion of the femoral shaft within the cup.

seen between the cup and the acetabulum; the femur moves within the cup and the cup moves within the acetabulum. A marked pelvic tilt is present, along with lumbar spine scoliosis and degenerative disc disease, at least in part due to the shortening of this patient's right leg; such shortening is inherent in shaft arthroplasty.

Radiographic Appearances

On a roentgenogram, the metallic cup can be identified. Unfortunately, the cup obscures the underlying remnant of the femoral head and much of the acetabulum. It should lie in the axis of the femoral neck and should be mobile on abduction views in relation to the acetabulum and, depending on the type of cup used, in relation to the femoral head as well. The extent of radiologically detectable widening of the acetabular joint space is variable (1,2,3).

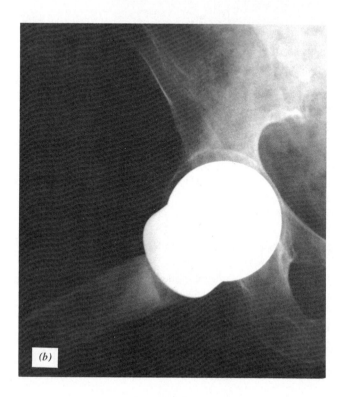

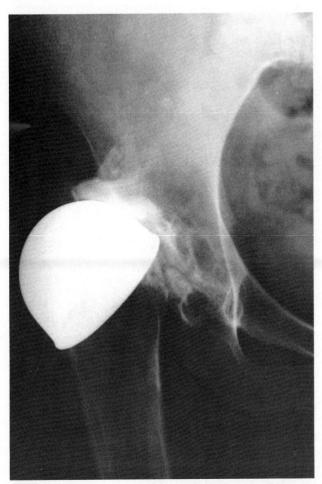

Figure 13-4. The cup used for this shaft arthroplasty has subluxed into valgus. There is sclerosis of the acetabular roof, suggesting degenerative arthrosis. Motion caused pain. The type of shaft cup shown in Figure 12-3 is used to decrease the chance of subluxation of a shaft cup arthroplasty.

Complications

Subluxation and Dislocation

The cup may dislocate or sublux with or without the femoral head (1,2). (See Figure 13-4).

Secondary Degenerative Arthrosis

Probably the most common causes of pain following cup arthroplasty are sclerosis and/or fragmentation of the femoral head, frequently associated with spotty areas indicating a lack of cartilage (1,2,3,4). Unfortunately, such areas cannot be evaluated by x-ray, since they are obscured by the metallic cup.

Example 13-3. This 35-year-old man was involved in a car accident six years ago, sustaining multiple lacerations and a posterior dislocation of the right hip. The dislocation was treated by closed reduction and traction immobilization for four weeks. His hip has become progressively painful since that time. Radiographs obtained two years following the injury (Figure 13-5a) disclosed a defect in the midportion of the posterior lip of the acetabulum (evidence of the prior posterior dislocation), superolateral joint space narrowing, and degenerative cysts in both the superomedial portion of the acetabulum and the superior aspect of the formal head. Osteophytes ring the base of the femoral head. Minimal ectopic bone formation is seen near the lateral acetabular rim. The changes are those of moderate posttraumatic degenerative arthritis.

A right hip arthroplasty was performed three months later. Radiographs one week postoperative (Figure 13-5b) disclose a properly positioned cup mold arthroplasty. The superomedially placed acetabular degenerative cyst is still present.

Three months postoperative, because of continued pain, the patient's hip was reoperated. At that time, the acetabulum was covered by fibrocartilage. The femoral head, however, showed several areas of eburnated bone on the weight-bearing surface. These areas were removed, the head reshaped, and the cup returned to its place. Two months following the second procedure (Figure 13-5c,d), the cup and the hip showed a normal postoperative appearance. The greater trochanter had not yet united with the femur.

The patient did well for three years but then developed progressive pain over the next three months. Radiographs at that time demonstrated increased acetabular sclerosis and a large, centrally placed degenerative cyst in the dome of the acetabulum (Figure 13-5e).

Because of the failure of the cup arthroplasty, a total hip replacement was performed. Because the patient was comparatively young, the Harris appliance, which permits easier replacement of the acetabular component, was used

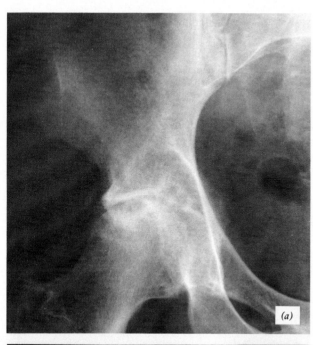

(a)

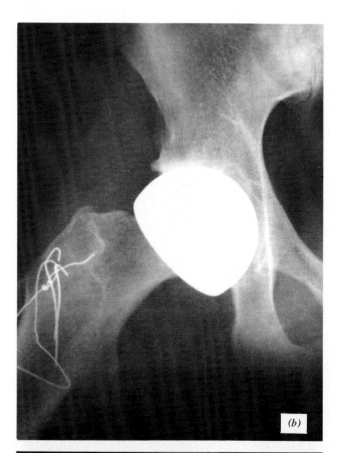

(b)

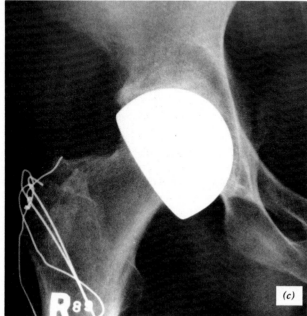

(c)

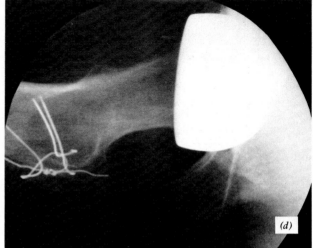

(d)

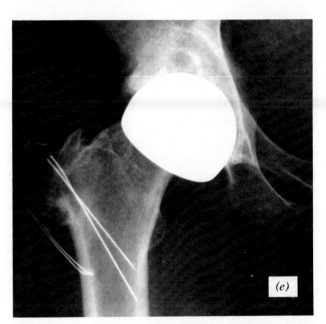

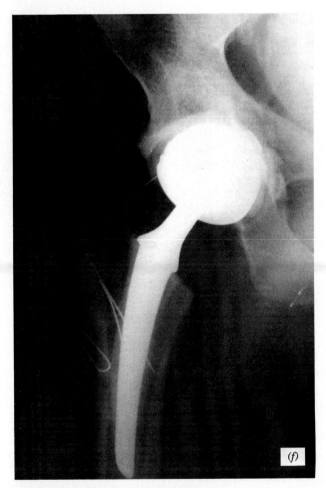

Figure 13-5. Example 13-3. Degenerative arthritis recurring following cup mold arthroplasty. (*a*) Two years following posterior dislocation of the hip, there are changes caused by moderate degenerative arthrosis, with cartilage narrowing and femoral head and acetabular degenerative cysts. A bony defect is present in the posterior acetabular rim, representing the residuum of the posterior dislocation. (*b*) One week following surgery, the cup appears properly placed. (*c,d*) Following reoperation at two months, the cup appears properly seated and the acetabular degenerative cyst is healing. The head is well seated on both frontal (*c*) and lateral (*d*) views, being moderately well centered on the axis of the femoral neck. (*e*) Three years following surgery, the pain has returned. Degenerative changes have recurred, and there is a degenerative cyst in the acetabulum. The wires for the greater trochanter osteotomy have broken. Breakage of the wires following healing of the greater trochanter osteotomy is not associated with symptoms; it represents a fatigue fracture of the wire due to repeated minor stress. (*f*) A Harris total hip replacement prosthesis. The acetabular component is made of two pieces; the plastic articulating insert is more easily replaced than the standard total hip replacement.

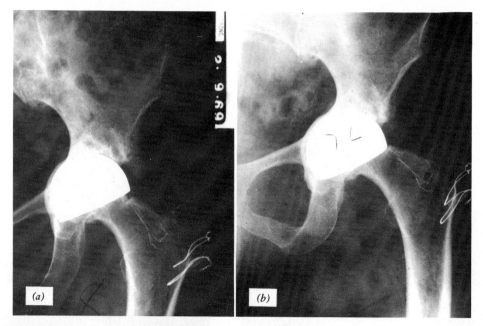

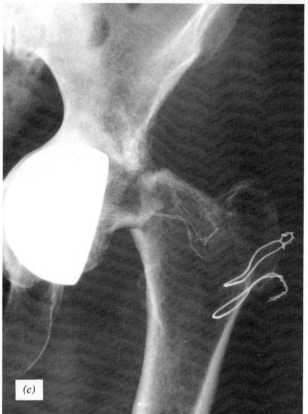

Figure 13-6. Breakage of the femoral neck due to recurrent impingement on it by the cup mold. Adduction (*a*) and neutral (*b*) views demonstrate indentation on the superior aspect of the femoral neck. (A similar indentation is seen in Figure 12-5*c*.) The cup is relatively fixed within the acetabulum. Lack of motion between the cup and the acetabulum can result in fracture. Motion between the femoral head and the cup varies with the type of cup prosthesis used. (*c*) A fracture of the femoral neck is now present and passes through the notch in the superior portion of the femoral neck. (Reprinted with permission, Radiologic Clinics of North America, April 1975.)

(Figure 13-5*f*). At the time of surgery, the femoral head was found to be fixed within the cup by granulation tissue, with no motion occurring between the cup and the femoral head. The femoral head showed evidence of degenerative arthritis.

This case demonstrates the problems with a painful cup arthroplasty. Because the metal of the cup cannot be adequately penetrated by x-rays, disease of the femoral head cannot be identified. It is only in those cases where acetabular disease is also present that an assessment of the cause or possible cause of pain following cup arthroplasty can be made.

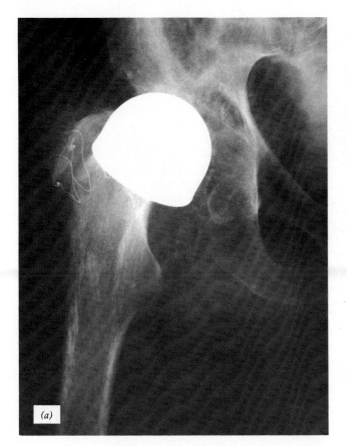
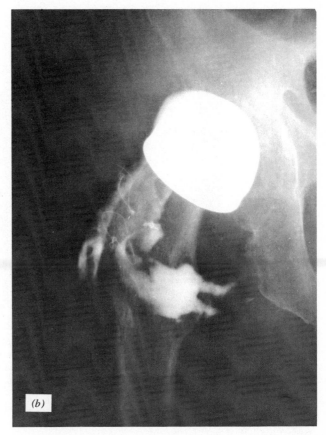

Figure 13-7. Infected cup mold arthroplasty. Shortly following a cup mold arthroplasty for post-traumatic arthritis, pus started to drain from the wound. (*a*) Three months following surgery, permeative lysis is present in the proximal femoral shaft, compatible with osteomyelitis. (*b*) A sinogram demonstrates communication of the infected sinus with the joint space.

Fracture

An immobile cup may cause fracture of the femoral neck by placing recurrent impressions on the neck (Figure 13-6a,b,c).

Infection

Infection occurring after a cup mold arthroplasty will show characteristic features of osteomyelitis with permea-

tive bone destruction and, occasionally, periosteal new bone formation (Figure 13-7a,b). The infection may be followed by extensive heterotopic bone formation, with markedly restricted motion (Figure 13-8a,b). Heterotopic bone formation is usually mild in the absence of infection, and, in one series where it occurred in 30% of the patients, restriction of motion was much less common, involving only about 3% of the patients (5).

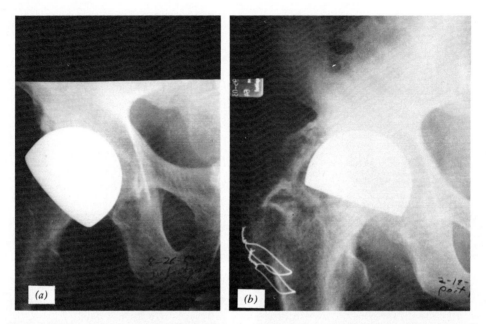

Figure 13-8. Infected cup arthroplasty. Extensive heterotopic bone. (*a*) Normal appearance of cup mold arthroplasty in a patient with a staphyloccus aureus infection one week following surgery. The patient was treated with reoperation, debridgement, replacement of the cup, and appropriate antibiotics. (*b*) Six months later extensive heterotopic bone is present. Hip aspiration at this time was sterile. (Reprinted with permission. Radiologic Clinics of North America, April 1975.)

SUMMARY

The cup mold arthroplasty has proved itself to be a useful procedure in patients with a variety of hip disorders. It results in a strong and stable, relatively pain-free, hip. Because of the prolonged rehabilitation necessary following this procedure, it is unlikely to be used today as a primary procedure, except, perhaps, in the young or unusually physically active person.

REFERENCES

1. Adams TC: A reconsideration of cup arthroplasty of the hip. *J Bone Joint Surg* 35B:199–208, 1953.

2. Aufranc OE: *Constructive Surgery of the Hip.* St. Louis, CV Mosby Co, 1962.

3. Gibson A: Vitallium cup arthroplasty of the hip joint. *J Bone Joint Surg* 31A:861–868, 1949.

4. Gibons A, Williams TH: Changes in the femoral head underlying a vitallium cup. *J Bone Joint Surg* 33B:119–121, 1951.

5. Hamblen DL, Harris WH, Rottger J: Myositis ossificans as a complication of hip arthroplasty. Presented at the British Orthopaedic Association Meeting, Belfast, April 1–3, 1971. Abstracted, *J Bone Joint Surg* 53B:764, 1971.

6. Smith-Petersen MN: Evolution of mold arthroplasty of the hip joint. *J Bone Joint Surg* 30B:59–75, 1948.

14
The Total Hip Replacement

INTRODUCTION

The concept that replacement of both the acetabular and femoral sides of the hip joint would be a worthwhile surgical invention dates back at least to the mid-1930s and, in some forms, back to the beginning of this century; however, these early attempts usually failed because of the difficulty in obtaining a solid bond between the prosthesis and the patient's bone. It was John Charnley's recognition of the safety and effectiveness of the methylmethacrylate interface, reported in 1960, that resulted in a great stride forward in the development of total hip replacements (5). The total hip replacement has now become one of the most common if not *the* most common elective operation performed on the hip. Because of this, the knowledge of the normal appearance of the total hip replacement and the ability to recognize its complications are of great practical importance.

COMMON TYPES

Although there are many varieties of total hip replacement, seven types are most often used. The Ring prosthesis (Figure 14-1) is the only one of those currently in use that does not use methylmethacrylate to help hold it in place. The Ring prosthesis consists of an acetabular component with a long screw placed in the axis of force through the pelvis, which articulates with a femoral component (33).

The McKee-Farrar prosthesis (Figure 14-2) is the result of many experimental designs by Dr. McKee and consists of two parts: an acetabular cup with many spikes on its outer surface. The cup is held to the acetabulum by methacrylate. The metal femoral component is similar to the Thompson prosthesis previously described (18).

The third type is the Charnley prosthesis (Figure 14-3), which is very popular in England but less often seen in the United States. This prosthesis has an acetabular component composed of high-density polyethylene marked by a hemispherical wire. The acetabular component is properly positioned medially, deep in the acetabulum. The femoral component consists of a modification of the Thompson prosthesis; it is unique in that the size of the femoral head is quite small compared to the other forms of total hip replacement. The small head decreases the chance of the prosthesis loosening.

The fourth type is the Charnley-Muller prosthesis (Figure 14-4a,b,c), a modification of the Charnley prosthesis. It uses a high-density polyethylene acetabular component, which is marked by a circumferential wire near its mouth and a Thompson-type femoral component. The major differences between this and the Charnley prosthesis are the appearance of the wire and the femoral head, which is larger than that used in the Charnley prosthesis. There are many variations of the Charnley-Muller prosthesis, but they need not be discussed here, with the exception of two kinds used in young patients (3). In the first, the Turner-Aufranc prosthesis (Figure 14-5a,b), the articular cavity in the acetabular component is placed eccentrically, closer to the feet, to permit a longer wear-life of the acetabular component. The second, the Harris

227

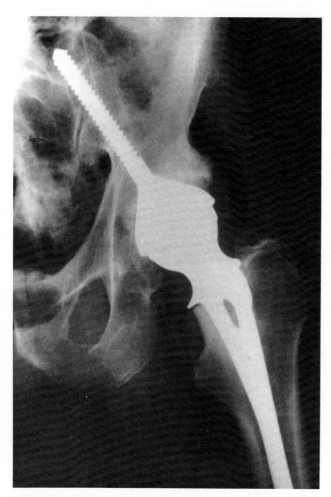

Figure 14-1. The Ring prosthesis, which is held to bone by the long acetabular screw and the long medullary stem of the femoral component. When properly placed, the acetabular component should be tightly fitted to a reshaped acetabulum. The flange should lie in contact with the femoral bone.

prosthesis (Figure 14-6), has a replaceable insert in the acetabular component, so that when the acetabular prosthesis wears out (in 10 to 15 years) it can be more easily replaced (10).

Type five consists of several prostheses not often used in the United States. They are nondislocatable; that is, the femoral head is held locked within the acetabulum component, preventing dislocation. Two types are illustrated in Figure 14-7a,b.

The sixth type is a multicomponent prosthesis that permits axial rotation of the femoral head component on the femoral prosthesis, in addition to the usual femoro-acetabular motion (Figure 14-8).

The last type uses a polyethylene acetabular component and a cup-shaped femoral component held to the femoral head by methacrylate. This is called a resurfacing prosthesis (Figure 14-9).

NORMAL POSITION

Highly important to the success of a total hip replacement are the positions of the acetabular and femoral components (35). Muscle weakness or laxness (24,31), combined with poor position, increases the chance of subluxation. No absolute positions can be applied for all prostheses and for all patients, but it is important to understand the reason for the variability and the limits of acceptable position. While not much can be done about an unacceptable position short of reoperation, some of the complications of improper positioning, such as dislocation, may be prevented by recognition of the abnormal position and the use of temporary postoperative external support.

ACETABULAR POSITION

The position of the acetabular component is of greatest importance in avoiding early dislocation of the total hip replacement. The placement must balance stability against motion and ease of surgery (28). The most stable position for the acetabular component for a patient in an upright position has the mouth of the component facing directly downward. This position allows adequate adduction and extension; however, the femoral component will impinge on the acetabulum in abduction and flexion. Conversely, if the acetabular cup is placed so as to gain maximum motion—that is, with the acetabular cup open laterally 60° and anteriorly 45° the ability to flex and abduct the hip will greatly increase, but the prosthesis will remain in position only if the muscles are powerful enough to hold it stable during adduction and extension.

Another factor in the balance between stability and mobility is the possible impingement of the neck of the

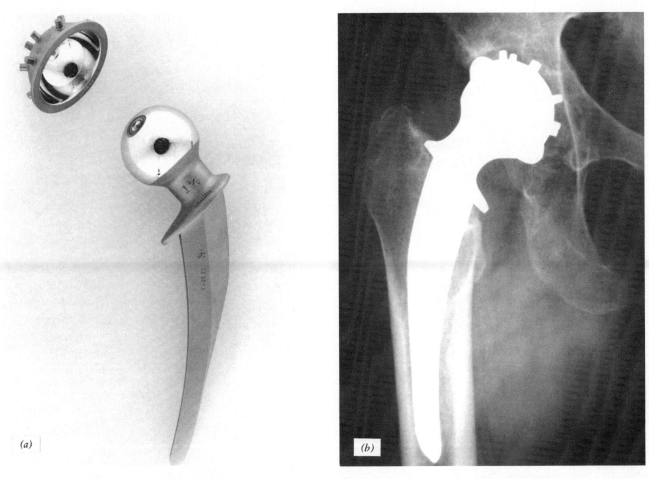

(a)

(b)

Figure 14-2. The McKee-Farrar prosthesis. There are several variants of this prosthesis. Initially designed for placement without methacrylate, it is now usually used with methacrylate. The metal-on-metal articulation is thought by some to result in slightly greater wear of the prosthesis. (a) Photograph of the appliance. (b) A radiograph of the McKee-Farrar prosthesis. It is surrounded by radiolucent methacrylate.

femoral component on the acetabular component at the extremes of motion. If the cup is placed with an inadequate anterior opening, the neck of the femoral component will impinge on it in flexion, and this recurrent trauma could be a cause of early loosening. Since the femoral neck of the prosthesis is curved rather than straight, the degree of anteversion or retroversion of the femoral component must be considered in determining the precise desired position for the acetabular component. In a patient with relatively poor mobility and weak muscles, the orthopedic surgeon will probably prefer to place the acetabular cup in a less open position to achieve greater stability; in the patient who requires greater motion at the hip, is physically more active, and has greater muscle power, the orthopedic surgeon may chose a more anteriorly and laterally open acetabular position.

Considering all these factors, there are still certain limits beyond which the position of the acetabular

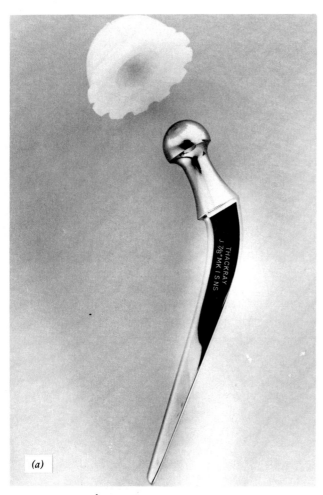

(a)

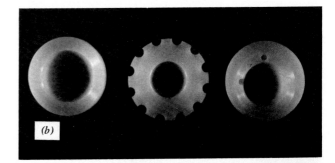

(b)

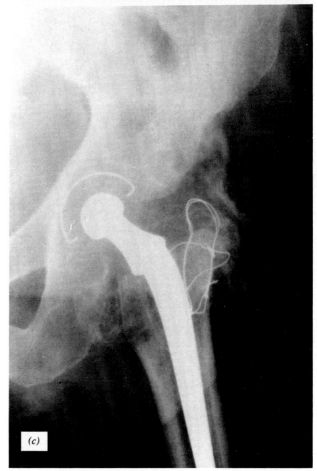

(c)

Figure 14-3. The Charnley prosthesis. (*a*) Photograph of the Charnley prosthesis. This prosthesis, still in use, is probably the grandfather of most current designs of prostheses. Charnley first recognized the safety and effectiveness of the methylmethacrylate interface and first popularized the use of a metal-on-plastic articulation. The prosthesis is properly placed quite deeply within the acetabulum. The prosthetic femoral head is purposely small. (*b*) Photograph of the articular surface of the polyethylene cups of the Charnley total hip (center). The Charnley-Muller total hip (left). The eccentric Harris total hip (right). (*c*) The Charnley prosthesis in use. Extensive ectopic bone is present.

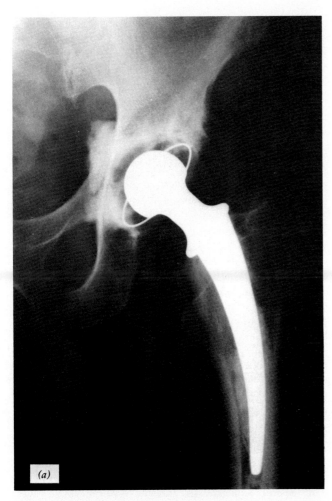

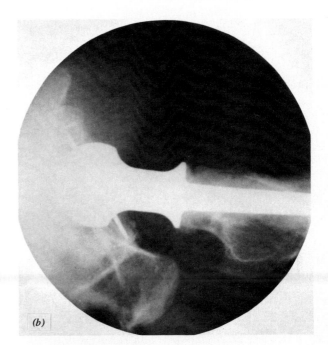

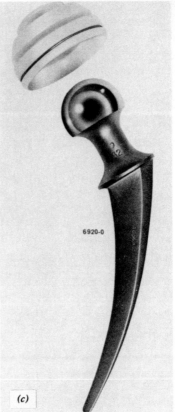

Figure 14-4. The Charnley-Muller prosthesis, placed in radiopaque methacrylate. Used in this patient as treatment of degenerative arthritis. (*a*) Frontal view, Charnley-Muller prosthesis. Placed in radiopaque methacrylate. (*b*) Lateral view, Charnley-Muller prosthesis. (*c*) Photograph of Charnley-Muller prosthesis. (Courtesy Howmedica®.)

231

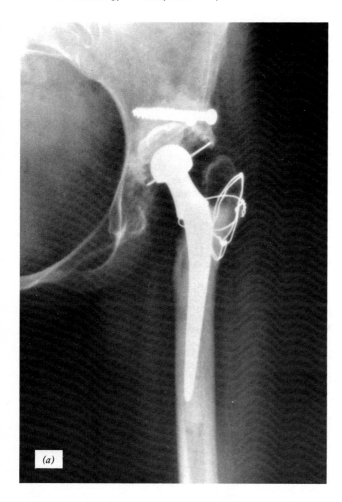

(a)

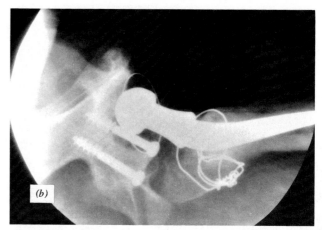

(b)

Figure 14-5. The Turner-Aufranc prosthesis. (a) On the frontal view, the femoral head is positioned eccentrically in the acetabular component to permit longer wear. (b) On the lateral view, the femoral head is centered within the acetabulum. The screws superior to the acetabulum, were used to reinforce this patient's pseudoacetabulum from late, chronic dislocation of the hip.

component becomes undesirable; Some of these undesirable positions are discussed below.

Lateral Opening Acetabular Component

If the lateral opening of the acetabular cup (including the effect of pelvic tilt) is greater than 50° (or especially 60°), the chance of subluxation or dislocation in the early postoperative period is greatly increased (10,12,31,43). If such a large lateral opening is seen on the first postoperative film, subluxation and/or dislocation may be prevented by instructing the patient not to adduct his/her leg for two to four weeks. In some cases, where the muscle power is

particularly weak, splints (only at night) or casts may be used to prevent dislocation during the early postoperative period. In Figure 14-10, the lateral opening is measured by drawing the angle between the acetabular wire ends and the horizontal axis of the pelvis.

Anterior Opening of the Acetabular Component

The desirable degree of anterior opening is variable. Certain authors recommend an anterior opening of 0°, compensating for this with an increased degree of anteversion in the placement of the femoral component, which will then permit adequate flexion (28,43). If anteversion is not used in the placement of the femoral component, 10 to 15° of anterior opening is usually suggested. The degree of anterior opening of the acetabular component of the Charnley-Muller–type prosthesis can be estimated roughly by measuring the distance between the superior and inferior portion of the wire ring. Each millimeter of separation between the two wires indicates a difference of approximately 1° in the range of 5 to 20° (Figure 14-10). The lateral view also provides a rough estimate (Figure 14-11).

Acetabular Retroversion

Posterior opening of the acetabular component is a major problem. When the acetabular component has its opening angled posteriorly, the patient will often experience subluxation or dislocation of the hip in flexion or in the sitting position. In the sitting position, the neck of the femoral component may impinge on the anterior lip of the acetabular component, resulting in subluxation and a predisposition to loosening (12,28,31,32,38). Anteversion of the femoral component partially counteracts this tendency. The choice of position of the acetabular

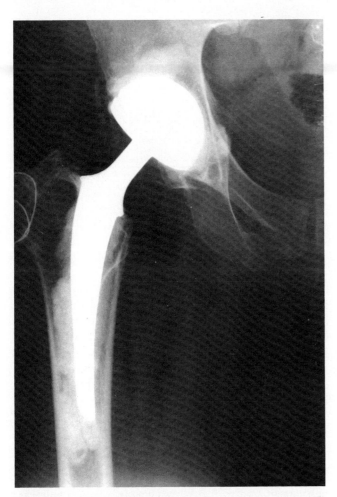

Figure 14-6. The Harris prosthesis. The acetabular component has a polyethylene insert to permit easier replacement.

component thus depends on a balance between the position of the femoral component, the degree of muscle power available to the patient, and the degree of motion desired for the patient.

POSITION OF THE NORMAL FEMORAL COMPONENT

The position of the femoral component is less critical than that of the acetabular component and is easier to achieve surgically. Surgeons have far greater experience with this type of placement from their experience with Moore and Thompson prostheses; also, landmarks on the femur are more easily defined than on the pelvis. Although the orthopedist must take into account the position of the acetabular component in considering his placement of the femoral component, in general the desired position is from 0° to several degrees of anteversion of the prosthesis (10,12,31,43). In the patient described in Example 14-11, the femoral component was initially placed in retroversion. This condition was recognized intraoperatively. As a result, dislocation was possible whenever the hip was flexed. A fracture of the femoral shaft occurred when an attempt was made to replace the femoral component.

A valgus position of the femoral component is preferred (12). Several of the later complications of the femoral component of a total hip replacement appear to be more common when the femoral component has been placed in a varus position. A varus position increases the stress on the component and on the methacrylate. Fracture of the stem of the femoral component and loosening of the prosthesis are more likely to occur in a prosthesis in a varus position than in one in maximum valgus position. Although it is preferable to place the prosthesis in a valgus position, it is not always possible to do so at the time of surgery because of variations in the shape of the femur.

NORMAL POSITIONING OF METHACRYLATE

Methylmethacrylate (9) is a plastic used to form a tight fit between the prosthesis and the surrounding bone. It is not a glue, but simply a space filler that can be molded to the

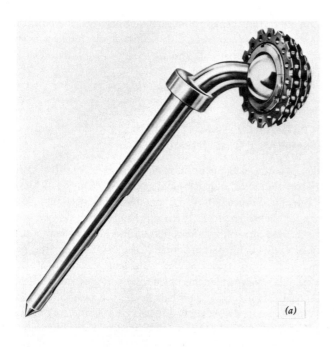

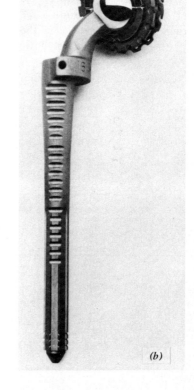

Figure 14-7. (*a*) Nondislocatable prosthesis; Russin-Silvash prosthesis. (*b*) A variant; the SRN prothesis.

irregularity of the bone in the femoral canal and acetabulum, thus preventing slipping (7,8) and providing a greater surface area for the transmission of force from the prosthesis to the bone (7,8). An exothermic reaction occurs as the methylmethacrylate is polymerized. The thicker the methacrylate, the greater the amount of heat given off (6). For this reason, many orthopedic surgeons prefer to use a thin layer of methylmethacrylate.

Because the methylmethacrylate diffuses the stress applied to the bone, it is important to have layers of methacrylate in those areas subjected to the greatest stress. For the femoral component, the methacrylate should be medial to the proximal aspect of the stem of the femoral prosthesis (12,31) and lateral to its more distal portion, as well as distal to its tip (Figure 14-12). Occasionally, when

looking at femoral component prosthesis loosening, the author has been impressed by his inability to identify methacrylate at the medial aspect of the proximal portion of the stem of the femoral component (Figure 14-13a,b). This finding may have prognostic significance. In patients whose femoral component sinks into the shaft, methacrylate may be lacking in the area distal to the tip of prosthesis (Figure 14-14a,b).

THE APPEARANCE OF THE NORMAL REACTION OF BONE TO METHACRYLATE

Methylmethacrylate is a radiolucent plastic; however, many orthopedic surgeons now mix it with a small amount of barium to make it radiopaque. Thus, the appearance of the methacrylate varies, depending on whether it is radiolucent (see Figure 14-2) or radiopaque (see Figures 14-4 and 14-6). In some patients the methacrylate appears to incite no reaction in the bone surrounding it, and one sees either the radiolucency of the methacrylate surrounded by

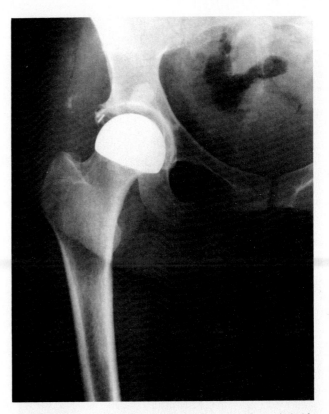

Figure 14-9. The resurfacing prosthesis. A metal cup is held to the reamed femoral head by methacrylate. The acetabular component is high-density polyethylene. These superficially resemble the cup arthroplasty, but have a polyethylene acetabular component and are a form of total hip replacement.

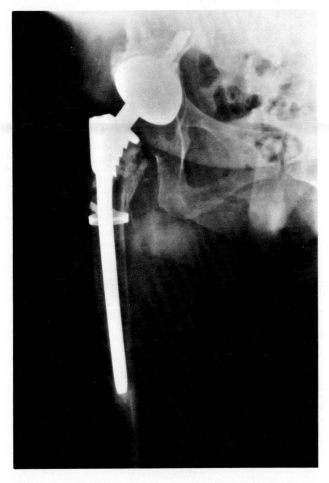

Figure 14-8. A multicomponent prosthesis—the Tronzo prosthesis. The femoral head is composed of plastic. It articulates axially with the strut of the femoral component and radially with the metal acetabular component. The metal band on the femur is not part of the prosthesis. It is a Pharm band, used to reinforce the bone. In this patient, the prosthesis was painful, cause undetermined.

normal cancellous bone (Figure 14-3c, femoral component) or the radiodensity of the opaque methacrylate surrounded by trabecular bone (Figure 14-6, femoral component). This is the normal appearance of methacrylate in the early postoperative months, but it may persist (6). Also common is the appearance of a thin zone of radiolucency separating radiopaque methacrylate from the surrounding bone (see Figures 14-4 and 14-6, acetabular component). In this situation, the gap, which ranges from a fraction of a millimeter to as much as 2½ mm wide, is filled in by a dense, fibrous tissue (42). While the presence of this fibrous tissue implies minimal motion, the ability of this tissue to distort without tearing permits

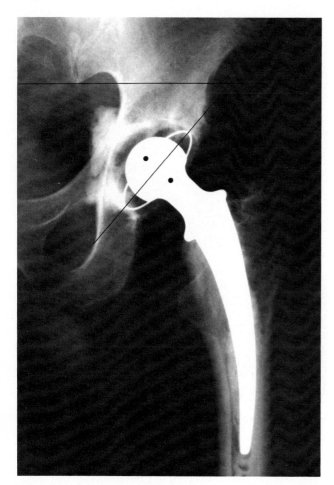

Figure 14-10. Charnley-Muller prosthesis with angle drawn for lateral opening. Dots indicate separation of wires used to estimate the degree of anterior opening. Each millimeter is equal to about one degree.

the slight difference in elasticity of the methacrylate and bone to occur without the development of progressive loosening (7,8). Both histologically and radiologically, this zone of fibrous tissue tends to be thicker in the proximal portion of the femoral component than in the distal portion of the component as shown in Figure 14-15 (6). Such a difference in thickness suggests a slightly greater degree of proximal motion than distal motion and may reflect the

weaker proximal support of the cancellous bone or the greater stress placed upon it. Often, the methacrylate incites a very thin band of condensed bone surrounding the zone of fibrous tissue. This may completely or incompletely surround the zone of radiolucency (Figure 14-16).

NORMAL OR EXPECTED RADIOGRAPHIC CHANGES

1. Drill hole near lower end of femoral component. This is a small vent hole introduced to decompress the femoral canal as the wad of methylmethacrylate is forced into it. Orthopedic surgeons can also use a thin catheter distal to the methacrylate to permit evacuation of air and

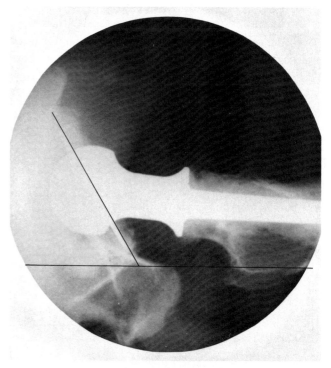

Figure 14-11. Charnley-Muller prosthesis. The angle of the wire compared to that of the estimated pelvis gives an estimate of the degree of anterior opening. Since this film is usually taken with the patient supine, it does not truly reflect the anterior opening when the patient is upright.

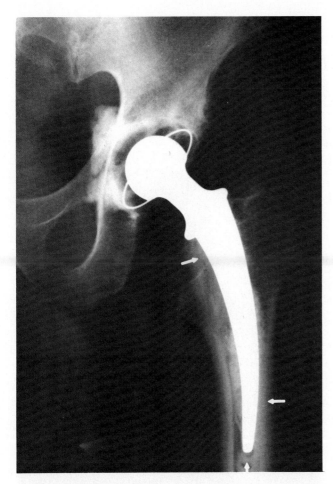

Figure 14-12. Charnley-Muller prosthesis with arrows marking areas of maximum stress.

debris distal to the methacrylate. The purpose is to prevent the fat emboli syndrome.

2. Resorption of the femoral neck. The surgical procedure for placement of the femoral component of the total hip replacement often results in damage to or stripping of the periosteum of the medial aspect of the femoral neck. Microfractures may occur at the same time. It is relatively common to see a small amount of resorption of the femoral neck following the placement of the prosthesis. As long as the prosthesis itself has not moved in relation to the trochanters, this resorption is of no significance (6). Resorption of the femoral neck associated with settling of the prosthesis into the femoral canal indicates loosening. In several instances this relationship was not recognized because the flange of the femoral component did not appear to be displaced from the femoral neck, since it was being resorbed at the same rate as the prosthesis sank (see Figure 14-13a,b). One step in the evaluation of a postoperative total hip replacement is the serial measurement of the distance of the flange to the top of the lesser trochanter to rule out the possibility that the prosthesis has settled.

3. A thin zone of radiolucency around the methacrylate. As mentioned above, it is normal to see a thin zone of radiolucency around the methylmethacrylate filled in by fibrous tissue. This thin zone of radiolucency will usually form within one year of the placement of the methacrylate and will not progress beyond that point. If the radiolucency does progress, loosening may be present. Although this zone of radiolucency is usually less than 1 mm, occasionally it is as great as 2 to 2½ mm, still without indicating loosening. When evaluating the significance of the radiolucency around the methacrylate, it is most important to have prior films available for comparison, for several reasons. The first is that a change in the thickness of the zone of radiolucency must be observed to be certain that loosening is present. The second is that there is no reason why the methacrylate must be forced into every convolution of its bony seat, and therefore it is possible, particularly with the acetabular component, to leave gaps between the bone and the methacrylate (43) (Figure 14-17). These gaps may be greater than 2.5 mm on the first postoperative film and may not change over many years; they do not indicate loosening. Only an increase in the gap is significant. Comparison films, however, must be interpreted with care because the author has seen several cases in which the gap between the methacrylate and bone appeared to increase and decrease on serial films. On reviewing these films, it quickly became apparent that the films were taken with the pelvis in different positions or with the x-ray beam centered differently. The effect of these changes was that the gaps between methacrylate and bone showed up on some films and not on others. Clearly,

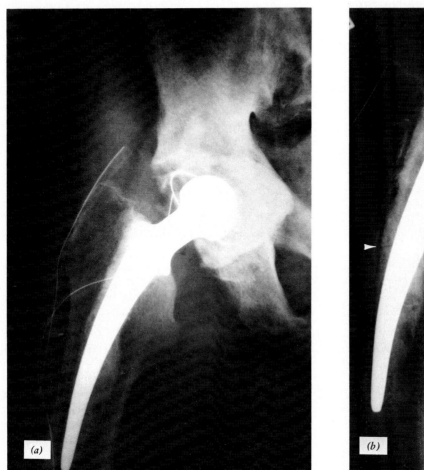

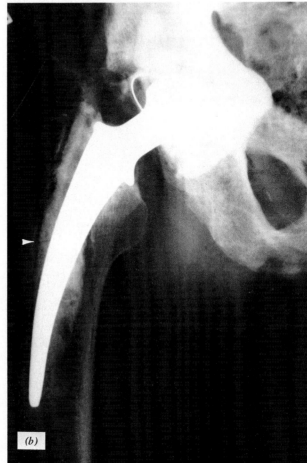

Figure 14-13. Loosening with varus shift of femoral component total hip replacement. No methacrylate medial to proximal portion of the femoral component. Minimal methacrylate lateral to distal portion of the femoral component. Charnley-Muller prosthesis. (a) Immediately following surgery, a drain is put in place. (b) Three years following surgery, the femoral component has shifted into varus. A gap is present between the proximal and lateral methacrylate and the prosthesis. The methacrylate is cracked (arrow). Proved loosening, but no evidence of infection.

if the patient were symptomatic, based on these films the physician might suspect that the gap indicated loosening, when in fact there had simply been projectional change.

4. On occasion a gap between the prosthesis and the methacrylate can be seen. Almost always, the methacrylate forms a radiologically close bond with the prosthesis, and

so loosening should not be suspected purely on the basis of radiolucency between methacrylate and prostheses. Histologically, a thin layer of fibroblasts is often present between the methacrylate and the prosthesis, but this layer is not visible radiologically (20). In general, when such a gap is visible, it is a reflection of a little bit of wobbling of the prosthesis as it is impressed into the methacrylate, leaving minimal gaps between the methacrylate and the prosthesis. Minimal shrinkage of the metal as it cools may occasionally cause a minimal gap. As far as the author can tell from serial observations, this kind of gap between the methacrylate and the prosthesis does not lead to loosening or other pathologic change. On occasion, however, the gap between the prosthesis and the methacrylate develops after the prosthesis has been placed; the gap is due to a shifting of the methacrylate at a loose methacrylate-bone interface (Figure 14-13). This combination then permits the fragments of methacrylate to shift away from the prosthesis. Thus, if the gap between the prosthesis and methacrylate is present in the immediate postoperative period, it is of no

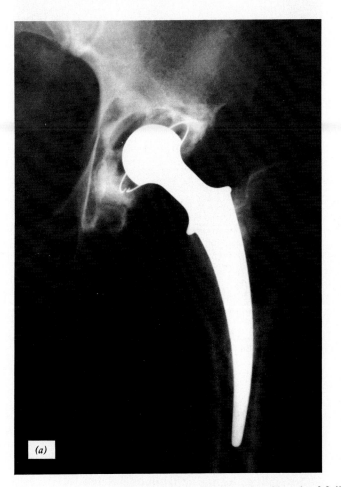

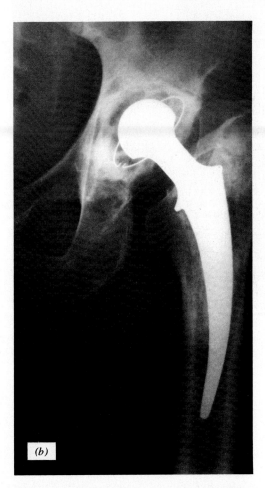

Figure 14-14. Settling of a Charnley-Muller femoral component. (*a*) Early postsurgical film. The flange of the prosthesis lies near a 5 mm segment of medial femoral neck. No methacrylate lies medial to the proximal femoral stem or distal to the tip of the prosthesis. (*b*) Two and one-half years later, the femoral component has telescoped into the femoral canal. The flange of the prosthesis now lies near the upper third of the lesser trochanter. Probable loose prosthesis, but no clinical evidence of infection.

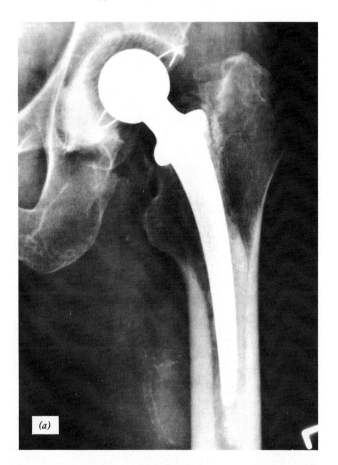
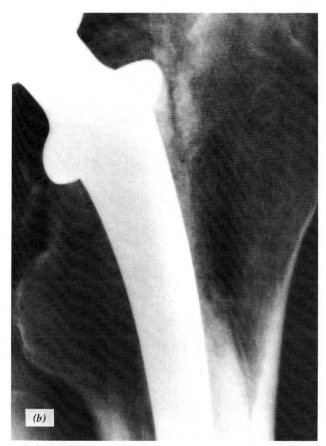

Figure 14-15. (*a,b*) A gap is present between the methacrylate and the bone, a normal response
to the placement of the total hip replacement. The gap is wider proximally than distally.

significance; however, when it occurs late in the course of
the postoperative period, the gap is a sign of loosening at
the methacrylate-bone interface.

5. Bone hypertrophy occuring near the tip of the
prosthesis. If the femur of a patient six months or more
after a total hip replacement is observed, it is often possible to note a slight thickening of the cortex near the tip or
just distal to the tip of the methacrylate or prosthesis of the
femoral component. This thickening probably occurs because the prosthesis prevents the normal flexibility of bone
in the proximal aspect of the femur; stress is then focused
in the area of the cortical thickening. This buildup of bone
is asymptomatic and indicates that the patient is using the

extremity to a greater extent than it had been used preoperatively.

PATHOLOGIC CHANGES

Abnormalities Resulting from or Related to Abnormalities of Positioning of the Components

Dislocation and Subluxation
The normal position of the acetabular and femoral
components has already been discussed. Although, given
sufficient stress, it is possible for appropriately placed

components to dislocate, subluxation and dislocation are more common either when the acetabular component is placed so that it is open laterally greater than 50° or when it is positioned so that it is open posteriorly (12,31, 32,35,37,38). Since there is a balance between muscle power and position in determining subluxation and dislocation, it is difficult to set hard and fast rules. In general, if an acetabular cup is more than 50° open laterally or the least bit open posteriorly, there is a good chance that dislocation may occur in the early postoperative period while

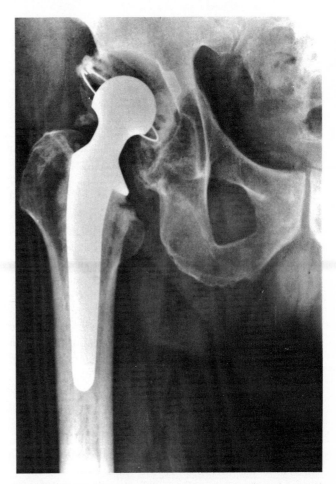

Figure 14-17. Gap between acetabular methacrylate and acetabular bone as seen on initial postoperative films.

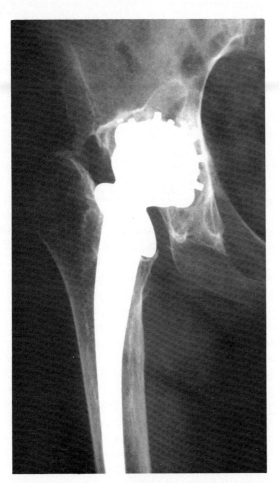

Figure 14-16. The use of radiolucent methylmethacrylate in this patient with a McKee-Farrar prosthesis permits clear visualization of the normal sclerotic reaction of bone to methacrylate.

muscle power remains weak. For this reason, if such a position is noted, it is helpful to warn the patient to avoid adduction of the leg, extremes of flexion of the hip, and unusual exertion. If these measures are carried out, occasionally accompanied by splinting or casting, many early postoperative dislocations may be prevented, provided the abnormality in positioning of the acetabular component is recognized. It is usually not necessary to go in and reposition the acetabular cup when one of these faults is present, since, with the improvement of the muscle power and postoperative scar healing, dislocation and subluxation become far less common. The author has seen a case where a patient debilitated by abdominal surgery then experienced a decrease in muscle power in the limb with a total hip replacement. This increased weakness of the muscles resulted in recurrent subluxation of the prosthesis when the patient was lying in bed (Figure 14-18). This complication should be watched for in anyone who has a total hip replacement.

Example 14-1. This older woman sustained a femoral neck fracture that was treated with a compression screw. Reduction was lost as the screw cut through the bone of the femoral head (Figure 14-19a). Because of continued pain, a Charnley-Muller total hip replacement prosthesis was placed. Initial postsurgical views (Figure 14-19b) demonstrated that while the prosthesis was located, the acetabular component (as marked by the acetabular wires) was open laterally by about 60°. Two weeks following surgery, sudden pain developed and radiographs disclosed dislocation (Figure 14-19c,d). Closed reduction with anesthesia was successful. Since healing of soft tissues and improved muscle power, additional dislocations have not occurred, and the patient was without symptoms in the hip six months following surgery (Figure 14-19e).

Early dislocation does not necessarily require reoperation. While the acetabular component in this case was too open laterally, the increasing muscular strength following surgery prevented recurrent subluxation and dislocation. Often, if this excessive lateral opening is recognized in the immediate postoperative period, extra external support may prevent dislocation until muscle strength has increased and soft-tissue healing has occurred. In this situation, dislocation may be prevented.

Recognition of Subluxation and Dislocation

The wire placed in the acetabular component of a total hip replacement is useful in determining the presence of subluxation and dislocation. Although the wire is not placed at the equator of the acetabular socket, it bears a constant relationship to this equator. The straight wires of the Charnley prosthesis, for example, when connected, form a line that lies 2 mm distal to the equator of the acetabular cup. Thus, with the Charnley prosthesis, if the center of the femoral head prosthesis lies outside of this wire ring, it is certain that the prosthesis is subluxed or

dislocated. In a similar manner the wire of the Charnley-Muller type prosthesis can be used to localize the equator of the acetabular cup. Again this wire has been placed to lie 2 mm distal to the equator. In evaluating the McKee-Farrar prosthesis, the markers are less well defined; however, the outer margin of the acetabular component should be concentric with the femoral head component. Thus, it is relatively easy to identify subluxation and dislocation. Although it is possible for the femoral head prosthesis to lie anterior or posterior to the acetabular cup and be superimposed exactly on the proper position of the wire ring, it is statistically unlikely and has never occurred in the author's experience.

Example 14-2. This patient was seen 10 years following open reduction of a fracture dislocation of the left hip. The patient had had increasing pain of the left hip over several preceeding years. A radiograph (Figure 14-20a) disclosed marked deformity, with sclerosis of the acetabulum and the remnant of a femoral head set high in a peudoacetabulum. Three screws were seen, with resorption around the screw adjacent to the femoral neck. Since there was no reason to suspect that a screw in the acetabular fragments might have any continuing force applied to it, the zone of lucency around this screw suggests that it was being pushed against by the femoral head as the hip moved, or that it was in an area of infection, or that there was a pseudoarthrosis between the fragments of the acetabular fracture.

At the time of surgery for total hip replacement, this screw could be seen protruding from the acetabulum and impinging on the femoral head. Deep erosion was present in the femoral head at the site of this impingment.

A Charnley-Muller total hip prosthesis was placed. At the time of surgery, it was noted that the position of the components was "somewhat stable" prior to the attachment of the greater trochanter fragment, and was quite stable after the greater trochanter had been attached. Radiographs (Figure 14-20b) showed a normally positioned hip joint replacement. The acetabular component was in the superiorly placed pseudoacetabulum.

Two months following the total hip replacement surgery, the patient returned complaining of hip discomfort. Radiographs (Figure 14-20c,d) demonstrated that the wires holding the greater trochanter fragment had broken

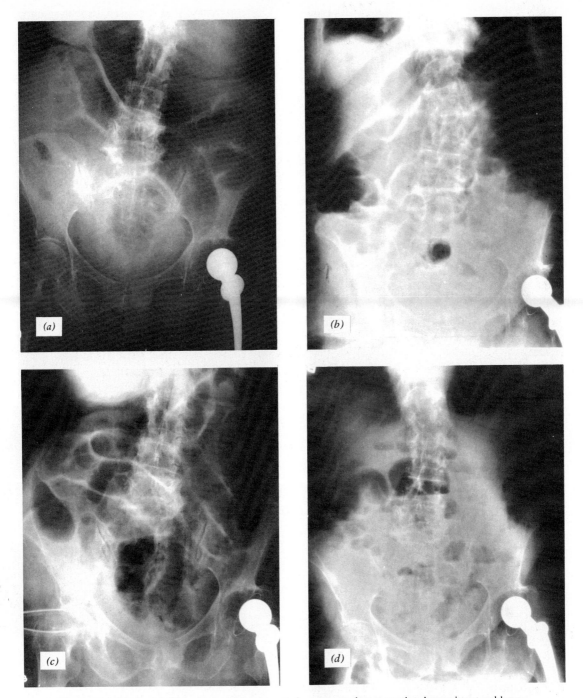

Figure 14-18. Serial films, each taken several days apart, demonstrating intermittent subluxation (*a,c*) and relocation of the femoral component (*b,d*) in a patient debilitated and disoriented following abdominal surgery. Subluxation is indicated by a shift of the relation of the acetabular wire to the central point of the femoral head component. Charnley-Muller prosthesis with moderate lateral opening of the acetabular component.

243

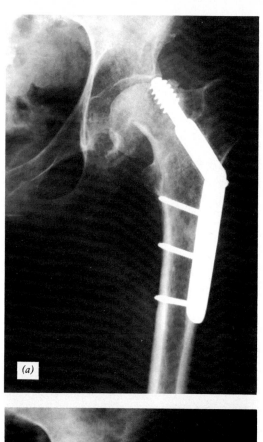

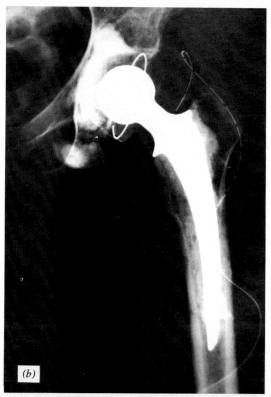

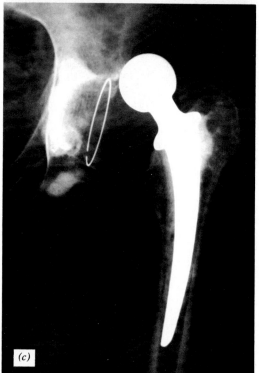

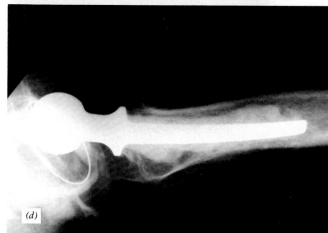

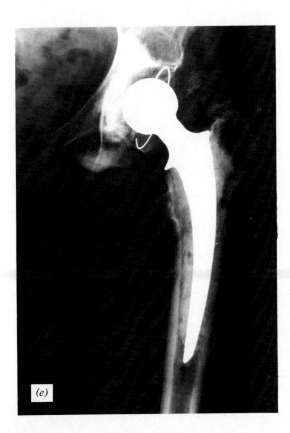

(e)

Figure 14-19. Charnley-Muller prosthesis showing excessive lateral opening of the acetabular component and dislocation. (*a*) Initial radiographs demonstrating the failed compression screw fixation of a proximal femoral neck fracture. (*b*) Initial postsurgical view shows a located joint with a markedly laterally open acetabular cup. A drain is in place. (*c*) Two weeks following surgery, dislocation is apparent. The femoral head no longer lies within the acetabular wire ring. (*d*) Lateral view demonstrates the dislocation. A normal amount of anterior opening of the acetabular cup is present. The widening of the wire loop reflects the marked lateral opening (in contrast to Figure 4-11). (*e*) Six months following closed reduction, the prosthetic hip remains located. The minimal periosteal reaction present along the medial and lateral femoral shaft is a normal finding following removal of an earlier appliance (the compression screw).

and the trochanter had been displaced superiorly. The center of the femoral head lay outside the circular wire of the acetabular component on both views, indicating dislocation.

The patient underwent an open-reduction operation to reposition the acetabulum.

The new position chosen for the acetabular component (Figure 14-20*e,f,g*) had much less lateral opening, only a minimal anterior opening, and was much more stable. The acetabular component was placed in the pseudoacetabulum. The femoral component was not changed.

The greater the degree of anterior and lateral opening, the greater is the degree of mobility possible at the hip, but the degree of stability is lowered. In this younger man, mobility was initially preferred, but when his prosthesis dislocated, a position of greater stability was sought.

The last two frontal films (Figure 14-20*e,g*) demonstrate a difference in the appearance of the acetabular ring. This is due to changes in the position of the pelvis (note the change in the appearance of the obturator foramen), not to a true shift in the position of the acetabular component.

The prosthetic femoral head should be positioned with its center 2 mm above the wire ring of the acetabular component. Even 2 mm of subluxation can be important, since it may indicate that debris or methacrylate is trapped within the prosthetic acetabulum. A fragment of methacrylate caught in the joint will rapidly erode the high-density polyethylene of the acetabular component, leading to a early failure of the prosthesis. (Example 14-12 is of a patient with initial minimal subluxation of the prosthesis due to interposed soft tissue.)

Dislocation of the hip is not always symptomatic.

Example 14-3. This middle-aged woman with severe bilateral hip disease had initial surgery on her right hip. Because of acetabular and femoral head disease, an Austin-Moore prosthesis was placed within a cup mold arthroplasty (this was an early form of total hip replacement). Although her hip remained relatively painful, the patient was satisfied with the result; however, when pain in her left hip became severe she sought treatment of left hip degenerative arthritis. A left total hip Charnley-Muller prosthesis was placed. Because of excessive bleeding from the acetabular roof, tantalum mesh was placed superiorly.

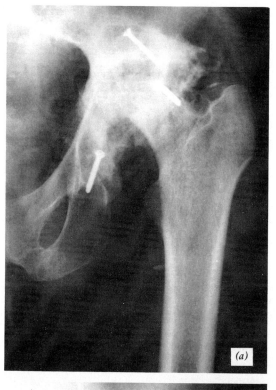

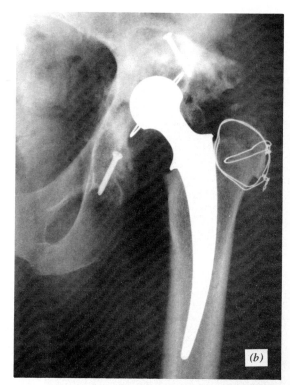

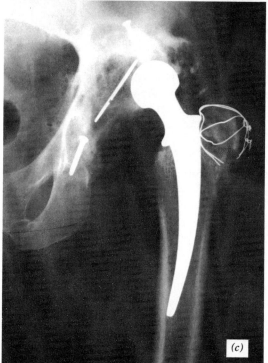

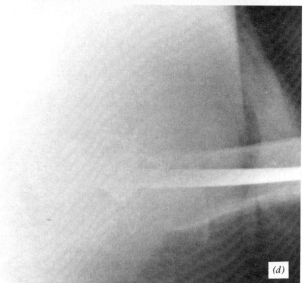

246

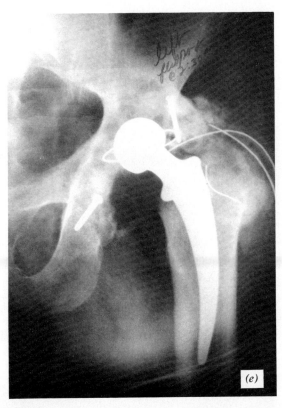

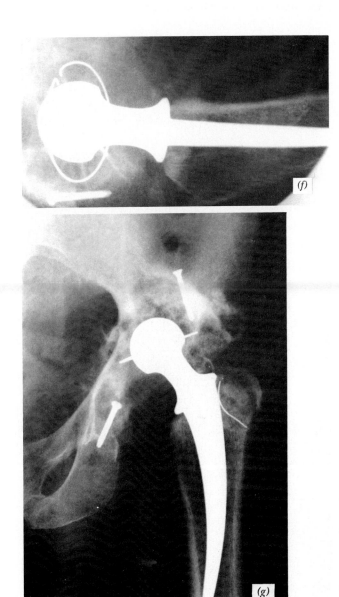

(e)

(f)

(g)

Figure 14-20. Dislocation of Charnley-Muller prosthesis, treated with repositioning of the acetabulum to decrease lateral opening. (a) Initial film. Ten years following fracture dislocation of the hip, severe secondary degenerative arthrosis is present. Extensive resorption of the femoral head may be due to avascular necrosis or degenerative arthrosis. Resorption surrounds the screw superimposed on the femoral neck. At the time of surgical exploration, this screw was found to impinge on the femoral head, indenting it—thus it was moving as the femoral head moved, causing resorption of bone around it. (b) Early postoperative view: Charnley-Muller prosthesis, normal postoperative position and appearance. (c) Two months following the total hip replacement, the wires holding the greater trochanter have broken and the femoral head now lies outside of the acetabular wires. The lateral opening of the acetabular component does not appear excessive: the anterior opening as demonstrated by the limited space between the wires is minimal. (d) The lateral view confirms the lack of anterior or posterior opening of the prosthesis and the lack of anteversion of the femoral component. This suggests that the two components are touching in flexion, perhaps contributing to the dislocation. (e,f) Following reposi-

tioning of the acetabulum, less lateral opening is present. There has been a slight increase in the anterior opening, demonstrated by a separation between the acetabular wires on the frontal view (e) and on the lateral view (f). (g) One month later, the position of the acetabular wire appears to have changed. This is a projectional artifact due to difference in position. Note the change in the appearance of the obturator foramen.

247

At time the patient was discharged from the hospital (Figure 14-21a), the left femoral head component was dislocated. The patient was unaware of this complication, and the surgeon apparently did not review the film. In follow-up examinations, hip motion was normal and the patient was satisfied with the result, so satisfied that 18 months later she returned, desiring the same procedure for her right hip. Views at that time (Figure 14-21b) showed the dislocation of the left hip, surrounded by extensive ectopic bone. The hip was fixed in position but asymptomatic. The right hip showed the presence of an Austin-Moore prosthesis within a cup mold arthroplasty.

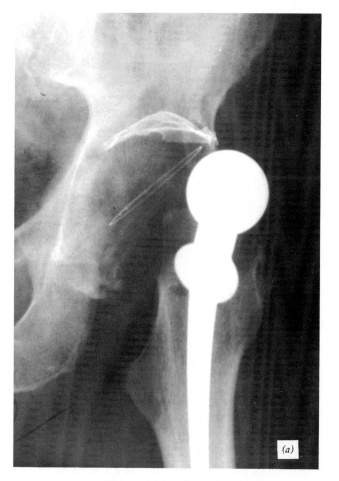

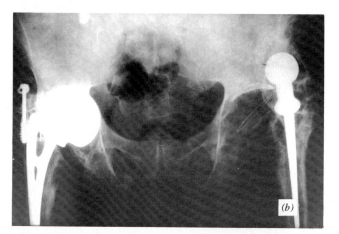

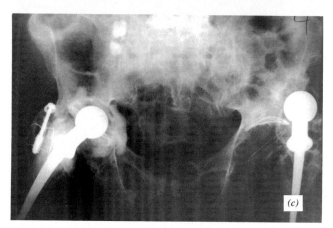

Figure 14-21. Example 14-3. Untreated dislocation of the femoral component of a Charnley-Muller prosthesis. (a) Early postsurgical film demonstrating dislocation. The femoral head lies outside of the acetabular component wire ring. Tantalum mesh was placed in the superior position of the acetabulum to aid in the control of bleeding. (b) Approximately 18 months following surgery, the dislocated left Charnley-Muller prosthesis is surrounded by ectopic bone. The right hip shows the Austin-Moore prosthesis placed in the cup mold arthroplasty. Note the prostrusio acetabuli with thin, medial acetabular wall. (c) Following placement of the Charnley-Muller prosthesis in the right hip. Extensive methacrylate in the pelvis is probably secondary to breakage of the medial acetabular wall. Patient has done well, as determined by in follow-up.

A right Charnley-Muller prosthesis was inserted (Figure 14-21c). Because of the lack of symptoms in the left hip, no treatment was indicated.

Penetration of the Cortex

Penetration of the cortex of the femur occurs occasionally. If the amount of protrusion of the tip of the femoral prosthesis is minimal, it does not seem to interfere with a good result (32). This protrusion is usually either in the posterior or posteromedial cortex. On occasion, when a large portion of the stem of the femoral component protrudes, pain develops in the femur, perhaps in some cases associated with the formation of a bursa and bursitis over the tip of the component. If symptoms develop, the prosthesis should be replaced. At least one author replaces the prosthesis prophylactically if he sees a large amount of protrusion (32).

Example 14-4. This 48-year-old man sustained an acetabular fracture with hip dislocation at age 46. An open reduction with screw fixation was performed but became infected with staphylococcus aureus. He was treated with antibiotics and immobilization in a spica cast. One year later the screws were removed. Culture at that time was negative. Because of severe pain, he was unable to use his hip and retired. Because of the severe pain, a total hip replacement was recommended. A preoperative view demonstrates the marked deformity (Figure 14-22a).

A Charnley-Muller prosthesis was selected. At surgery, great difficulty was encountered in placing the prosthesis because of dense adhesions. A short neck femoral prosthesis was unstable, but a long neck femoral prosthesis proved to be stable. At the time of surgery, the protrusion of the stem from the femur was noted but was not thought significant enough to warrant prolonging an already lengthy procedure. Postsurgical views demonstrated the medial and posterior cortical penetration (Figure 14-22b,c).

Six weeks following surgery, the patient came in to the emergency room of the hospital with sudden highly painful swelling of this thigh, which was thought to be the result of a bleeding muscle or vascular rupture. Three months later, the hip and thigh were asymptomatic.

Protrusion of the stem of the femoral component is more common in certain situations than in others (16). It is slightly more likely to occur if the operation follows the removal of a femoral plate. Often the screw holes are enlarged in order to remove the metal of the screws from the femur. When this occurs, a hole is left in the femur, which permits easy passage of the femoral stem out of the femur. There is often a problem in placing the femoral component when the total hip replacement is used following a failed McMurray-type displacement osteotomy of the proximal femur. In this procedure, a subtrochanteric osteotomy is performed with medial displacement of the femoral shaft. This sharply alters the angle of alignment of the femur, and a curved femoral prosthesis placed in this femur will often protrude medially (Figure 14-23a,b,c,d). Once this problem was recognized, the prosthesis was redesigned to provide a femoral component with a straight stem for such cases. When this special straight-stem prosthesis is used, protrusion of the stem is unlikely to occur.

Example 14-5. This 60-year-old man had severe *left* hip pain five years following prior *right* hip surgery (Figure 14-24a). At age 55, because of increasing right hip pain, the patient had an intertrochanteric right femoral osteotomy with medial displacement of the shaft. Pain was completely relieved. At age 60 the patient returned with *left* hip pain; a radiograph (Figure 14-24b) showed severe cartilage narrowing, osteophyte proliferation, and the formation of degenerative cysts compatible with degenerative arthrosis. A left total hip replacement with a Charnley-Muller prosthesis was performed, resulting in complete relief of pain. Four months following his left hip surgery, the patient returned complaining about his right hip and seeking a right total hip replacement. A straight-stem Charnley-Muller prosthesis was used (Figure 14-24c).

The straight-stem femoral prosthesis is used when prior surgery or fracture has resulted in valgus deformity or a straighter alignment of the proximal femur. If a straight-stem prosthesis is not used, difficulties with placement may occur, the most common being difficulties with insertion and positioning of the prosthesis. Occasionally, the stem of the prosthesis may protrude from the shaft medially (see Figure 14-23c).

It is not uncommon for a patient who is satisfied with the results of prior hip surgery to have a total hip replacement on the opposite hip and then realize that this

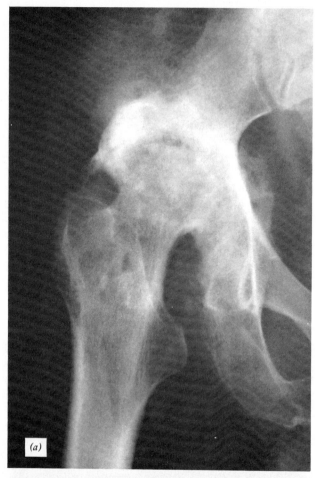

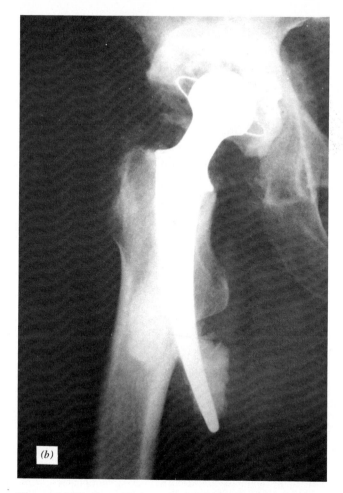

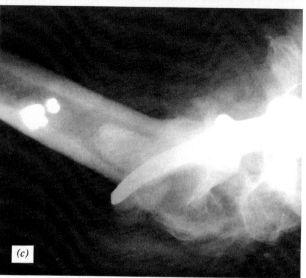

Figure 14-22. Example 14-4. Protrusion of femoral component; Charnley-Muller prosthesis with probable delayed muscle bleed. (a) Initial view. Healed traumatic dislocation with acetabular fracture and staphyloccus aureus infection. The acetabulum is shifted superiorly. There is extensive sclerosis and deformity of the acetabulum. The joint cartilage is markedly narrowed. The femur is in external rotation (shown by the position of the lesser trochanter), simulating valgus deformity of the proximal femur. (b) Postsurgical view demonstrates the protrusion of the femoral stem medially. The gap between the acetabular methacrylate and acetabular bone is probably because the plastic was not adequately pressed into the gap at the time of surgery. (c) The lateral view demonstrates the posterior protrusion.

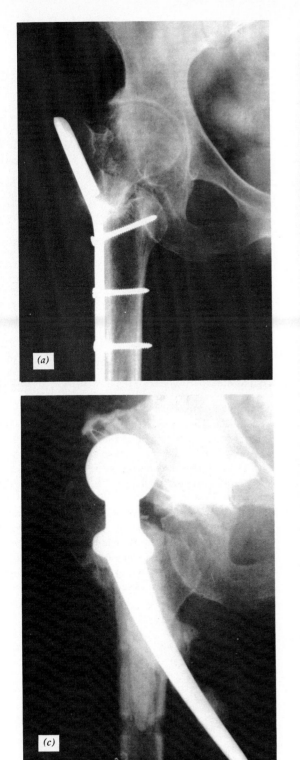

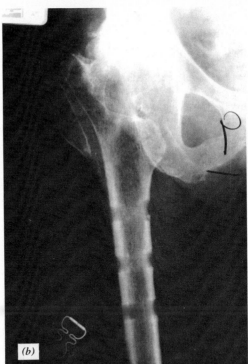

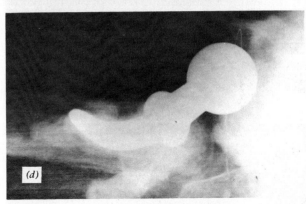

Figure 14-23. Medial protrusion of the femoral component used following McMurray medial displacement intertrochanteric osteotomy. (*a*) Deformity of healed McMurray osteotomy with medial displacement of the shaft. (*b*) Following removal of the spline and overdrilling of the screws, large gaps are left in the femoral cortex. (*c,d*) The femoral component protrudes through one of the cortical holes medially. Because of the abnormal position of the femoral component, the acetabulum had to be placed in a pronounced lateral position. The medial protrusion of the stem was not recognized until the postoperative period. The patient has had a slight soreness in the area of protruded stem, with no significant disability.

251

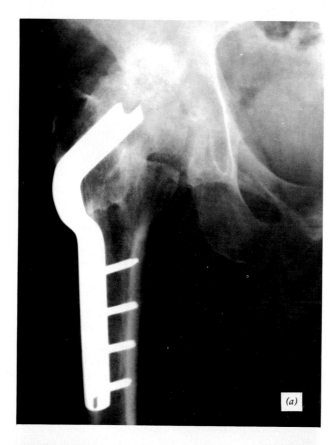

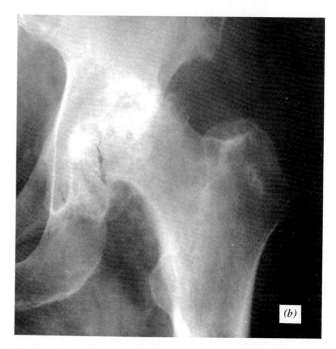

Figure 14-24. Example 14-5. Standard Charnley-Muller prosthesis in the left hip, and straight-stem Charnley-Muller prosthesis used on right hip following late failure of McMurray osteotomy. (a) Changes five years following McMurray osteotomy. There is medial displacement of the shaft; the position is held with an angled blade plate. Sclerosis, joint cartilage narrowing, and degenerative cysts reflect the severe degenerative arthrosis. (b) The left hip prior to the total hip replacement demonstrates marked osteophyte formation and extensive cartilage narrowing. A few degenerative cysts are present. (c) Following the bilateral Charnley-Muller total hip replacements, the appearances of the straight-stem (right) and standard (left) Charnley-Muller components can be contrasted.

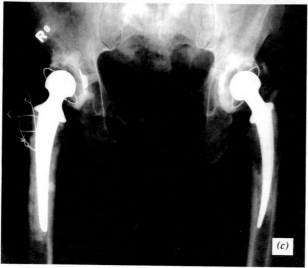

procedure gives him or her greater mobility and less pain than the earlier surgery on his other hip. The patient will then often seek a total hip replacement for the originally operated hip. Patients will accept some pain and stiffness without complaint until they realize this discomfort can be eliminated by a total hip replacement.

A straight-stem prosthesis need not be used following a McMurray osteotomy if care is taken at surgery and if the degree of medial displacement of the shaft is limited.

Example 14-6. This middle-aged woman sustained a subcapital fracture of the femoral neck, which was treated by open reduction and internal fixation with three pins. One year later bone graft was placed from the trochanteric region into the femoral head because of developing avascular necrosis. This procedure did not prevent the collapse of the femoral head, and five years later a McMurray medial displacement and varus osteotomy was performed, with removal of osteophytes (Figure 14-25a,b). Although the osteotomy healed in three months (Figure 14-25c), the pain persisted for about a year. Following that there was moderate pain relief for six years, coupled with improvement in the appearance of the joint and femoral head (Figure 14-25d). Because of recurrence of pain, in the seventh year following the osteotomy, a Charnley-Muller total hip prosthesis was placed (Figure 14-25e,f). A standard femoral component was used.

Penetration of the Acetabular Bone

On occasion the acetabular component has been noted to migrate through the medial acetabular cortex into the pelvis (10). This problem is likely to occur in two situations. In the first, a total hip replacement is used following fracture of the acetabulum (24). In this situation, the bone of the medial aspect of the acetabulum is incomplete and may provide insufficient support for the acetabular component, thus permitting migration. For this reason several authors have recommended placing a bone graft in the medial aspect of the acetabulum when the bone is deficient or extremely thin because of a previous fracture.

Displacement of the acetabular component may also take place when the bone of the acetabulum is either soft, moldable, or highly osteoporotic, as in patients with rheumatoid arthritis (24). Acetabular protrusion may occur in Paget's disease and in osteomalacia.

In these situations, it is possible for the acetabular component to migrate into the pelvis. In the patient with Paget's disease, this migration tends to occur slowly as the bone remodels and, although it may restrict motion, acetabular migration is usually of no significance otherwise. In patients with rheumatoid arthritis, however, the displacement of the acetabular component may occur rapidly and may produce symptoms of pain and limited motion. For this reason, some authors have advised taking special care in shaping the acetabulum at the time of placement of the acetabular component in patients with rheumatoid arthritis.

Example 14-7. This 61-year-old woman was initially treated for severe right medial protrusion of the acetabulum with a right cup arthroplasty. During the six months of rehabilitation, the patient did well; however shortly after rehabilitation was completed, the bone within the acetabulum disappeared and the cup protruded into it. When the patient seen two years later (Figure 14-26a), there was marked protrusion of the cup mold into the pelvis, with fracture and resorption of the femoral neck. (The femoral head still remained within the cup but was not visible.)

At the time of total hip arthroplasty, the acetabulum was reinforced with bone graft. A long-neck Charnley-Muller prosthesis was used (Figure 14-26b). The femoral component was placed with moderate anteversion (Figure 14-26b,c), demonstrated by the gap between the wires on the frontal view and by the position on the lateral view. Wires were used to reattach the greater trochanter. Because of the weakness of the acetabulum, the patient was kept on crutches.

Ten months following surgery, the patient was found to have tenderness over the greater trochanter. The radiograph demonstrated breakage of the wires (Figure 14-26d). The patient was kept on crutches.

Twenty-two months following surgery (Figure 14-26c), the patient was almost pain free. Additional bone was present in the medial wall of the acetabulum. There was no shift of the prosthesis. Partial weight bearing was continued.

Acetabular protrusion may also be prevented by reinforcing the acetabulum with wire mesh or metalic appliances (Figure 14-26f,g,h).

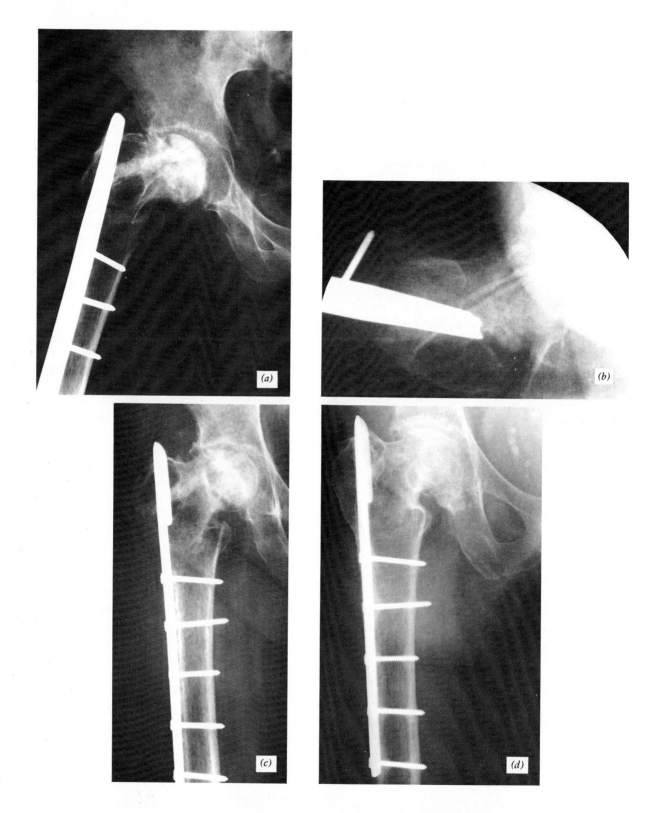

254

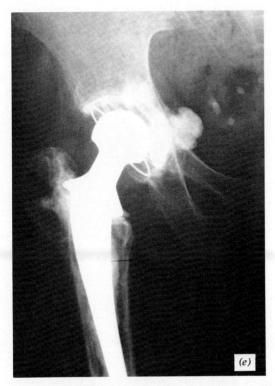

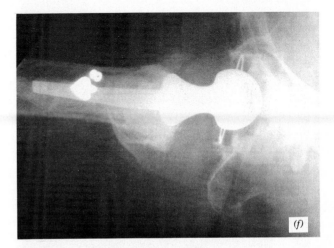

Figure 14-25. Example 14-6. Standard Charnley-Muller prosthesis used in treatment of avascular necrosis following earlier treatment with bone graft, and McMurray medial displacement and varus osteotomy. (*a*) Frontal and (*b*) lateral views following McMurray medial displacement and varus osteotomy. The tubular bone graft can be seen running from the region of the greater trochanter to the femoral head. A spline holds the position of the fragments. Sclerosis of the femoral head is due to avascular necrosis. (*c*) Three months following the osteotomy, trabeculae are seen to cross the osteotomy line. (*d*) Six years following the osteotomy, the femoral head was reformed. There is a moderate joint space. There is only minimal medial displacement of the shaft and slight lateral displacement of the medial femoral neck. (*e*) A standard Charnley-Muller prosthesis has been placed. the remnant of the laterally displaced medial femoral neck cortex has been resected to permit the placement of the prosthesis. There is slight anterior opening of the acetabular component. Minimal periosteal reaction along the femoral shaft is due to the reoperation and does not represent infection. (*f*) The lateral view shows that the femoral prosthesis has been placed with little anteversion. The acetabular component has been inserted with minimal anterior opening.

Intraoperative and Stress Fractures

Occasionally fractures of the femur and, less often, fractures of the acetabulum occur during total hip replacement. Some of these fractures are associated with the preparation of the bone for receiving the component (24) or during its placement; others occur during relocation of the femoral acetabular relationship. Although these fractures heal normally, their early recognition is important to prevent displacement of the components and of the fracture. The femoral fractures the author has seen have tended to be almost undisplaced and very difficult to recognize prior to displacement. It is thus important that every

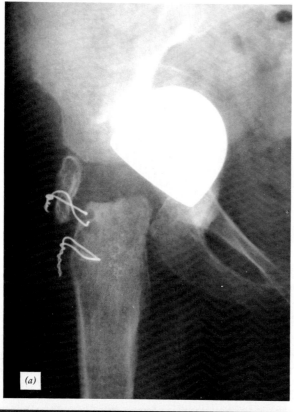

(a)

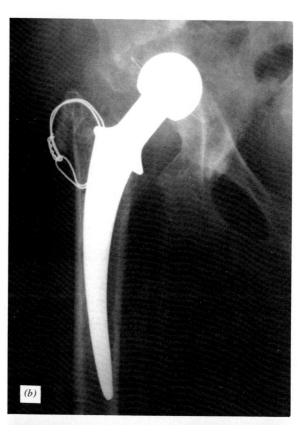

(b)

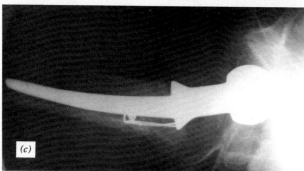

(c)

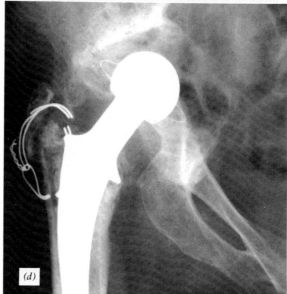

(d)

256

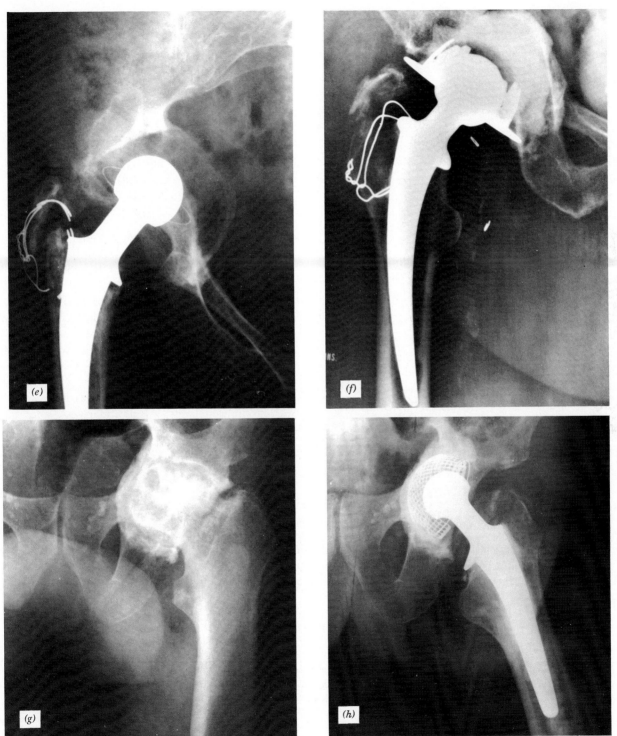

257

(*Legend on next page*)

postoperative film be screened carefully for the presence of possible fracture, and the orthopedist should be warned that such a fracture is present. In general, these fractures will not be found by a cursory examination of the area, but only by a most careful search of the bone of the cortex. It is interesting that many of these presumably intraoperative fractures escape notice at the time of surgery. This is presumably because they are undisplaced at that time. Fractures may also occur in the early postoperative period (24). When a patient has received a total hip replacement, the joint feels so good that it is difficult to prevent him or her from bearing full weight on it in the early postoperative period. The bone, however, is often weakened (osteoporotic) by years of chronic hip disease; it cannot bear the stress placed on it by this sudden increase in activity and either fractures or develops a stress fracture. Stress fractures have been seen in the femur just distal to the prosthesis (27), in the acetabulum, and in the ischium just inferior to the acetabulum (14,29). In the patient with onset of unexplained pain after a total hip replacement, such subtle fractures and stress fractures should be suspected.

Despite the presence of the prosthesis, there is no reason why the bone of the femur or pelvis cannot fracture when subjected to sufficient force. Thus, fractures of the pelvis and of the femur have occurred following total hip replacement, when the bone was subjected to sufficient force (24). The article by McElfresh (27) is a summary of nine such cases. In general, these fractures are readily recognized and their traumatic etiology easily established.

Example 14-8. This 45-year-old woman had dull, aching pain in her right hip for at least a year, aggravated by activity. A radiograph demonstrated severe degenerative arthrosis (Figure 14-27a). During the reaming of the femoral canal for the prosthesis, the femur fractured. An intraoperative radiograph confirmed the fracture (Figure 14-27b). Vitallium wires were used in a circlage, and the placement of the femoral component was completed. Following surgery, the patient was put on a treatment of three weeks of bed rest followed by limited weight-bearing ambulation. Two months following surgery, the hip was pain free; the patient was permitted full weight bearing on the hip and has done well since (Figure 14-27c).

Example 14-9. This 69-year old man with bilateral degenerative arthrosis of the hips had a left cup arthroplasty. He did well for one month, at which time sudden acute pain occurred and continued (Figure 14-28a). During surgical exploration, the femoral head was found to have fractured within the metal cup. A left Charnley-Muller prosthesis was placed. Films obtained several days following surgery disclosed an unsuspected fracture of the femoral shaft (Figure 14-28b). The patient was kept nonweight bearing for six weeks and was then permitted partial weight bearing. The patient has done well since, with no hip complaints; it is now four years since surgery (Figure 14-28c).

Example 14-10. This patient had an unsuccessful cup arthroplasty, replaced by a straight-stem Charnley-Muller

---

Figure 14-26. Example 14-7. Total hip replacement with thin acetabular bone. (a) Traction view of cup mold arthroplasty demonstrating the acetabular protrusion of the cup, the thin acetabular bone, and the fracture and resorption of the femoral neck. (b) Appearance following total hip arthroplasty with a long-neck Charnley-Muller femoral component. The acetabulum has been reinforced by bone graft (not visible). There is a very small anterior opening of the acetabular component, as shown by the separation of the acetabular wires. (c) The lateral view shows that the femoral component has been positioned with moderate anteversion. (d) Ten months following surgery, the wire holding the greater trochanter fragment has broken and the trochanteric fragment has displaced superiorly. The acetabular bone remains quite thin. (e) Twenty-two months following surgery, the position of the prosthesis is unchanged. There has been a slight thickening of the bone of the acetabulum. (f) A Muller ring helps support the acetabular component in another patient with acetabular protrusion. (g,h) Another patient with acetabular protrusion and degenerative arthrosis in whom wire mesh is used to reinforce the acetabular methacrylate.

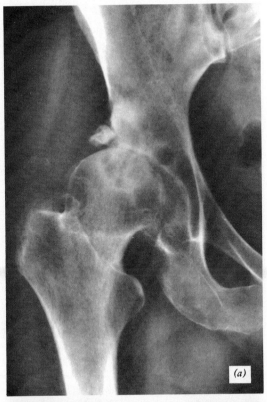

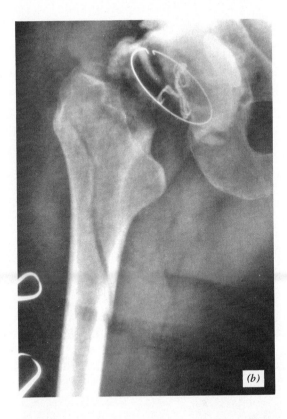

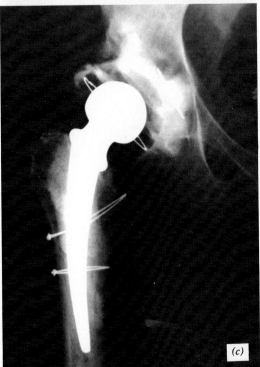

Figure 14-27. Example 14-8. Intraoperative fracture occurring during reaming for the femoral component of a Charnley-Muller prosthesis. (*a*) Presurgical view. There is severe degenerative arthrosis with cartilage narrowing, lateral subluxation of the femoral head, and degenerative cysts of the femoral head and the acetabulum. (*b*) Intraoperative view. The acetabular component has been inserted. The inter- and sub trochanteric fracture is identified. (*c*) Two months following surgery, the fracture is not visible. Two circlage wires are present. A small amount of radiopaque methacrylate lies within the fracture line in the medial femoral cortex.

259

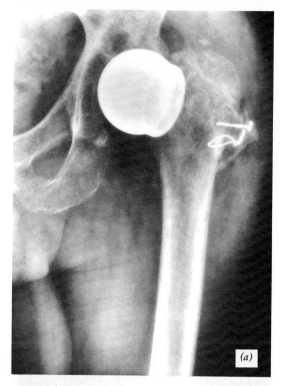

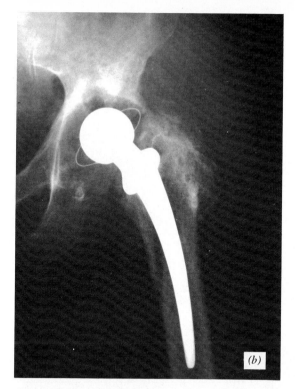

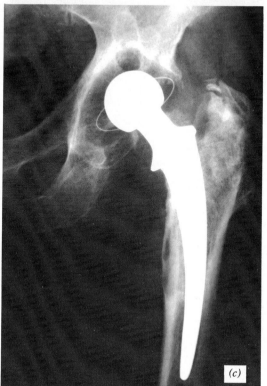

Figure 14-28. Example 14-9. Intraoperative fracture recognized several days following surgery. Charnley-Muller prosthesis. (*a*) Failed cup arthroplasty. Fracture of the femoral head within the metal cup is not detectable. (*b*) A fracture through the medial femoral shaft is present. (*c*) A focal radiolucency is present in the medial femoral cortex, due to radiolucent methylmethacrylate that extended through the fracture line.

prosthesis (Figure 14-29a). This procedure was successful. The patient then sustained severe trauma, with traumatic dislocation of the acetabular component (Figure 14-29b).

Problems with the Greater Trochanter

In performing total hip replacement operation, it is sometimes desirable to remove the greater trochanter temporarily to simplify surgery. The greater trochanter is then often either replaced in its normal position or transferred distally to increase the power of the gluteus medius muscle (43) and to prevent laxity in the joint, which might lead to subluxation (24). This osteotomy and reattachment may lead to problems associated with the trochanter. Nonunion associated with distraction of the trochanter occasionally occurs and may result in some disability, possibly requiring reoperation in certain patients (31). Other patients have no problems related to the greater trochanter nonunion (10). On occasion fibrous union develops between the trochanter and the remainder of the femur. This does not appear to be of clinical significance but ap-

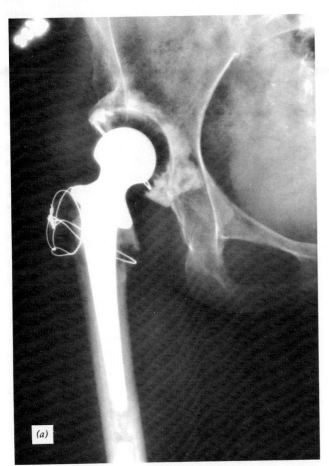 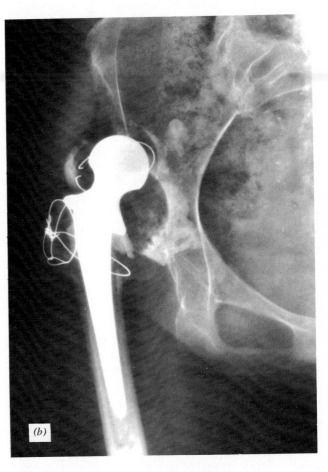

Figure 14-29. Example 14-10. Traumatic dislocation of the acetabular component of a straight-stem (Charnley-Muller prosthesis. (a) View three months after placement of the Charnley-Muller prosthesis. Normal position, with the acetabular cup in a superiorly placed pseudoacetabulum. (b) Following severe trauma, the acetabular component has broken free from the methacrylate.

pears as a radiolucent line between the trochanter and the remainder of the femur (31,43). It is not uncommon for wires used to attach the trochanter to the femur to break after months or years in the presence of an apparently solid union of the trochanter and femur. The breaking of the wire presumably results from recurrent microstress but is usually of no clinical significance (31,43). In a radiographic evaluation of the placement of the trochanter, it is important that the trochanter be apposed to the bone of the femur; the trochanter should not be apposed to methacrylate, since bone will not fuse to methacrylate (see Example 14-11). If the trochanter has been apposed to methacrylate, nonunion is possible (24,31). Since many cases of nonunion show minimal symptomatology (10), reoperation is not necessary for trochanteric problems unless symptoms are present (31).

Example 14-11. As an infant, this 68-year-old woman was treated with casts for congenital displacement of the left hip. At age 22 she had surgery on her left hip, probably a shelf procedure. The radiograph (Figure 14-30a) taken at age 46 demonstrated fusion of the left proximal femur to the superior displaced pseudoacetabulum. The shape of the pseudoacetabulum and of the left iliac crest suggested that a shelf operation had been performed many years before. There was a moderate adduction deformity of the right hip. The fusion was thought to be spontaneous.

At age 59, surgery was performed on the left hip, resulting in a Girdlestone-type arthroplasty (Figure 14-30b) (See Chapter 15).

At age 68, because of increasing left hip pain and instability, a left total hip replacement was advised. The preoperative radiograph (Figure 14-30c) demonstrated the Girdlestone type arthroplasty, with resection of the femoral head and neck, articulation with the pseudoacetabulum, and marked osteoporosis of the femoral shaft.

Surgery was quite difficult because of the extensive deformity and the moderate soft tissue contractures. An extensive muscle release was necessary to bring the femur down to the level of the true acetabulum. After the femoral component was inserted, it was found to be in approximately 20° of retroversion, an unacceptable position.

When the femoral component was repositioned, the proximal femur fractured. Tantalum mesh was used to help support the methacrylate (22). Large quantities of methacrylate were used to supplement the highly osteoporotic bone (Figure 14-30d).

Acetabular placement was also difficult. The lateral opening of the acetabulum is approximately 60°. The medial wall of the acetabulum appears to have fractured at the time of placement (Figure 14-30d,e,f). Because of the extensive loss of bone, it was necessary to suture the trochanteric fragment to the tantalum mesh and methacrylate. Because of the problems encountered, the patient was kept in traction and only gradually allowed up. A left foot drop developed during surgery. Slightly more than three weeks following surgery, the patient was in physical therapy and experienced discomfort in her left hip. Radiographs disclosed dislocation of the prosthesis (Figure 14-30e). The dislocation was recognized because the femoral head was no longer seated within the acetabular ring.

The dislocation was reduced under anesthesia the next day (Figure 14-30f). However the trochanteric fragment had separated from the femur. The reduction was stabilized in a spica cast to permit soft-tissue healing, and the patient was seen to be doing well at a short follow-up examination.

This case illustrates some of the problems associated with the positioning of a total hip replacement in a patient with a dislocated hip, and also the problem of converting a Girdlestone arthroplasty to a total hip replacement (19). Dr. Tronzo (39) and Drs. Dunn and Hess (15) have treated late congenital hip patients by resecting enough femur to place the acetabular component in the true acetabulum without subjecting the adjacent muscles and nerves to excessive traction. It is also possible to place the acetabular component in the pseudoacetabulum (Figure 14-29a).

In the patient who had extensive muscle release, it may not have been possible to provide sufficient stability, and the cautious postoperative management chosen was appropriate. An acetabular prosthesis that was less open laterally would have added a measure of stability.

If the femoral component had been placed in retroversion initially, it would have impinged on the acetabular component during hip flexion (as in sitting or climbing stairs), an unsatisfactory situation, which, if not corrected, could have resulted in recurrent subluxation in flexion; also, its impingement on the acetabulum might have led to early loosening.

Breakage of the Prosthesis

As noted elsewhere in this book, a prosthesis does not substitute totally for normal bone. The resilience of a prosthesis to recurrent microstress is less than that of normal bone, since it cannot repair itself (21). On rare occasions breakage of the components of a total hip replacement does occur. The breakage usually occurs in the metallic parts of the prosthesis usually within the femoral component, since most of the acetabular components are composed of high-density polyethylene. The femoral components have been repeatedly redesigned to increase their resilience to this recurrent stress. The usual history of a patient whose femoral prosthesis has fractured is that the patient has been getting along with minimal or no symptoms and then has a sudden onset of pain in the hip, thigh, or knee. The pain appears only during motion and weight bearing (21). Since the prosthesis is held firmly in its distal portion and is only minimally loose in its proximal portion, there is often only minimal displacement at the breakage line of the prosthesis. Thus, for any patient who experiences pain following total hip replacement, the radiologist must carefully scrutinize the femoral stem on both frontal and lateral views (Figure 14-31d,f). While different parts of femoral prosthesis have been known to break, such breakage most often occurs at the junction of the distal and middle thirds of the prosthesis (Figure 14-31c,d). This preferential breakage is partially due to the manufacturing process, which results in a slightly weaker area at this location than elsewhere in the prosthesis. Radiographs of patients who have fractured fractured femoral prostheses consistently reveal the same two conditions. The first is that the prostheses have often been placed in a varus position (21), which increases stress on the stem of the femoral component (Figure 14-31a,b). Second, there often appears to be little or no visible methacrylate medial to the proximal portion of the stem of the femoral prosthesis (21) (Figure 14-31b). As a result, this area is less well supported in these cases than in more

successful total hip replacements. Fortunately, most patients who have a femoral component in varus position and minimal or no methacrylate medial to the proximal portion of the stem of the femoral component do not experience fracture or other problems of the prosthesis. However, if the postoperative films do show the prosthesis in varus position and little or no methacrylate, it is advisable to look for a possible fracture of the prosthesis. Reoperation is not indicated prior to the development of symptoms.

Loosening

Early designs for total hip replacement, before it was known that methylmethacrylate could be used as a filler, frequently failed after a number of years because of loosening of the component. The Ring prosthesis, for example, which is not fixed with methacrylate, often shows good early results, but with the passage of time loosening occurs and pain results in these hips (18).* We have already discussed the characteristic observations of the loosening of prostheses not held by methacrylate in the section on femoral head replacements. The appearance associated with loosening in patients whose prostheses are fixed with methacrylate is slightly different (25). It is important to note that most patients with loosening of the prosthesis have minimal or no symptoms (10,30). Thus, the presence of signs of loosening does not necessarily indicate a clinical failure of the prosthesis. We have previously reviewed the normal reaction of the bone to the presence of methacrylate and the prosthesis. Briefly, it is important to remember there are two forms of methacrylate: one that is radiolucent and one that has barium added to make it radiopaque. Normally, when radiolucent methacrylate is used, a radiolucent gap is visible between the prosthesis and the bone, with normal bone adjacent to the radiolucent area. However, there will often be a thin zone of bony sclerosis at the margin of the methacrylate. Both of these appearances are normal. When barium (radiopaque) methylmethacrylate is used either the methacrylate will lie next to the bone, with normal bony trabeculae starting at the edge of the methacrylate, or a thin (1 to 2.5 mm) zone of radiolucency will surround the methacrylate, which in

---

* Ring (33,34) does not find late deterioration or loosening.

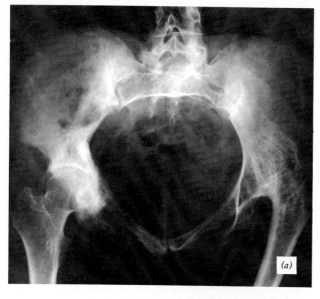

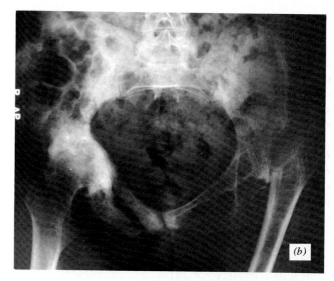

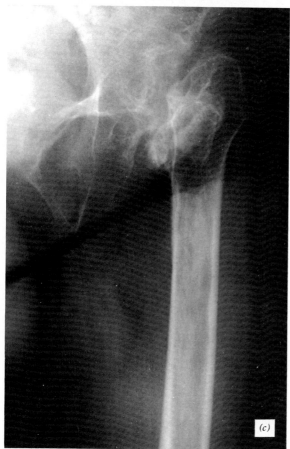

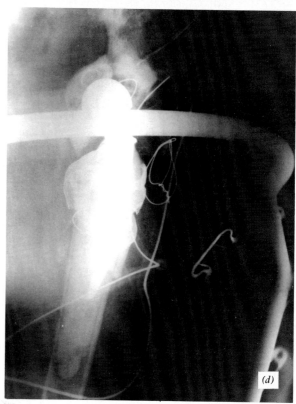

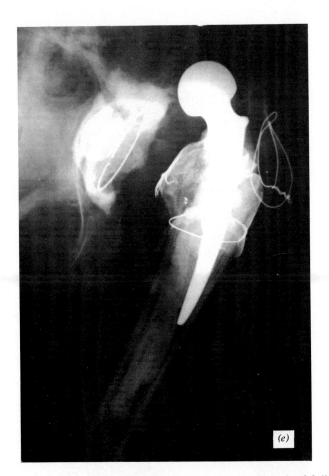

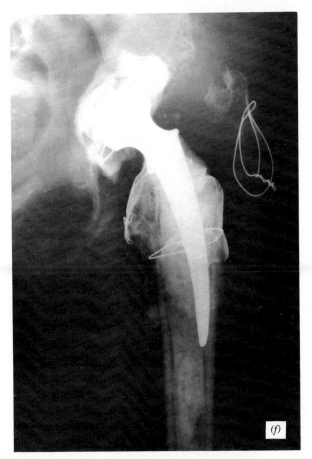

Figure 14-30. Example 14-11. Charnley-Muller prosthesis placed in osteoporotic bone. Extensive methacrylate. Trochanteric wires attached to methacrylate, with loss of position. Intraoperative fracture. (*a*) Patient age 46. The left hip is fused to the pseudoacetabulum. Paget arthritis of the right hip is present. (*b*) Following the left Girdlestone arthroplasty, a gliding articulation is present between the femur and the pelvis. (*c*) Severe osteoporosis of the femur is apparent: Girdlestone arthroplasty. (*d*) Charnley-Muller prosthesis. The femur fractured during adjustment of the femoral component. Tantalum mesh is used as reinforcement, as is abundant methacrylate. The medial wall of the acetabulum has also fractured. The greater trochanter fragment is sutured to the methacrylate and tantalum mesh. (*e*) Dislocation of the femoral component. (*f*) Following relocation of the component, the trochanteric wires have pulled out of the methacrylate.

turn will be separated from the surrounding normal bone by a very thin zone of bony sclerosis.

The earliest indication of loosening is a progressive widening of this radiolucent zone around the methacrylate. Although there are no absolute measurements to use on a single film, a space greater than 1 mm may be suspicious, and a space greater than 2 mm is moderately suggestive of loosening (37). A distance 3 mm or greater strongly indicates loosening, particularly if the space encircles much of the margin of the methacrylate (Figuer 14-13*a,b*).

The second sign of loosening is a settling of the prosthesis from its original position deeper into the medullary

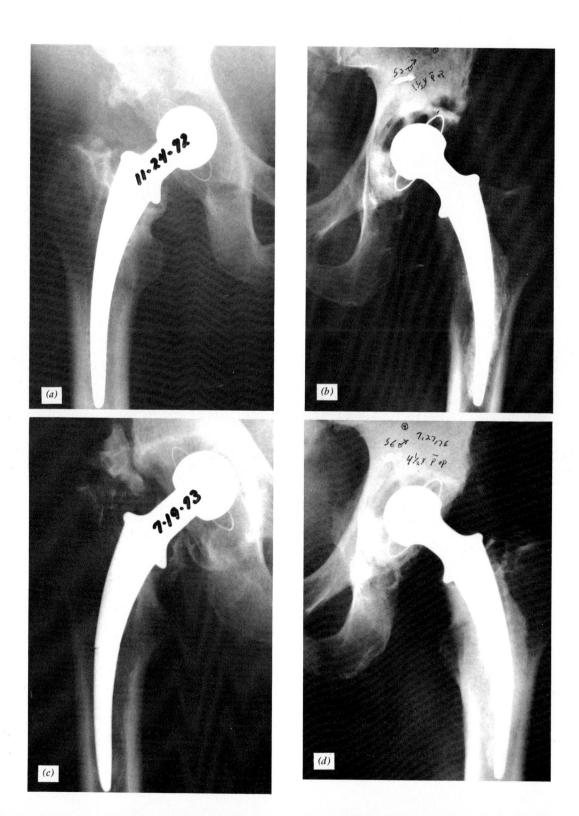

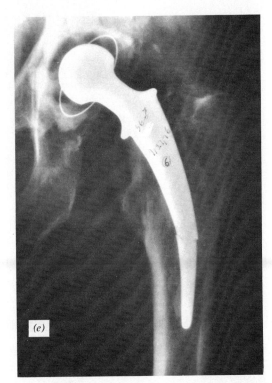

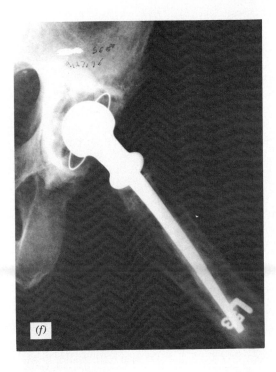

Figure 14-31. Breakage of femoral components of total hip replacements. (*a,b*) Two patients whose femoral components later broke. Both are placed in varus. The component in (*b*) is place in radiopaque methacrylate; no methacrylate lies medial to the proximal stem. (*c*) Fracture of the stem of the prosthesis at the distal portion of the middle third of the stem. (*d,e,f*) Fracture of the distal third of the stem. (*d*) In the earlier films, the fracture can be detected by a slight change in curvature, but escaped observation at the time. (*e,f*) Two months later, the breakage of the femoral stem is now obvious.

cavity (Figure 14-13*a,b*). This was discussed briefly in the section on resorption of the femoral neck as a normal finding. If the femoral neck resorbs, the prosthesis should maintain its prior relationship with the lesser trochanter. Often the sinking of the prosthesis is not recognized because the prosthesis sinks at the same rate that the femoral neck is being resorbed. As the prosthesis settles, it may become firmly impacted and stable (40). The slow sinking of the prosthesis occasionally leads to an increased area of intramedullary bone formation near the tip of the prosthesis, resulting in a slight intramedullary sclerosis of the bone in this area (6). When this condition appears, and particularly when it is progressive, loosening may have occurred.

Separation of a piece of methacrylate from the bulk of the methacrylate at the tip of the prosthesis is also an indication of settling (40) (Figure 14-32*a,b,c,d,e,f*). As the loosening becomes more severe, the degree of resorption around the methacrylate increases, and eventually a larger and larger area of radiolucency appears around the prosthesis, often with progressive resorption of the endosteal surface of the cortex and sometimes with penetration of the cortex itself (Figure 14-33*a,b,c*). Often the zone of radiolucency appears nonuniform and suggests the presence of a pivot point or toggle point of the prosthesis, resulting in an hourglass-shaped radiolucency around the methacrylate (Figure 14-34). This was more common in early total hip

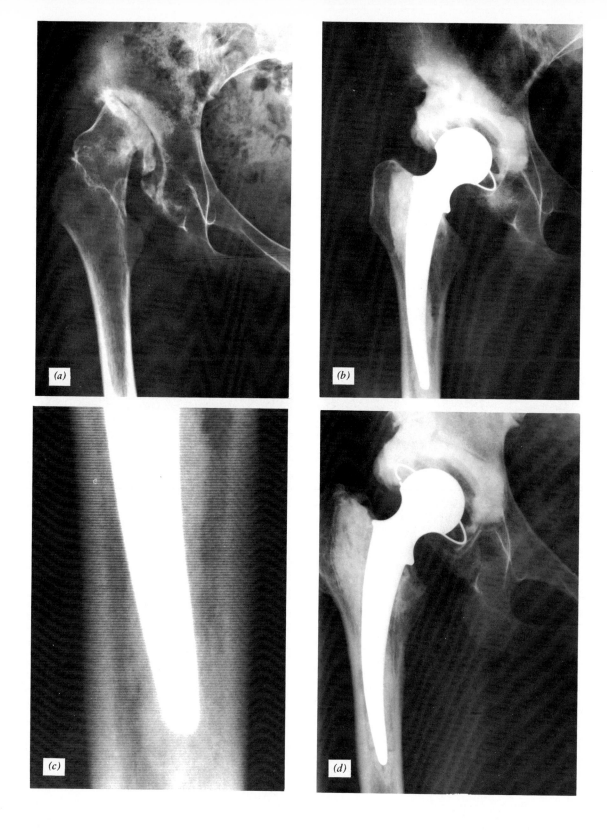

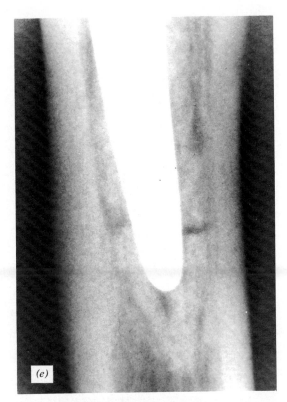

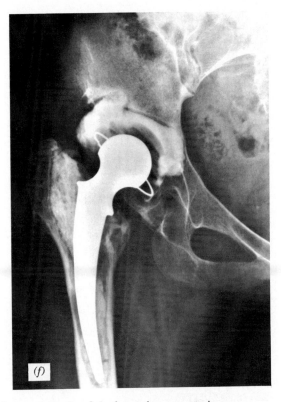

Figure 14-32. Separation of a piece of methacrylate near the tip of the femoral component is an early indication of sinking of a loose prosthesis. (*a*) Presurgical appearance. Late findings in congenital dislocation of the hip. The deformed femoral head articulates with a gliding pseudoacetabulum. (*b*) Early postsurgical view demonstrates placement of the Charnley-Muller prosthesis. The acetabular component is placed in the pseudoacetabulum. A small amount of radiolucency is present around the acetabular component super laterally, representing the lack of a tight impression of methacrylate into the cavity. (*c*) A close-up of (*b*) shows no cracks in the opaque methacrylate. (*d*) Four years following surgery, the prosthesis is loose. A crack is present in the distal femoral methacrylate, indicating a slight settling. A gap between the acetabular and femoral methacrylate and the bone has formed and is moderately wide. There is also a gap between the proximal femoral stem and the methacrylate lateral to it. (*e*) Close-up of the tip of the femoral component. The crack in the methacrylate is apparent. Thickening of the lateral femoral cortex is present. This thickening may occur as a normal postprosthesis reaction. (*f*) Six years following surgery, there has been increasing resorption of bone around the methacrylate. The medial wall of the acetabulum has buckled (fractured).

replacements, where the early signs of loosening were not recognized and where early reoperation was not contemplated. It is unusual to see such severe degrees of resorption now, since these patients usually undergo reoperation earlier to permit the maintenance of adequate bony stock for good fixation of the replacement prosthesis. Loosening may also be indicated by a shift in the position of the prosthesis. Clues to this shift are a change in the degree of anteversion of the femoral component or a shift in the degree of lateral or anterior opening of the acetabular

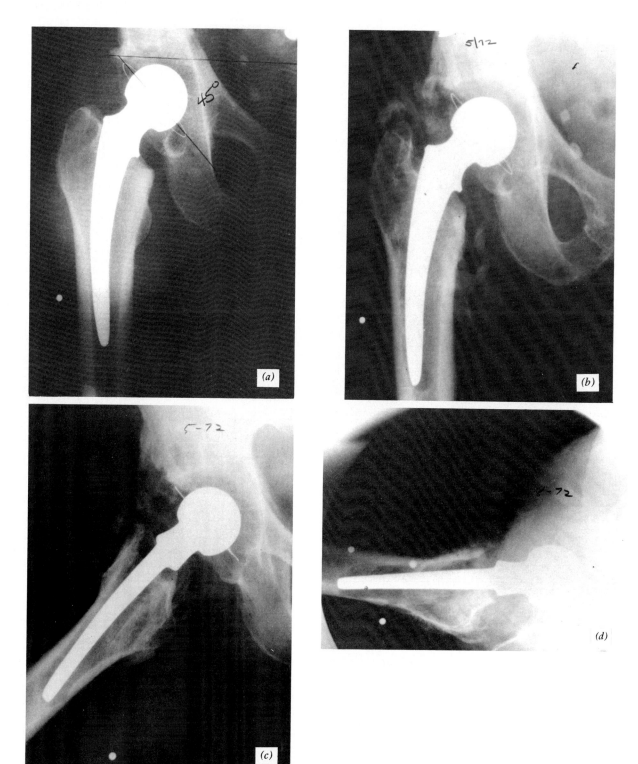

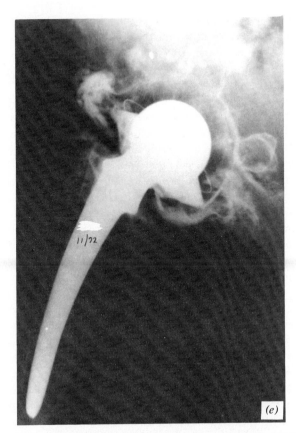

(e)

methods of confirmation include intraoperative examination (which is on occasion indicated as a primary diagnostic procedure because of the presence of continued pain in the area of the arthroplasty) and arthrography. In general, arthrography is used as the initial procedure to confirm the presence of loosening and to evaluate the presence of unexplained pain in prosthesis (32,37). In this procedure a needle (the author, prefers a 3½ -inch, 22-gauge spinal needle) is passed under fluoroscopic control

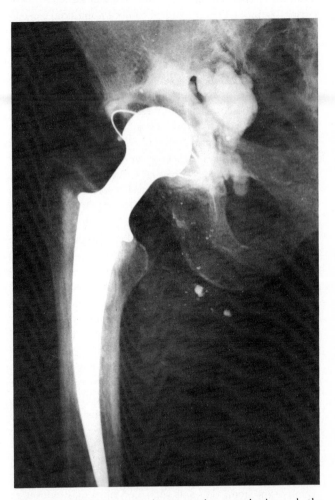

Figure 14-33. Progressive loosening of a Charnley-Muller prosthesis. (*a*) Early postoperative view demonstrating the Charnley-Muller prosthesis in radiolucent methylmethacrylate. (*b*) One year later there is moderate ectopic bone formation. The zone of radiolucency around the prosthesis is apparent (this could simply be due to demarcation of the radiolucent methacrylate; however, the lateral cortex is also resorbed, suggesting a focal increase in pressure lateral to the distal portion of the stem). (*c*) The lateral view demonstrates the extent of cortical resorption. (*d*) Three months later, the cortex is almost penetrated by the resorption. (*e*) An arthrogram confirms loosening of the acetabular and femoral components.

component as observed in serial films. Although these changes are relatively uncommon, it is important to look for them.

The changes that appear when loosening occurs are obvious when they are extreme but may seem normal when they are mild in degree. It is therefore important to be able to confirm the presence of loosening. The available

Figure 14-34. The gap between the prosthesis and the methacrylate, proximally and distally, is wider than that near the midportion of the stem of the femoral component, suggesting a pivot point of toggling in this patient with a loose femoral prosthesis.

into the pseudocapsule of the joint. The pseudocapsule is often quite firm and difficult to penetrate and a twisting motion is often necessary as the joint is approached. The author has found it most useful to attempt to enter the joint either just inferior to the acetabular component or along the medial aspect of the neck of the femoral component close to the femoral head. When the joint has been entered, joint fluid is aspirated. If no joint fluid can be aspirated, a single drop of contrast is injected to confirm position. Irrigation of the joint with nonbacteriostatic normal saline is then attempted to obtain material for culture. In general, if the prosthesis is loose or infected, joint fluid for culture can be obtained without irrigation. It is usually not possible to recover fluid injected into the joint; however, an attempt should be made to do so. Following this procedure, approximately 10 to 15 cc of 50 to 60% water-soluble contrast material is injected. If the methylmethacrylate is radiolucent, films are taken in neutral position, internal rotation, external rotation, and following longitudinal traction on the extremity. If the methylmethacrylate has been made radiopaque by barium, a useful trick is to obtain a subtraction series of films. This is explained and illustrated in Chapter 3. The sign of loosening is the tracking of the radiographic contrast material around the methacrylate. In general, the loose symptomatic prosthesis will permit the contrast to be tracked most of the way around the methacrylate. Occasionally the contrast tracks only minimally around the prosthesis. In the author's experience, in cases where such minimal tracking appears, the patients involved have not been symptomatic enough to warrant surgical intervention. Thus, although some degree of loosening is probably present in these cases, surgical confirmation was not obtained (30). The Salvati series (36) demonstrated only one false negative using this procedure; it is a most useful method of evaluating the presence of loosening, when properly performed.*

Stress films may be helpful in evaluating loosening. Push-pull films, where the prosthesis is first compressed and then distracted by longitudinal traction on the extremity, and abduction and adduction films may be used to test for loosening. These will appear positive only if the

* Murray (30) had many false positives using arthrography and disagrees with other authors.

degree of loosening is marked, but they may be helpful nevertheless (36). When traction is placed on the femur in an attempt to distract the joint and demonstrate loosening or to demonstrate trackage of contrast material around the prosthesis during arthrography, it is important to remember that if a painful hip is pulled rapidly, the muscles of the thigh will go into reflex contraction and, overpower the ability of most physicians to distract the prosthesis. In order to demonstrate distraction of the prosthesis, particularly if it is painful, it is important that slow steady, and continuous traction be applied to the extremity. The ideal length of time is about 10 minutes, but this is often impractical in a busy fluoroscopic schedule. Traction is therefore usually applied for only three to five minutes prior to obtaining film. An important measure of the effectiveness of longitudinal traction is the ability to sublux the femoral component minimally out of the acetabulum. This shift can be demonstrated on the arthrogram by the presence of contrast material within the articular cavity between the metal femoral prosthesis and the polyethylene acetabular prosthesis (similar to that seen in Figure 14-36h). When no contrast has been injected, this shift can be detected by relating the position of the center of the femoral head to the wire of the acetabulum and occasionally by the presence of a vacuum phenomenon (Figure 14-35). If no shift is seen, the traction has probably been ineffective and the film should be repeated.

Example 14-12. This 68-year-old man experienced severe hip pain due to degenerative arthritis many years following childhood Legg-Perthes disease. A radiograph (Figure 14-36a) at that time showed minimal protrusio acetabuli, moderate joint narrowing, marked osteophyte proliferation, and many degenerative cysts. (Barium was present in colonic diverticulae).

A Charnley-Muller prosthesis was inserted, and radiographs taken one month following surgery demonstrated the Charnley-Muller prosthesis in radiolucent methacrylate (Figure 14-36b,c). Note the normal appearance of the femoral cortex and the lack of demarcation around the methacrylate (it had not yet had time to develop). Close observation discloses that the femoral head is minimally subluxed. The equator of the prosthetic femoral head should lie 2 mm above the center of the wire

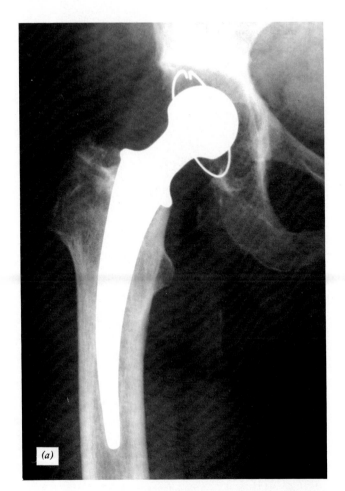

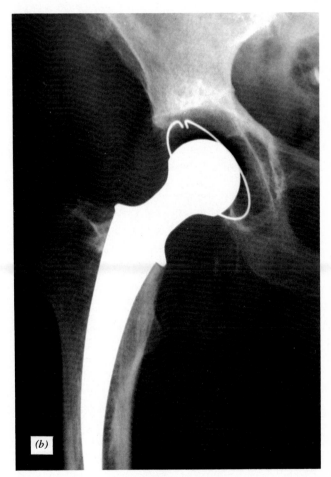

Figure 14-35. Effective, negative push-pull films. (*a*) Push (longitudinal compression film) normal. (*b*) Pull (longitudinal traction film). Air (vacuum phenomenon) in acetabular prosthetic cavity. The femoral head has shifted distally in relation to the acetabular marker wire. Clinically, no evidence of loosening. Pain was transitory and probably due to irritation of the lateral femoral cutaneous nerve.

ring. In this case the wire ring is at the equator. This suggests the presence of foreign matter within the prosthetic joint space.

The following winter, the patient was working in his garden and developed pain in his left thigh. Radiographs (Figure 14-36*d*) at that time disclosed the femoral prosthesis to be properly seated in the acetabular component. Demarcation of the radiolucent methacrylate had occurred, with a thin rim of sclerosis around the methacrylate in the greater trochanteric region. Minimal erosion of the inner portion of the cortex just distal to the lesser trochanter had occurred. This would be unusual in a firmly seated prosthesis and suggests the development of focal granulation tissue (possibly due to infection) with or without loosening. Because symptoms were minimal, no additional workup was done.

One year later, because of continued minimal symptomatology, the patient was reevaluated. At that time push-

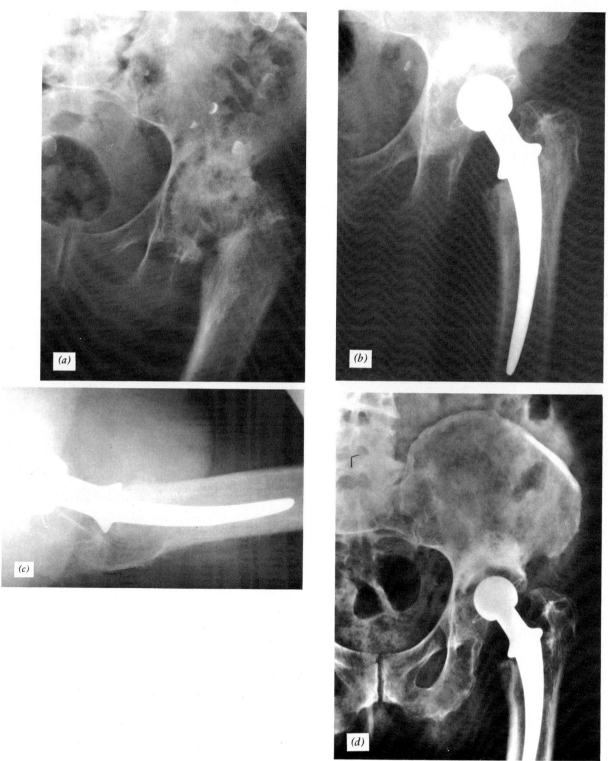

274

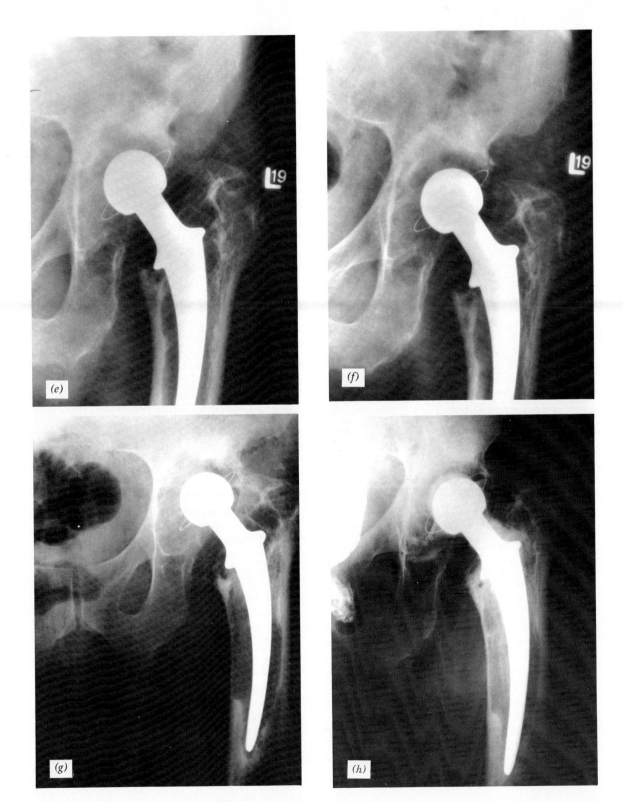

275

(*Legend on the next page*)

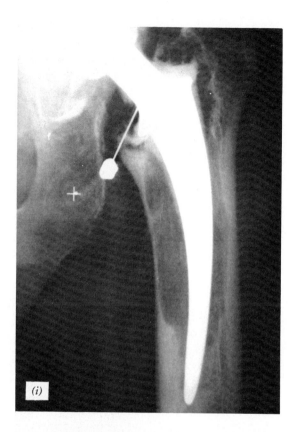

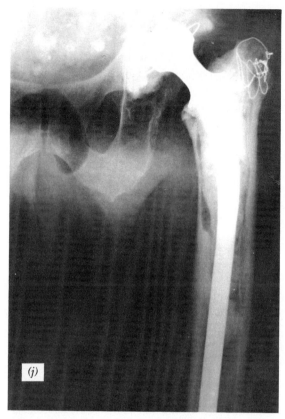

Figure 14-36. Example 14-12. Loosening of total hip replacement. (*a*) Presurgical view demonstrates severe degenerative arthrosis with marked osteophytes, cartilage narrowing, and degenerative cysts. (*b,c*) After one month the Charnley-Muller prosthesis appears well seated, with moderate lateral and minimal anterior opening. Moderate anteversion is identified on the lateral view. The head is minimally subluxed, with its central point lying at the center of the acetabular wire loop rather than at the normal position 2 mm inside of it (see text, page 242). This suggests the presence of foreign matter within the articular cavity of the acetabular component. (*d*) Seven months following surgery, there is demarcation of the methacrylate from the medullary bone, a normal finding. Erosion of the inner surface of the proximal medial femoral cortex has also appeared. This suggests the presence of focal granulation tissue. (*e,f*) Twenty-one months following surgery, longitudinal compression (*e*) and distraction (*f*) views show no evidence of loosening. Effective traction is demonstrated by the shift of the femoral head within the wire acetabular prosthesis marker. Increased endosteal resorption of the medial femoral cortex suggests the presence of granulation tissue or loosening. (*g*) Four and one-half years following surgery, extensive cortical resorption is present. The femoral head remains minimally subluxed. The prosthesis has settled slightly. There is sclerosis of bone at the tip of the prosthesis. (*h*) An arthrogram demonstrates the tracking of contrast around the lateral femoral methacrylate and between the acetabular cup and the minimally subluxed femoral head (nontraction view). (*i*) Contrast also tracks between the femoral prosthesis and the radiolucent methacrylate, medially and laterally. (*j*) Replacement with a long-stem Charnley-Muller femoral component.

pull films (longitudinal compression and distraction films) were obtained (Figure 14-36*e,f*). These radiographs demonstrate additional resorption of the inner portion of the medial cortex. The shift of the femoral head prosthesis in relation to the acetabular wire indicates that adequate traction was applied. No shift of the prosthesis was seen.

Two years later, four years following the total hip replacement, the patient fell and developed severe and continuous pain in his left hip and thigh. Radiographs at that time demonstrated marked resorption of the endosteal cortex (Figure 14-36*g*). The prosthesis had settled (note its relation to the line of condensed bone crossing the greater trochanter), and increased sclerosis was seen at the tip of the prosthesis. These are all signs of loosening. The prosthetic femoral head also lay with its equator at the center of the acetabular wires, indicating minimal subluxation.

Because of these findings, an arthrogram was done (Figure 14-36*h,i*) and showed tracking of contrast between the methacrylate and the prosthesis. Minimal contrast is also seen between the femoral head prosthesis and the acetabulum and could not be eliminated by pressure.

Because of the severe symptomatology, the total hip replacement was replaced with a long-stem Charnley-Muller prosthesis (Figure 14-36*j*). At the time of surgery, the methacrylate surrounding the femoral component had fragmented, extensive granulation tissue was present, and some of the granulation tissue had grown between the femoral head prosthesis and the acetabular component.

William Harris (23) has described a series of cases in which extensive localized bone resorption within the femur occurred following total hip replacement. As in this case, the extensive resorption suggested the presence of tumor or infection. During surgery, in these cases, the prostheses were found to be only slightly loose, but there was extensive granulomatous reaction, this author has seen similar cases (Figure 14-37*a,b,c,d*).

Early total hip replacement prostheses, which used Teflon in the acetabular cup (Figure 14-38), have also shown intense focal areas of resorption, presumably the result of a reaction to fragments of Teflon.

The minimal subluxation of this prosthesis that is visible on the initial film and several of the subsequent films suggested the presence of foreign matter within the prosthetic joint. In this case, tissue debris was probably present, and the separation of the components permitted the ingrowth of granulation tissue. On occasion, such separation is due to fragments of methylmethacrylate, and these fragments can cause rapid erosion of the acetabular polyethylene.

A gap (as shown by arthography) between the prosthesis and the methacrylate may occur in two situations. The first is the result of a small amount of wobbling at the time of placement of the prosthesis and does not seem to have clinical significance; in the second, displacement of fragments of methacrylate develops because of loosening of the methacrylate-bone interface, with resorption of bone and displacement of the methacrylate. When radiopaque methacrylate is used a gap caused by wobbling of the prosthesis on insertion should be apparent on the first postoperative study; if loosening is the cause of the gap, it should appear after the first film. With radiolucent methacrylate, one must be far more cautious in evaluating the significance of this finding.

Erosion of the inner surface of the cortex is not usually the result of the operative procedure. Loosening or infection are more usual causes of erosion of the inner cortex.

Increasing sclerosis at the tip of a prosthesis placed in methacrylate is usually a sign of loosening. Where prostheses are inserted without a methacrylate interface, sclerosis may be seen in asymptomatic patients; it is a normal finding, reflecting the greater stress placed on the bone near the tip of a prosthesis in which the methacrylate does not serve as a diffuser of the force applied to the bone.

Infection

Infection of a total hip replacement is unfortunately a common problem and may result in serious morbidity. In several series of cases, the overall incidence of infection has reached 8% of all hips replaced. About half of these are early infections, occurring in the immediate postoperative period. They are usually readily recognizable clinically either as wound infections or because of onset of pain in the area of the prosthesis in the early postoperative period. These symptoms are associated with fever, increased sedimentation rate, and signs of sepsis. In general, this kind of early infection shows little or no radiographic changes. To a radiologist, the late infection is far more important.

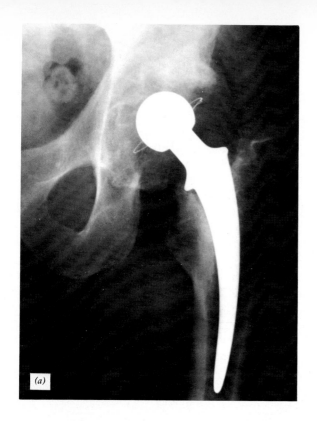

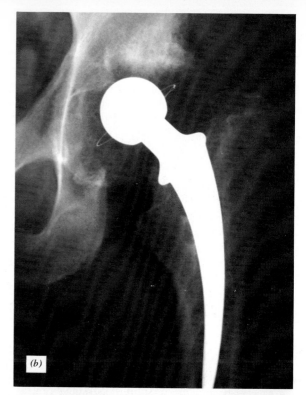

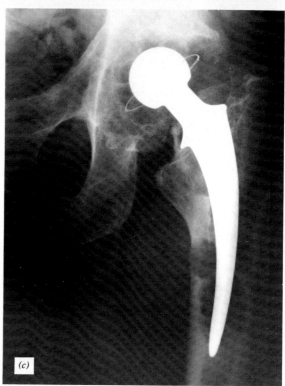

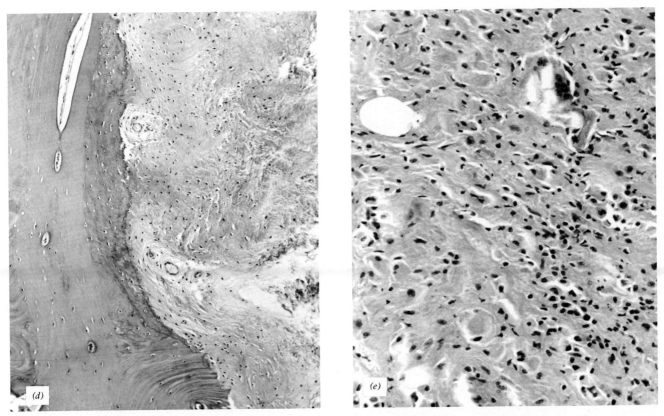

Figure 14-37. Extensive granulatomatous response to total hip replacement with methacrylate. (a) Eighteen months following total hip replacement, there is demarcation of the radiolucent methacrylate from the femoral medullary bone. (b) Thirty months following surgery, focal areas of resorption bone are noted medial to the proximal portion of the prosthesis. Minimal settling is present. (c) Five and one-half years following surgery, these focal areas of resorption have enlarged and new areas have developed. The patient has only minor symptoms of pain. Additional settling of the prosthesis has occurred. (d,e) Histologic sections reveal histiocytes with a granular acidophillic cytoplasm. Some giant-cell reaction is present. An iron stain showed finely divided iron in numerous macrophages. (Photomicrographs courtesy of Dennis Noe, M.D.)

There is a difference of opinion in the orthopedic literature as to whether these infections are infections by low-virulence organisms contracted during surgery and not recognized for some time after or whether they are de novo infections occurring in the area of surgery. There are clinical and theoretical reasons to suggest that both mechanisms can be active. It is not uncommon to find that the patient who, several years postoperatively, has a definite hip joint infection is the patient who, from the early postoperative period on, had symptoms of mild discomfort in the hip (10). Although the symptoms were present so early, they had never been intense enough to warrant a diagnosis or further analysis to find their cause. On the other hand, occasionally there are patients with definite postoperative infections in their hip who have been asymptomatic and then experience a relatively rapid onset of symptoms associated with infection. Cruess (75) suggests that some of these infections may be secondary to

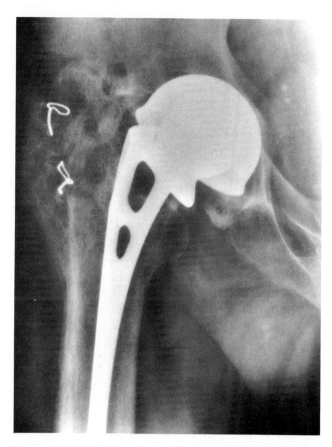

Figure 14-38. The Press-fit total hip prosthesis. An early design that used a Teflon cup and no methacrylate. The teflon wore rapidly and often resulted in extensive granulomatous reaction with erosion of bone.

spread from another focus of infection and suggests that prophylactic antibiotics be used during dental work—similar to the method used in the patient with rheumatic heart disease. In general these late postoperative infections are associated with low-virulence organisms and often present as unexplained pain.

Radiographically, the plain films of the hip may be normal, may show signs of loosening as previously described (11,31,43), or on occasion may show areas of focal bone resorption at the methacrylate-bone interface. One difference between septic and aseptic loosening is that

the widening of the methacrylate bone interface in plain loosening is usually symmetrical, whereas in septic loosening one often sees some variation in the thickness of the zone of resorption (2), often wider near the joint and narrower distal from the joint (6), or with radiolucency surrounding the trochanteric wires (2). Only rarely are there classical changes of true osteomyelitis such as permeative resorption of bone or periosteal reaction, and usually in these cases the infection is so severe that the clinical diagnosis is not in doubt. Hip arthrography can be useful in determining the presence of hip joint infection. First, a sample can be aspirated for culture. Since some of these organisms are quite fastidious in their growth requirements and because some of them are anaerobes, careful culture techniques should be used. Depending on the laboratory used, it is often desirable to transfer the material aspirated from the hip joint directly into anaerobic culture media and to look for fastidious and unusual anaerobes as well as the more common pyogenic organisms. The arthrogram in such instances may show only the presence of loosening or may show areas of abscess formation communicating with the joint. On occasion sinus tracts are identified.

Example 14-13. This 75-year-old woman had a total hip replacement at age 74. She did well for two months, but then developed progressive pain and the wound started to drain. A superficial debridement of the wound was done, without relief of symptoms. In preparation for the second surgery, films were taken 11 months following surgery. The frontal view (Figure 14-39a) demonstrated a Charnley-Muller-type total hip prosthesis. The femoral component appears normal otherwise. Examination of the acetabular cup discloses an uneven 2 to 3 mm band of radiolucency surrounding both the superolateral and inferomedial portion of the methacrylate. This radiolucency also extends around the methacrylate placed in the inferior keyhole previously drilled in the acetabular bone. The superior keyhole demonstrates no similar zone of radiolucency.

The radiolucency around the methacrylate of the acetabulum enveloped it incompletely and thus probably did not represent loosening. There are two possible explanations for this radiolucency. First, at the time of placement, methacrylate may not have been forced tightly against the acetabular bone. Although this can occur, it is unlikely to involve both the superior and inferior portions of the acetabulum. Second, infection and granulation tissue may be causing this resorption of bone.

Sinography was then performed, with the injection of contrast material into one of the draining sinuses (Figure 14-39b,c). The sinogram showed communication with the base of the femoral neck of the prosthesis.

At surgery, the prosthesis seemed to be firmly fixed, but, when pressure was exerted on the acetabular component, pus exited from the superolateral portion of the acetabulum—methacrylate interface. The acetabular component was removed, and a purulent-looking membrane lay between the methacrylate and the bone. The junction between the methacrylate and the bone of the femur was normal, with no evidence of infection. Cultures were negative, but pathologic evaluation disclosed evidence of acute and chronic inflammation.

Because of the infection, the prosthesis was removed and the patient was left with a Girdlestone-like arthroplasty (see Chapter 15) (Figure 14-39d). The broad, linear radiolucency in the femoral shaft resulted from a window cut in the femoral cortex to aid in the removal of the methacrylate.

Infection may be suspected from the presence of focal resorption between the methacrylate and the bone. If resorption is progressive but does not encircle the prosthesis, infection is probable. If the prosthesis is encircled by radiolucency, the probable diagnosis is loosening, possibly with infection. If there is only a single set of films to evaluate, the possibility that the radiolucency results from failure of firm impressing of the methacrylate into the bony acetabulum may explain the observations. Usually, when there is a failure of approximation of the methacrylate to the bone, it is limited in extent and is in the inferomedial portion of the acetabulum.

In this case, injection into the sinus tract demonstrated that the infection did reach the joint space. The failure of a sinus tract injection to reach the joint space, on the contrary, does not mean that the joint is uninvolved by the infection. If uncertainty exists, a needle should be placed into the joint and the joint aspirated and injected with contrast.

The presence of periosteal reaction around the femur following total hip replacement usually does not indicate the presence of infection; rather it indicates that the total hip replacement was performed as a secondary procedure, replacing some earlier appliance (Figure 14-40). (Also see Figure 14-19, 14-23, 14-25, and 14-36d.) Following surgery the periosteal reaction is relatively active for two to four weeks in the postoperative period and then becomes quiescent (nonprogressive) after that. In most causes of periosteal new bone, once the process has stabilized, the gap between the cortex and the periosteal new bone fills in with more normal bone. For some unexplained reason, following replacement of a hip appliance with a new prosthesis, this periosteal reaction remains as a lamellar periosteal reaction for many years and does not fill in in the expected manner. If this condition is observed, with no previous films available for comparison, the periosteal reaction might be mistaken for an active periosteal reaction rather than a stable, chronic, inactive response to the surgery. Rarely is periosteal reaction due to infection. However, periosteal reaction in the absence of a second surgical procedure on the hip is suspect (Figure 14-41).

Recently, a number of medical centers have been experimenting with a new method of treating the infected total hip replacement. In this new procedure, the infected prosthesis is removed, sterilized, the joint and infected tissue debrided, and the prosthesis replaced, all as a single procedure. Thus it may not be necessary to deny the patient the benefits of a total hip replacement because of prior infection (16).

In certain patients whose clinical symptomatology and radiographic findings strongly suggest infection, no organism has appeared in culture. The author feels that poor bacteriologic techniques are at fault; therefore it is inadvisable to change a diagnosis of infection because of the failure to culture an organism (11).

Abnormal Locations of Methacrylate

Although methylmethacrylate is essential as a filler between the prosthesis and bone, its placement in other locations may result in problems: intrapelvic protrusion (Figure 14-42) can result in sciatic nerve entrapment (4), and methacrylate placed near nerves may lead to sciatic and femoral nerve palsies. These palsies may also occur as

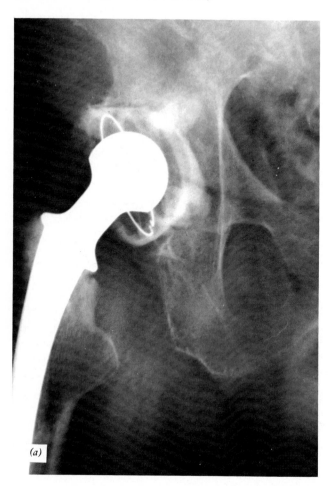

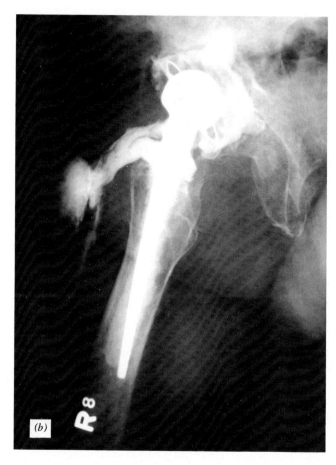

a result of operative trauma (41). Declan Nolan (31) reports several cases in which methacrylate in unusual places was associated with continued pain; this pain was relieved by removal of the extra methacrylate. Although we have not recognized this problem in our patients, methacrylate in a nonperioprosthetic location should be considered as one of the potential causes of unexplained pain following total hip replacement.

Unexplained Pain

In general, the patient who has had a total hip replacement is asymptomatic or largely asymptomatic following this replacement. The degree of pain relief is remarkable.

When such a patient returns with unexplained pain, it is necessary to discover the possible causes. We have already mentioned many causes of unexplained pain, such as loosening, infection, fracture of the prosthesis, and problems with the greater trochanter. Stress fractures must also be considered as the source of such unexplained pain (25,29). Another abnormality that should be looked for is the presence of trochanteric bursitis (37). This is not uncommon following any surgical procedure on the hip. Clinically, tenderness localized to the greater trochanter may be an indication of trochanteric bursitis. Such a condition may be detected radiographically by the presence of distrophic calcification in the area of the bursa overlying

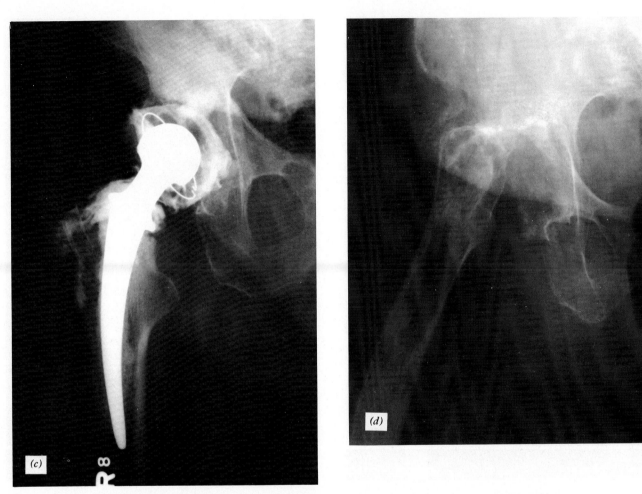

Figure 14-39. Example 14-13. Infection surrounding the acetabular component of a Charnley-Muller prosthesis. (*a*) A wide band of radiolucency surrounds the inferior and superior portions of the acetabular methacrylate. There is no radiolucency surrounding the superior plug of methacrylate. This asymmetric resorption suggests infection. (*b,c*) Sinus tract injection demonstrates communication with the joint space. Contrast surrounds the inferomedial acetabular methacrylate. (*b*) Lateral view, (*c*) Frontal view. (*d*) Following removal of the prosthesis and the methacrylate, the patient is left with a Girdlestone-type arthroplasty.

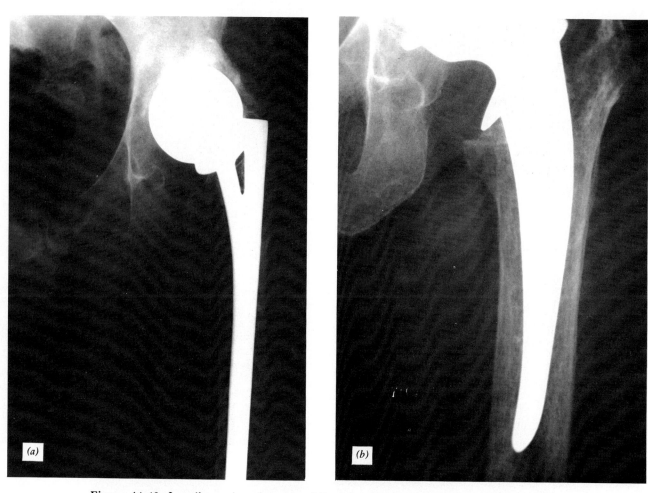

Figure 14-40. Lamellar periosteal reaction following replacement of a long-stemmed Austin-Moore prosthesis with a McKee-Farrar prosthesis. (*a*) Long-stem Austin-Moore prosthesis, showing moderate ectopic bone. (*b*) Lateral Lamellar periosteal reaction McKee-Farrar prosthesis in radiolucent methacrylate.

Figure 14-41. Periosteal reaction of the lateral femoral cortex due to infection following total hip replacement. (*a*) Presurgical view shows sclerotic demarcation within the femoral head, due to avascular necrosis. The joint space is narrowed and irregular because of the secondary degenerative arthrosis. (*b*) Four months following Charnley-Muller total hip replacement, the prosthesis is normally seated. No periosteal reaction is present. (*c*) Six years following surgery, there is extensive periosteal reaction along the lateral femoral cortex. (*d*) An arthrogram shows asymmetric tracking of contrast around the acetabular component inferomedially; also visible is a sinus track adjacent to the infected lateral femoral cortex.

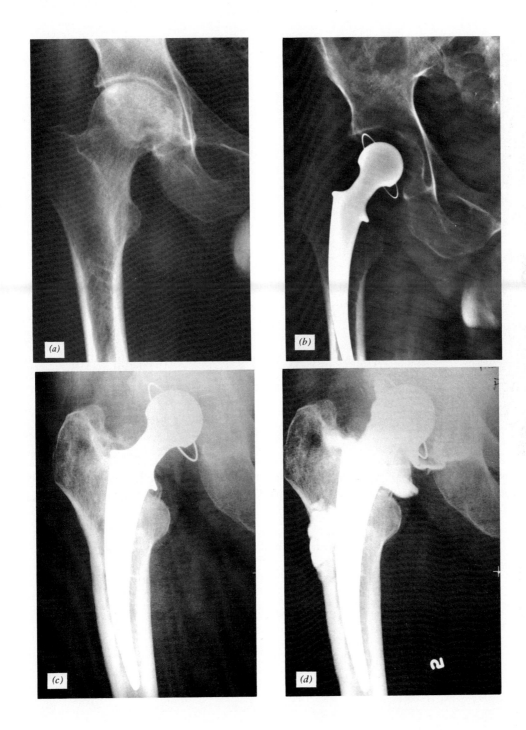

(a)

(b)

(c)

(d)

285

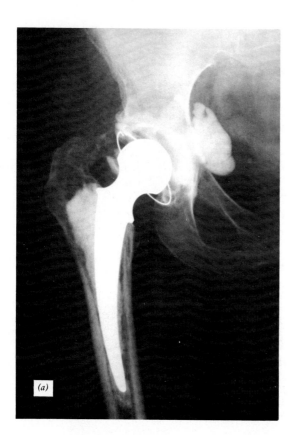 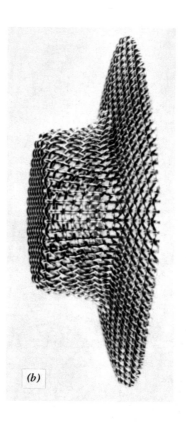

Figure 14-42. (*a*) Marked intrapelvic protrusion of methacrylate. Sometimes this results in sciatic nerve damage. To prevent this, a small, hat-shaped piece of mesh is often used to limit the protrusion of methacrylate into the pelvis (Figure 14-43). (*b*) A close-up of the hat-shaped mesh used to prevent intrapelvic protrusion of methacrylate.

either the lateral aspect or the proximal aspect of the greater trochanter (Figure 14-43). When a patient has unexplained pain following total hip replacement, both bone and good soft-tissue radiographs should be obtained in an attempt to find the etiology of this problem. If none of the possible causes already mentioned are identifiable on the plain film, it is often helpful to proceed to a hip arthrogram, which may show changes due to loosening or infection.

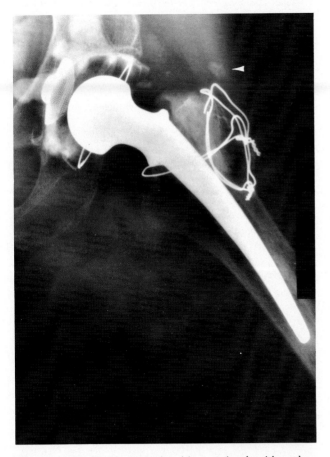

Figure 14-43. Trochanteric bursitis associated with a loose femoral component of a Charnley-Muller prosthesis. Calcification superolateral to the wires of the greater trochanter corresponded to the site of tenderness in this patient. Treatment of the trochanteric bursitis substantially decreased, but did not eliminate, the pain in this patient.

SUMMARY

In this chapter we have reviewed the common types of total hip replacements and features of their normal and abnormal positions. We have also dealt with the appearance of and the reaction of the body to methylmethacrylate, the filler used to fix the total hip replacement. It is important to remember that there are normal x-ray changes following total hip replacement, as well as those that suggest disease. Resorption of the femoral neck, the presence of a thin zone of radiolucency around the methacrylate, reinforcement of the bone of the femoral cortex near the tip of the prosthesis, and the presence of a small gap between the methylmethacrylate and the prosthesis are all usually normal. In evaluating the total hip replacement it is necessary to look for the radiographic changes indicating poor positioning, which can, in turn, predispose the prosthesis to dislocation and subluxation, the presence of intraoperative fractures, problems with the greater trochanter, stress fractures, loosening, infection, fracture of the prosthesis, and trochanteric bursitis.

REFERENCES

1. Anderson GBJ, Freeman MAR, Swanson SAU: Loosening of the cemented acetabular cup in total hip replacement. *J Bone Joint Surg* 54B:590–599, 1972.

2. Bergstrom B Lidgren L, Lindberg L: Radiographic abnormalities caused by postoperative infection following total hip arthroplasty. *Clin Orthop* 99:95–102, 1974.

3. Bisla R, Inglis A, Chitranjan RS: Joint replacement surgery in patients under 30. *J Bone Joint Surg* 58A:1098–1104, 1976.

4. Casagrade P, Danahy P: Delayed sciatic nerve entrapment following use of self-curing acrylic. *J Bone Joint Surg* 53A:167–169, 1971.

5. Charnley J: Anchorage of femoral head prosthesis to the shaft of the femur. *J Bone Joint Surg* 42B:28–30, 1960.

6. Charnley J: The bonding of prosthesis to bone by cement. *J Bone Joint Surg* 46B:518–529, 1964.

7. Charnley J: A biomedical analysis of the use of cement to anchor the femoral hip prosthesis. *J Bone Joint Surg* 47B:354–363, 1965.

8. Charnley J, Kettlewell J: The elimination of slip between prosthesis and femur. *J Bone Joint Surg* 47B:56–60, 1965.

9. Charnley J: *Carylic Cement in Orthopedic Surgery.* Edinburgh and London, E and S Livingstone 1970.

10. Charnley J: The long-term results of low-friction arthroplasty of the hip performed as a primary intervention. *J Bone Joint Surg* 54B:61–76, 1972 A.

11. Charosky C, Bullough P, Wilson P: Total hip replacement failures: A histologic evaluation. *J Bone Joint Surg* 55A:49–58, 1973.

12. Coventry MB, et al: 2,012 total hip arthroplasties: A study of postoperative course and early complications. *J Bone Joint Surg* 56A:273–284, 1974.

13. Cruess RL, Bickel Wm S, Von Kessler Kirby LC: Infection in total hips secondary to a primary source elsewhere. *Clin Orthop* 106:99–101, 1975.

14. Dandy DJ, Theodorou BC: The management of local complications of total hip replacement by the McKee-Farrar technique. *J Bone Joint Surg* 57B:30–35, 1975.

15. Dunn HK, Hess WE: Total hip reconstruction in chronically dislocated hips. *J Bone Joint Surg* 58A:838–845, 1976.

16. DuPont J, Charnley J: Low-friction arthroplasty of the hip for the failure of previous operations. *J Bone Joint Surg* 54B:77–87, 1972.

17. Eftekhar MS: Dislocation and instability complicating low friction arthroplasty of the hip joint. *Clin. Orthop* 121:120–125, 1976.

18. Evarts C, et al: The Ring total hip prosthesis. *J Bone Joint Surg* 54A:1677–1682, 1972.

19. Ferrari A, Charnley J: Conversion of hip joint pseudoarthrosis to total hip replacement. *Clin Orthop* 121:12–19, 1976.

20. Fornasier VL, Cameron HU: The femoral stem/cement interface in total hip replacement. *Clin Orthop* 116:248–252, 1976.

21. Galante JO, Rostoker Wm, Doyle JM: Failed femoral stems in total hip prostheses. A report of six cases. *J Bone Joint Surg* 57A:230–236, 1975.

22. Harris Wm H, Jones Wm N: The use of wire mesh in total hip replacement surgery. *Clin Orthop* 106:117–121, 1975.

23. Harris Wm H, Schiller AL, Scholler JM, Freiberg RA, Scott R: Extensive localized bone resorption in the femur following total hip replacement. *J Bone Joint Surg* 58A:612–618, 1976.

24. Luck J Vernon, Brannon EW, Luck James V: Total hip replacement arthroplasties: Causes, orthopedic management, and prevention of selected problems, abstracted. *J Bone Joint Surg* 54A:1569–1571, 1972.

25. Marmon L: Stress fracture of the pubic ramus simulating a loose total hip replacement. *Clin Orthop* 121:103–104, 1976.

26. Marmon L: Femoral loosening in total hip replacement. *Clin Orthop* 121:116–119, 1976.

27. McElfresh EC, Coventry MB: Femoral and pelvic fractures after total hip arthroplasty. *J Bone Joint Surg* 56A:483–492, 1974.

28. McKee GK, Watson-Farrar J: Replacement of arthritic hips by the McKee-Farrar prosthesis. *J Bone Joint Surg* 48B:245–259, 1966.

29. Miller AO: Late fracture of the acetabulum after total hip replacement. *J Bone Joint Surg* 54B:600–606, 1972.

30. Murray WR, Rodrigo JJ: Arthrography for the assessment of pain after total hip replacement. *J Bone Joint Surg* 57A:1060–1065, 1975.

31. Nolan DR, Fitzgerald RH Jr, Beckenbaugh RD, Coventry MB: Complications of total hip arthroplasty treated by reoperation. *J Bone Joint Surg* 57A:977–981, 1975.

32. Patterson FP, Brown S: The McKee-Farrar total hip replacement. *J Bone Joint Surg* 54A:257–275, 1972.

33. Ring PA: Complete replacement arthroplasty of the hip by Ring prosthesis. *J Bone Joint Surg* 50B:720–731, 1968.

34. Ring PA: Total replacement of the hip joint. *J Bone Joint Surg* 56B:44–58, 1974.

35. Ritter M: Dislocation and subluxation of the total hip replacement. *Clin Orthop* 121:92–94, 1976.

36. Salvati E, Freiberger R, Wilson PD: Arthrography for complications of total hip replacement. *J Bone Joint Surg* 53A:701–709, 1971.

37. Salvati E, et al: Radiology of total hip replacement. *Clin Orthop* 121:74–82, 1976.

38. Stauffer RN, Sim FH: Total hip arthroplasty in Paget's disease of the hip. *J Bone Joint Surg* 58A:476–478, 1976.

39. Tronzo RG, Okin EM: Anatomic restoration of congenital hip dysplasia in adulthood by total hip replacement. *Clin Orthop* 106:94–98, 1975.

40. Weber FA, Charnley J: A radiological study of fractures of acrylic cement in relation to the stem of a femoral head prosthesis. *J Bone Joint Surg* 57B:297–301, 1975.

41. Weber ER, Daube JR, Coventry MB: Peripheral neuropathies associated with total hip arthroplasty. *J Bone Joint Surg* 58A:66–69, 1976.

42. Willert HG, et al: Reaction of bone to methacrylate after hip arthroplasty. *J Bone Joint Surg* 56A:1368–1382, 1974.

43. Wilson PD, et al: Total hip replacement with fixation by acrylic cement. *J Bone Joint Surg* 54A:207–236, 1972.

15
Salvage Procedures— The Girdlestone Arthroplasty

Salvage procedures are those performed after another method has failed. The Girdlestone arthroplasty, first reported in 1849 (6) and popularized by F. R. Girdlestone (2,3) for the treatment of septic (particularly tuberculous) arthritis, is one of the more commonly performed salvage operations on the hip. Though it may sometimes be used as a primary procedure on a badly damaged hip joint, it is usually performed following failure of some other procedure on the hip, particulary if the prior procedure resulted in infection. The Girdlestone arthroplasty is used as one of the salvage procedures following failed cup, failed femoral head replacement, and failed total hip replacement arthroplasties (6).

The Girdlestone procedure consists of a resection of the femoral head and neck along the intertrochanteric line. The resection may be coupled with debridement or reaming of the acetabulum. On occasion, the superolateral margin of the acetabulum is smoothed to create a better gliding surface for the femur, but this is usually not done nor does it seem necessary for the success of the procedure. Following resection of the femoral head and neck, the patient is usually treated in traction until wound healing has occurred.

The articulation, after weight bearing has been resumed, is between the proximal portion of the femur and the buttock muscles, with some support coming from the lateral wall of the pelvis. Some pistoning is always present, giving the patient an uncosmetic but relatively

pain-free gait. In a series of failed total hip replacements in which 17 Girdlestone procedures were performed for loose or infected prostheses, 16 of the 17 resulted in decreased pain, and 12 of the 17 were at least as good as they were prior to the total hip replacement (7). In

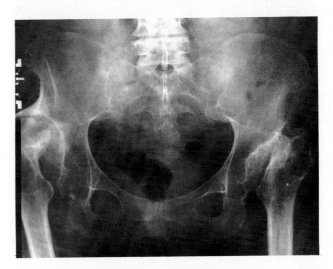

Figure 15-1. Example 15-1. Girdlestone arthroplasty as late treatment for congenital dislocation of the hip. A right hip shelf procedure is present; the shelf is over the pseudoacetabulum. A left Girdlestone arthroplasty is present. The left femoral head and neck are resected, and the superolateral rim of the acetabulum is smoothed.

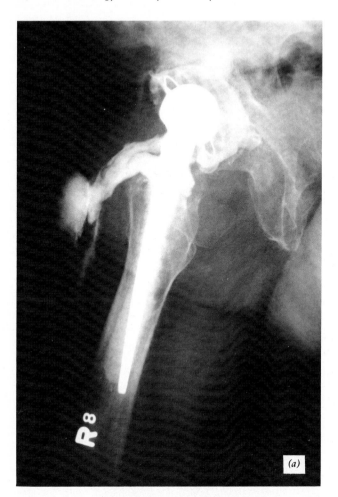

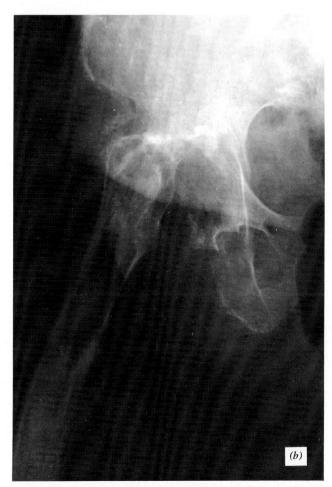

Figure 15-2. Example 15-2. Girdlestone arthroplasty as part of treatment for infected total hip replacement. (*a*) Sinus tract injection showing communication of the sinus tract with the region of the prosthetic femoral neck. (*b*) Following removal of the prosthesis and the methacrylate, and joint debridement, the patient is left with a Girdlestone variant arthroplasty.

another series (6) of 41 patients, only 18% of those who had a unilateral procedure were dissatisfied with their result.

Because of the leg shortening inherent in the arthroplasty, most of the patients with a Girdlestone arthroplasty benefit from a shoe lift, and many are helped by one or two canes with the shoe lift (1,6,9).

Those patients with bilateral procedures usually do quite poorly and have an awkward, unstable gait; therefore bilateral procedures are not recommended in bi-

lateral hip disease (6). Unilateral Girdlestone with a contralateral fusion or more stable arthroplasty may be satisfactory, except, as noted by Zabihi (9), for Moslems, who require hip mobility for their traditional prayers and who prefer bilateral Girdlestone arthroplasties to a fused hip on one side and a Girdlestone procedure on the other.

Example 15-1. This 61-year-old woman, at the age of 2½, had bilateral congenital dislocation of the hip. She was initially treated with closed reduction and casting. At age 11 a right shelf procedure was performed with good results, lasting until age 61, at which time a total hip replacement was placed. The left hip did well until age 43, when increasing pain due to secondary degenerative arthrosis was treated with a reshaping of the femoral head and acetabulum (see Chapter 6). This did not succeed in relieving pain, and at age 53 a left Girdlestone arthroplasty was performed, resulting in partial relief of pain (Figure 15-1). Following the right total hip replacement, the pain in the left hip was not considered sufficient to warrant additional surgery. The patient now uses one cane, is able to walk two to three blocks, and can climb stairs using the banister. She can also enter public buses.

Example 15-2. This 75-year-old woman had a total hip replacement, which did well for two months and then began to drain pus. Because of increasing pain and drainage, a sinus tract injection was performed, demonstrating communication with the joint space (Figure 15-2a). The prosthesis was removed and the patient was left with a Girdlestone-type arthroplasty (Figure 15-2b).

The Failed Girdlestone Arthroplasty

Some Girdlestone arthroplasties are painful. Often, no radiologic abnormality is apparent, but occasionally an irregularity of the gliding surface of the proximal femur is seen; sometimes sclerosis suggestive of a degenerative arthrosis is also present.

Modifications of the Girdlestone Arthroplasty

In order to overcome some of the gait abnormalities associated with the Girdlestone arthroplasty, several modifications are available. These include an intertrochanteric osteotomy designed to give better mechanical length to the gluteal muscles (4) and angulation osteotomies to improve the support given by the lateral pelvic wall (1,5,6). These angulation osteotomies are similar to or modifications of the Shantz osteotomy (see Chapter 4 and Figure 15-3). The resection angulation arthroplasty may be combined with the shelf procedure (8). These variations improve stability but decrease motion moderately.

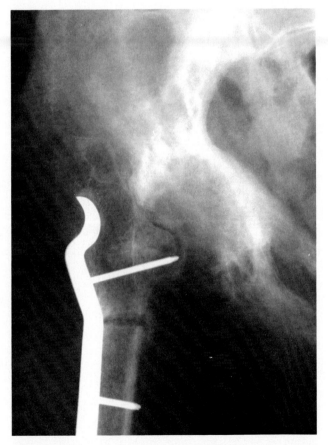

Figure 15-3. A Milch osteotomy performed as treatment for Paget arthritis of the hip. The femoral head and neck have been resected. A valgus subtrochanteric osteotomy has been performed. The valgus osteotomy is thought to permit the proximal fragment to transfer some force directly to the lateral pelvic wall.

REFERENCES

1. Batchelor JS: Excision of the femoral head and neck in cases of ankylosis and osteoarthritis of the hips. *Proc R Soc Med* 38:689–690, 1945.

2. Girdlestone GR: Actue pyogenic arthritis of the hip *Lancet* 1:419–421, 1943.

3. Girdlestone GR: Discussion on treatment of unilateral osteoarthritis of the hip-joint. *Proc R Soc Med* 38:363, 1945.

4. Gruca A: The treatment of quiescent tuberculosis of the hip joint by

excision and dynamic osteotomy. *J Bone Joint Surg* 32B:174–182, 1950.

5. Milch H: Resection angulation operation for arthritis of the hip. *Bull Hosp Joint Dis* 9:187–196, 1948.

6. Parr PL, et al: Resection of the head and neck of the femur with and without angulation osteotomy. *J Bone Joint Surg* 53A:935–944, 1971.

7. Patterson FP, Brown CS: McKee-Farrar total hip replacement. *J Bone Joint Surg* 54A:257–275, 1972.

8. Stamm TT: Arthroplasty in discussion of treatment of unilateral osteoarthritis of the hip-joint. *Proc R Soc Med* 38:366–367, 1945.

9. Zabihi T, et al: A modified girdlestone operation in the treatment of complications of fractures of the femoral neck. *J Bone Joint Surg* 55A:129–136, 1973.

16
Hip Fusion

Several diseases of the hip result in progressive stiffness and spontaneous fusion across the hip joint. When the hip finally fuses, pain is usually relieved. Surgical fusion results in a strong, stable, and painless hip. Whether used as a primary procedure or as a salvage procedure following the failure of other treatment for hip disease, hip arthrodesis may be the procedure of choice for selected patients. While motion at the hip is lost, there is sufficient mobility of the spine and opposite hip to provide 40 to 50° of flexion and 30 to 40° of combined adduction-abduction (18).

The patients best suited for arthrodesis are those for whom a total hip replacement is not feasible. Those patients with stiff hips prior to surgery are usually the ones most satisfied with the procedure, since they have already learned to compensate for the loss of hip motion. Arthrodesis is preferable to total hip replacement in patients who have a previously infected hip (2) (this is no longer an absolute contraindication to total hip replacement), and in those patients who need a strong and totally dependable hip: construction workers, seamen, and the like. Following successful fusion, patients can walk 5 to 10 miles without pain, or they can function high on a building scaffold without the fear that their hip will give way.

TYPES OF FUSION

The two basic types of hip fusion are the intra-articular and the extra-articular. These two procedures can be combined in the same hip (15,10,11). A variety of procedures are available for both intra- and extra-articular fusion, which in part reflects the difficulty that may be en-

countered in achieving healing to solid fusion. The best results yield approximately 90% solid fusion and 8% fibrous union.

The Intra-Articular Fusion

The earliest fusions performed were the intra-articular type. These were done by debriding the joint cartilage on both the femoral head and acetabulum and then fixing the hip in its desired position by a spica cast. The successful rate of fusion following this procedure was 40% (18). This low success rate was thought to be due to the lack of adequate immobilization; the spica cast permits some motion at the hip (18). Because of the high failure rate, other procedures evolved. Spica casting in the infected hip often leads to fusion (Figure 16-1). Historically, the next procedures to evolve were the extra-articular fusions, which will be described later.

Modifications of the intra-articular fusions, which incorporated the use of hip nails, were subsequently developed. The simplest was the placement of a hip nail across the joint into the acetabulum (Figure 16-2). Although this procedure occasionally succeeded (17,18), it was usually associated with inadequate stabilization, loosening of the nail, and recurrent pain in patients with limited hip motion prior to surgery. Two hip nails, placed at different angles, had a somewhat greater rate of success when used in older patients who did not put much strain on the hip (16).

Debridement of the joint cartilage combined with the use of a hip nail across the joint has an even higher success rate (12,18). In these patients, the hip is immobilized in a

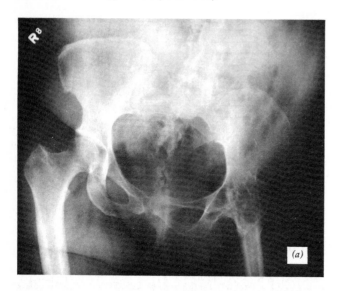

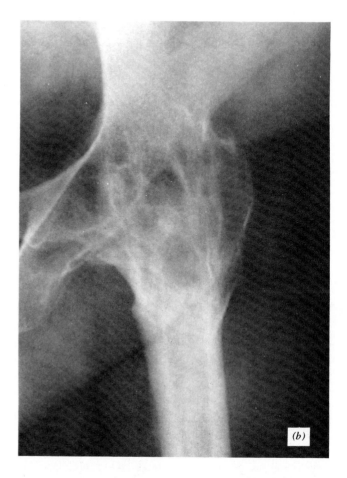

Figure 16-1. Infected hip treated with a spica cast, leading to intra-articular fusion. In late childhood, this woman had pus draining from her left hip and was treated for two years in a spica cast, resulting in fusion of the hip. She did well until age 36, at which time back pain occurred. A femoral osteotomy was done to improve the position of the femoral shaft. (*a*) At an 18-year follow-up of the osteotomy, the patient was doing well, with no complaints related to the hip, but was disturbed because her left leg was four inches shorter than her right. (*b*) A close-up view demonstrates the site of the subtrochanteric osteotomy.

spica cast for approximately seven weeks following surgery. Partial weight bearing is then permitted.

Complications of Intra-Articular Fusions
All of the above methods of intra-articular fusion have similar complications. Delayed union and nonunion may occur. Fibrous union is usually asymptomatic. Where hip nails are used, the nail may break or the bone may fracture at the site of penetration of the nail through the lateral femoral cortex (12).

Variations of the Intra-Articular Fusion—Charnley's Modification
Charnley devised a variation of the intra-articular fusion to provide increased stability of the hip. In his procedure,

the medial wall of the acetabulum is removed to permit central dislocation of the femoral head. This is transfixed with a single screw and gives a high degree of union. Stress fractures of the femoral neck, however, occur in about 5% of these patient (5,13,14).

Barmada (2) describes two similar fusion procedures; in one, a Charnley-type central femoral head dislocation is combined with an extra-articular plate. In the other, a transverse osteotomy of the innominate bone is performed with medial displacement of the acetabulum (similar to the Chiari osteotomy described in Chapter 4). A compression plate is then used to hold the position of the bone fragments. Because of the improved stabilization, patients are permitted to ambulate with crutches after the second week. In a series of 16 patients, 100% fused.

from the ilium. Bone graft for the ischiofemoral arthrodesis can be obtained either from the tibia or from the iliac crest. The performance of either of these arthrodeses involves the debriding of a broad, raw, bony surface where the graft will be placed. In one popular

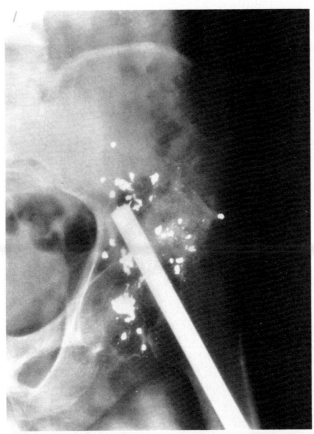

Figure 16-2. A long Smith-Petersen nail has been used for an intra-articular fusion of this hip. Many metal fragments are present, but the exact nature of the original injury is uncertain.

Extra-Articular Fusions

Extra-articular fusions are of two kinds. The first is an iliofemoral fusion (Figure 16-3), superior to the hip joint; the second is an ischiofemoral fusion (Figure 16-4a,b), inferior to the hip joint. Both of these methods have a good success rate. When these extra-articular procedures are performed for intra-articular inflammatory disease (for example, tuberculosis or septic arthritis), the rate of healing is better than that obtained in intra-articular fusion (9); and often, when the extra-articular fusion has healed, intra-articular fusion proceeds spontaneously (6). The bone graft for iliofemoral arthrodesis is usually obtained

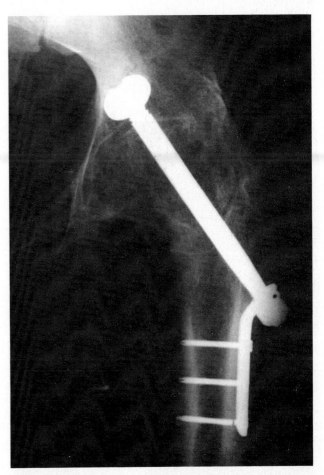

Figure 16-3. Iliofemoral fusion associated with a bolt placed across the hip joint. As a teenager, this 31-year-old man had hip drainage (possibly caused by TB). Because of increasing hip pain, a McMurray osteotomy was performed when the patient was 29. Dense adhesions were present, and a progressive loss of motion recurred following the osteotomy. This was associated with pain, and the hip was fused when the patient was 31. Iliofemoral extra-articular bone graft lies superolateral to the acetabulum. A bolt has been placed across the undebrided hip joint.

method, the Brittain procedure, osteotomies are cut through both the subtrochanteric portion of the femur and the ischium, with bone graft placed between. The osteotomies provide a broad surface for healing. The Brittain arthrodesis is often coupled with medial displacement of the proximal femur (3,4,7).

Although Brittain did not realize the value of the subtrochanteric osteotomy at the time he initially reported his procedure, many authors have subsequently discussed the value of this subtrochanteric osteotomy in promoting fusion, no matter which method of joint fusion is used (1,4,11,15,17). The major impediment to healing of a fusion is continued motion at the joint. A great deal of stress is placed on a fused hip joint. The lever arm of the femur produces a force magnification of approximately 25 to 1 if the knee is flexed and approximately 50 to 1 if the knee is straight (17); thus minimal force on the distal femur exerts great force across the attempted fusion. The subtrochanteric osteotomy prevents these forces from being transmitted to the head of the femur, thus permitting fu-

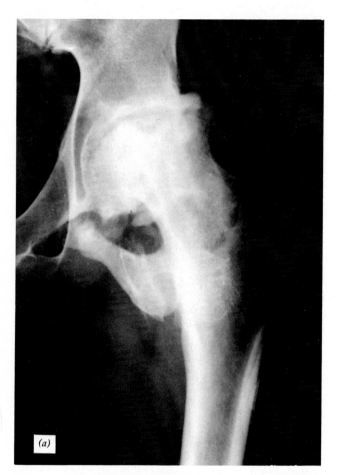
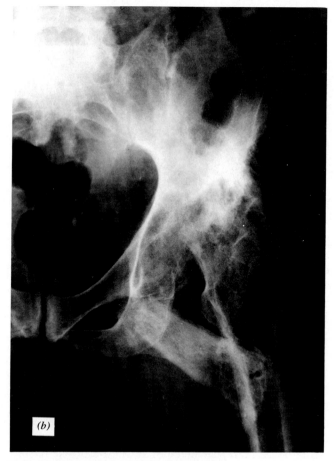

Figure 16-4. Ischiofemoral, extra-articular fusion. Two different patterns. Bone graft has been placed from the ischium to the femur, near the lesser trochanter. (*a,b*) Severe degenerative arthrosis of the hip is present. This patient has combined ischiofemoral and intra-articular fusion.

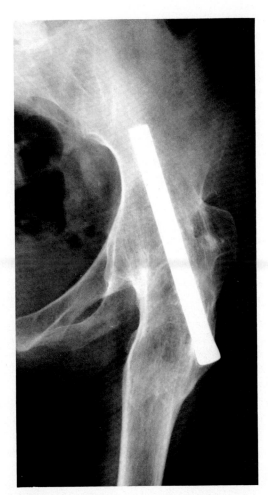

Figure 16-5. An intra-articular fusion held with a Smith-Petersen nail. The site of the subtrochanteric osteotomy can be identified.

sion of the proximal fragment. Because of differences in bony structure and blood supply, subtrochanteric osteotomies essentially always heal, and thus the subtrochanteric osteotomy, initially used by Brittain, greatly increases the chance of obtaining a firm union at the hip with any fusion procedure (Figure 16-5). An additional advantage of the subtrochanteric osteotomy is that it permits a delayed positioning of the distal femoral fragment, simplifying and shortening the initial surgery (15) (See Figure 16-1.)

Complications of Extra-Articular Fusions

The bone grafts used in the extra-articular arthrodesis will occasionally fracture or resorb. These changes may appear in follow-up radiographs of the hip fusion (4). Fractures may occur in the tibia at the bone graft donor site (9). Hip fusion in children often results in leg length discrepancy. Epiphyseal plate fusion in the distal femur and proximal tibia may occur spontaneously following proximal leg surgery, resulting in severe leg length discrepany (8).

Appearance of the Hip at Long-Term Follow-up

Following hip arthrodesis, progressive hypertrophy of both the bone graft and the femur may occur because of the additional stress placed on the painfree leg. Fibrous unions can occur but are usually painless and of no consequence. One should always watch for the development of delayed stress fractures, as these may occur a long time after the original surgery.

Spinal Changes Associated With Hip Fusion

There is a great deal of disagreement in the orthopedic literature as to whether there is any increased incidence of degenerative spondylosis following hip fusion. Although this condition is common in patients with hip fusion, in several studies where the incidence of degenerative spondylosis has been compared in patients with and without hip fusions, who are otherwise matched for age, no difference in the appearance between the two groups was reported. Indeed, Watson-Jones (18) reports on a series of patients in whom back pain was relieved by the improved position achieved by hip fusion compared to the abnormal preoperative positioning, which had resulted in scoliosis and marked lordosis.

SUMMARY

Hip fusion is an effective approach to the management of unilateral hip disease. It is particularly helpful in the treatment of the infected hip but can also be used for other hip disease. It may be the best procedure to provide a stable, painless, strong, and reliable hip.

Hip fusions may be intra-articular, extra-articular, or a combination of the two. The extra-articular arthrodesis may be either iliofemoral or ischiofemoral. Intra- or extra-articular arthrodeses may be coupled with subtrochanteric osteotomy to improve the chance of fusion and to improve the eventual position.

REFERENCES

1. Apley AG, Denham RA: Osteotomy as an aid to arthrodesis of the hip. *J Bone Joint Surg* 37B:185–190, 1955.
2. Barmada R, Abraham E, Ray RD: Hip fusion utilizing the cobra head plate. *J Bone Joint Surg* 58A:541–544, 1976.
3. Brittain HA: Ischio-femoral arthrodesis. *J Bone Joint Surg* 30B:642–650, 1948.
4. Chan KP, Shin JS: Brittain ischio-femoral arthrodesis for tuberculosis of the hip. *J Bone Joint Surg* 50A:1341–1352, 1968.
5. Charnley J: Stabilization of the hip by central dislocation, abstracted. *J Bone Joint Surg* 37B:514–515, 1955.
6. Dobson J: Arthrodesis in tuberculosis of the hip joint. *J Bone Joint Surg* 30B:95–105, 1948.
7. Foley WB: Ischio-femoral arthrodesis of the hip by posterior open approach. *J Bone Joint Surg* 31B:222–226, 1949.
8. Gill GG: The cause of discrepancy in length of the limbs following tuberculosis of the hip in children. *J Bone Joint Surg* 26:272–281, 1944.
9. Hahn D: Ischio-femoral arthrodesis for tuberculosis of the hip. *J Bone Joint Surg* 45B:477–482, 1963.
10. Howard RC: V-arthrodesis of the hip, abstracted. *J Bone Joint Surg* 32B:282, 1950.
11. Kirkaldy-Willis WH: Ischio-femoral arthrodesis of the hip in tuberculosis. *J Bone Joint Surg* 32B:187–192, 1950.
12. Lam SJS: Arthrodesis of the hip. *J Bone Joint Surg* 50B:14–23, 1968.
13. Morris JB: Charnley compression arthrodesis of the hip. *J Bone Joint Surg* 48B:260–279, 1966.
14. Piggot J: Charnley stabilization of the hip. *J Bone Joint Surg* 42B:476–479, 1960.
15. Sharp N, Guhl J, Sorenson R, Voshell A: Hip fusion in poliomyelitis in children. *J Bone Joint Surg* 46A:121–133, 1964.
16. Somerville EW: Two-nail fixation of the hip. *J Bone Joint Surg* 51B:648–653, 1969.
17. Thompson FR: Combined hip fusion and subtrochanteric osteotomy allowing early ambulation. *J Bone Joint Surg* 38A:13–22, 1956.
18. Watson-Jones R: Nail arthrodesis for unilateral osteoarthritis of the hip joint in discussion on treatment of unilateral osteoarthritis of the hip-joint. *Proc R Soc Med* 38:363–366, 1945.

17
Tracer Imaging and Computed Tomography in Disease of the Hip

The plain radiograph and the arthrogram are the traditional and standard methods for evaluation of the hip and its diseases. Tracer imaging techniques using Gallium citrate Ga 67 and technetium phosphate Tc 99m complexes are useful in selected patients. Computed tomography has, at present, only a limited role in the evaluation of hip disease. This chapter will briefly discuss these additional imagining techniques.

TRACER IMAGING TECHNIQUES

Selected radioactive agents may be of use in the imaging of portions of the skeleton. Of the available compounds, phosphate complexes of technetium Tc 99m are the agents most widely used. These agents localize to bone; the degree of accumulation is proportional to regional blood flow and to the degree of extraction of the agent from the blood. Extraction is increased in regions of recent or current bone deposition (9).

Gallium citrate Ga 67 accumulates in regions of inflamation. Four mechanisms are involved in this localization. On injection, gallium Ga 67 binds to transferrin. In regions of inflamation, plasma (including transferrin) can leak into the tissues. Gallium Ga 67 also localizes in the leukocytes that are attracted to regions of inflamation. Increases in

local vascularity and a possible accumulation of gallium Ga 67 in bacteria are additional causes for focal accumulation (9,15).

These two radioactive agents, sometimes used together, may be useful in the determination of hip disease. They are most often used for the evaluation of Legg-Perthes disease and the painful total hip prosthesis.

Legg-Perthes Disease

Tracer imaging techniques may be used in the diagnosis and follow-up of patients with Legg-Perthes disease (6,14). Early in the course of the disease, imaging with technetium phosphate Tc 99m complexes may show decreased tracer uptake in a portion of the femoral head epiphysis. This decreased activity may be detected before the development of radiographic abnormalities. When the radiograph is abnormal, the tracer image may help to demonstrate the full extent of the ischemia, which may have some prognostic value. When the femoral head epiphysis enters the phase of reconstitution, increased activity develops in the epiphysis and adjacent metaphysis (6).

In the child with suspected Legg-Perthes disease whose radiographs are normal, tracer imagining may make an early diagnosis possible. Although the author knows of no cases of early Legg-Perthes disease that showed a normal tracer image, it is a good idea to follow the cases of these children to be sure the diagnosis was not missed.

Avascular Necrosis

Tracer imaging techniques are useful in the early diagnosis of avascular necrosis of the femoral head and in differentiating between degenerative arthritis and avascular necrosis with degenerative arthritis. The disease may be diagnosed prior to radiographic changes. Early in the course of the disease, activity is decreased (9), while later in the course of the disease, activity in the femoral head is increased (2,5,9).

Septic Arthritis

Imaging with gallium citrate Ga 67 may be useful in the evaluation of possible septic arthritis. In the normal hip, gallium citrate Ga 67 will permit the identification of the bone ends and joint space. In the patient with septic arthritis, gallium citrate Ga 67 can accumulate in the synovium, making it impossible to see the joint space (9).

Total Hip Replacement Prosthesis

Following placement of a total hip prosthesis and the use of a technetium Tc 99m tracer, increased radioactivity can be detected at the surgical site. This activity decreases over a period of three to nine months (3,4,7). The presence of increasing radioactivity in that period or the persistence of radioactivity beyond it is abnormal.

Three processes can result in abnormal increased technetium Tc 99m activity: heterotopic bone formation, loosening, and infection. In heterotopic bone formation, the increased activity is usually located lateral and superior to the greater trochanter (1,11); with loosening of the femoral component, increased radioactivity is usually seen near the distal tip of the prosthesis, corresponding to the location where increased intramedulary bone might be

seen radiographically (8) (Figure 17-1a,b). When a loose prosthesis is involved, increased technetium Tc 99m activity may be present in other periprosthetic sites (7,8). When infection is present, sharp increase in the activity of this tracer can be detected (1,3,4) (Figure 17-1c). Gallium citrate Ga 67 activity may also be increased in regions of infection. The sequential use of both agents can show that the increased activity seen with technetium phosphate Tc 99m is due to inflamation probably secondary to infection (9).

Comparisons of standard radiographic and arthrographic techniques with the results of tracer imaging studies are limited; in the one available comparative study (8), in the diagnosis of loose prostheses, the plain radiograph was accurate in 70% of the cases, the tracer study in 85%, and the arthrogram in 94%.

In the patient with unexplained pain following total hip replacement, tracer imaging studies provide valuable data when the radiograph is normal or equivocal. When the radiograph is suggestive or positive for loosening or infection, arthrography with bacteriologic culture of any fluid obtained is preferable.

COMPUTED TOMOGRAPHY IN DISEASE OF THE HIP

Computed tomography has limited uses in the patient with disease of the hip. The tomography permits the imaging of transverse sections through the body and can demonstrate details of the bony- and soft-tissue anatomy of the pelvis and upper femurs (13). It can also be used to evaluate the bony integrity of the pelvis; femoral anteversion can be measured directly because of the transverse image, and major muscle groups can be visualized and their size determined.

The major limitations of computed tomography are the relatively high radiation dose (10), which usually restricts its use in children to those with neoplastic disease and the image distortion and reverberation that occurs when a metal object is in the imaged section.

Detailed transverse imaging of the pelvis permits the demonstration of alterations of normal anatomy and the delination of the extent of lytic metastatic disease involving

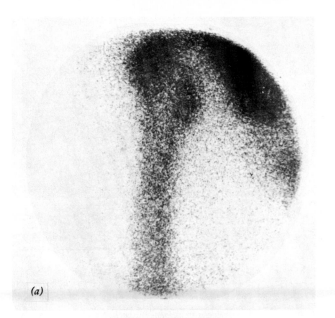

(a)

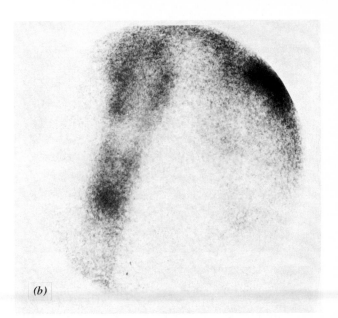

(b)

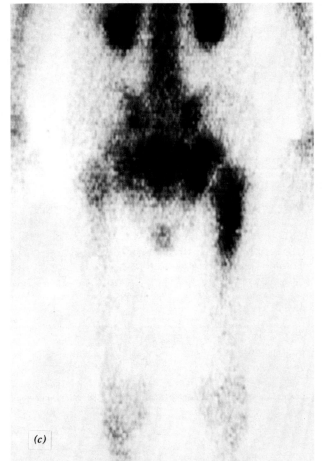

(c)

Figure 17-1. Tracer imaging in patients with total hip prothesis using technetium phosphate TC 99m complexes. (Courtesy Robert Katz, M.D.) (*a*) Normal total hip prothesis. There is decreased tracer activity in the region of the methacrylate. Increased radioactivity near the lesser trochanter is normal. Tracer activity near the greater trochanter is due to a healing trochanteric osteotomy. (*b*) A loose femoral component of a total hip prothesis. Increased radioactivity is present near the tip of the femoral component. The plain radiograph and arthrogram were also positive in the patient. The loosening of the component was proven surgically. (*c*) Osteomyelitis of the femur surrounding a total hip prothesis femoral component. The plain radiograph and the arthrogram were also positive in the patient. The osteomyelitis was proven surgically.

the pelvis (12,13). This information gathered from these observations could be used for planning the radiation field or surgical approach for treatment.

Femoral anteversion can be altered in patients with congenital displacement of the hip and in patients with neurologic disease affecting the hip. Computed tomography might be used to measure the degree of femoral anteversion directly by imaging the femoral neck with the femur in a standard position—the patella pointing at the ceiling (Figure 17-2*a*).

Computed tomography can also show the size of the major muscle groups of the hip—the iliacus, the psoas,

301

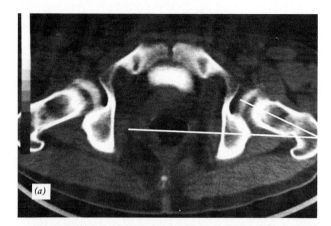

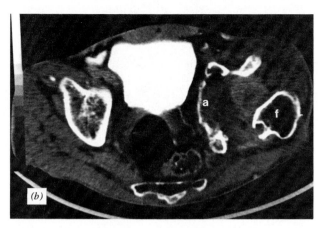

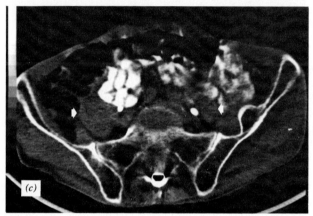

Figure 17-2. Computed tomographic sections (American Science and Engineering scanner). (Courtesy Stanley S. Siegelman, M.D.) Transverse section through the femoral neck. the femur is positioned so that the patella is pointing up. Femoral anteversions can be measured directly. (*b,c*) Transverse sections through the pelvis of a patient with a healed central acetabular fracture and Girdlestone arthroplasty. The medial displacement of the left acetabular wall (a) and superior displacement of the proximal femur (f) can be identified. The psoas muscle on the side of the fracture is smaller than on the normal side (arrows).

and the glutei (Figure 17-2*b,c*). In certain hip diseases these muscles may be smaller than normal. In patients with tumor, tumor invasion of these muscles can be demonstrated (13). Abscesses in these muscles can also be identified.

SUMMARY

Although the precise role of tracer imaging and computed tomographic techniques has not yet been defined, each of these two techniques can be of use in selected patients, and it is by their use that a precise role for these studies may be defined.

REFERENCES

1. Bauer CH, Lindberg L, Naversten Y, Sjostrand LO: ^{85}Sr radio-nuclide scintimetry in infected total hip arthroplasty. *Acta Orthop Scand* 44:439–450, 1973.

2. Cameron RB: Strontium 85 scintimetry in nontraumatic necrosis of the femoral head. *Clin Orthop* 65:243–261, 1969.

3. Campeau RJ, Hall MF, Miale A Jr: Detection of total hip arthroplasty complications with Tc 99m pyrophosphate, abstract *J Nucl Med* 17:526, 1976.

4. Creutzig H: Bone imaging after total replacement arthroplasty of the hip joint. *Eur J Nucl Med* 1:177–180, 1976.

5. Crutchlow WP: Sr^{85} scintimetry of the hip in osteoarthritis and osteonecrosis. *Amer J Roentgenol* 109:803–812, 1970.

6. Danigelis JA, Fisher RL, Ozonoff MB, Sziklas J: ^{99m}Tc-polyphosphate bone imaging in Legg-Perthes disease. *Radiology* 115:407–413, 1975.

7. Feith R, Sloof TJJH, Kazem I, Rens ThJG van, Nigmegen, Strontium ^{87m}Sr bone scanning for the evaluation of total hip replacement. *J Bone Joint Surg* 58B:79–83, 1976.

8. Gelman MI, Coleman R Edward, Stevens Peter M, and Davey BW: Radiography, radionuclide imaging, and arthrography in the evaluation of total hip and knee replacement. *Radiology* 128:677–682, 1978.

9. Lisbona R, Rosenthall L: An update on radionuclide imaging in benign bone disorders, review article. *J Can Assoc Radiologists* 29:188–192, 1978.

10. McCullough EC, Payne J: Patient dosage in computed tomography *Radiology* 129:457–463, 1978.

11. Mall J, Hoffer P, Murray, W, Rodrigo J, Anger H, Samuel A: Heterotopic bone, a potential source of error in evaluating hip prosthesis by radionuclide techniques. *J Nucl Med* 18:604, 1977.

12. Naidich DP, Freedman MT, Bowerman JW, Siegelman SS: Computerized tomography in the evaluation of the soft tissue component of bony lesions of the pelvis. *Skeletal Radiol* 3:144–148, 1978.

13. Naidich DP, Freedman MT, Bowerman JW, Siegelman SS: The ten section approach to computed tomography of the pelvis. Exhibit, annual meeting of the Radiologic Society of North America, December, 1978.

14. Paul DJ, Gilday DL, Gurd A, Bobechko W: A better method of imaging the abnormal hip. *Radiology* 113:466–467, 1974.

15. Staab, EV, McCartney WH: Role of gallium 67 in inflammatory disease. *Semin Nucl Med* 3:219–234, 1978.

Postscript

The hip and its diseases are complex, and this complexity has led to the development of many different and competing procedures. No one current procedure can be considered totally successful or applicable to all patients. While the search for new procedures continues, older techniques are reevaluated and some are restored to use. It is likely that many of the procedures discussed in this book will continue to be utilized in selected patients, and a knowledge of them and their radiographic patterns will continue to be important. Though new procedures will be devised, most will continue to show the same patterns of change as the body responds to the surgery. Details may change, but the general radiographic patterns of success and failure will continue.

Index

Abduction, 62, 64
  sustained, 65, 67
Absorption, Legg-Perthes disease, 89, 91, 92
Acetabular angles, 61-62
Acetabular bone penetration, 253, 257-258
Acetabular position, *see* Total hip replacement
Acetabular profusion, 152, 157
Acetabular replacement, 2, 3, 7
Acetabular sclerosis, *see* Sclerosis
Acetabuloplasty, 70-72
  Pemberton, 71, 72
Active tenodesis, 82
Acute cartilage necrosis, 115
Adduction, contracture, 64
Adduction deformity, 212, 213. *See also* Osteotomy
Adduction tenotomy, 64, 79, 83
Adult, hip surgery in, *see* Hip surgery, adult
Anatomic reduction, 185, 190
  in external rotation stress, 191
Andren Von Rosen view, 60, 61
Angulation of bone, 4, 5, 6, 8
  osteotomies, 291
Anterior opening of acetabular component, 232, 236
Appliance:
  orthopedic, 4-7
  principles, 9-10
  radiologic evaluation, 29-45
  response of bone to:
    adult, 29, 31, 32, 33, 34
    child, 29, 30, 31, 32, 33, 34
    radiolucency, bone resorption, 29-31, 35, 36, 37
      line around radiopaque methylmethacrylate, 31-32, 41, 42
      shift in bone fragments, 30-31, 38, 39
    see also Methylmethacrylate
  See also entries under individual appliances; Femoral neck
      fractures; and Intertrochanteric fractures
Arthritis of hip:
  degenerative, 156, 160, 224
  secondary, 141, 143
  See also Cup mold arthroplasty; Girdlestone arthroplasty: Hip

fusion; and Intertrochanteric osteotomies, degenerative
    arthrosis
Arthrodesis, 4. *See also* Hip fusion
Arthroplasty:
  Colonna capsular, 71, 73
  definition, 4
  see also Cup mold arthroplasty; Femoral head replacements; and
    Total hip replacement
Arthrosis, *see* Intertrochanteric osteotomies, degenerative arthrosis
Aseptic loosening, 380
Aseptic necrosis, 105, 108
Austin-Moore prosthesis, 45, 49, 51, 245, 248
  femoral head replacement, 152, 154, 156, 159-160, 161, 166, 219
    breakage, 168
    description, 144, 149
    in methylmethacrylate, 145, 150
    placed in cup arthroplasty, 169, 170
    replacing Jewett, 145, 150
    size, 145-147
  femoral neck fracture, 32, 34
  long stem, 284
  prosthetic replacement of diseased bone, 204, 205
  see also Femoral head replacements
Avascular necrosis, 20, 115, 165, 225
  predispose to degenerative arthritis, 156, 160
  use of tracer imaging, 300
  see also Femoral neck fractures

Barlow's test, 59
Barmada, R., 294
Barr bolt, 14
Batchelor plate, 76
Bilateral cup mold arthroplasty, 218, 220
Blade plates, 6, 20
  splines, 20
Bolts, 5, 14
  lag, 5, 15
Bone density, increased, 151, 154
Bone resorption, 29-31, 35
  infection as cause, 30, 36, 37

motion between bone and appliance as cause, 30, 35
Brittain procedure, 296, 297
"Broomstick plaster," 89, 103
Brotherton, B. J., 98
Buttress plate, 189

Capital femoral epiphysis, slipped, *see* Slipped capital femoral
        epiphysis
Cartilage necrosis in femoral head replacement, 156, 160, 166
Caterall, A., 93, 98
    criteria, 99-100, 101
Caterall's groups, 93, 98
Catto, Mary, 125, 133
Center-edge angle, Wiberg's, 99, 100
Cerebral palsy, *see* Neurogenic dysfunction of hip, surgery in
Charnley, John, 227
Charnley-Muller prosthesis, 147
    acetabulum opening, 47
    description, 44
    loosening, 48, 50, 53
    radiopaque methylmethacrylate, 27, 28, 43
    straight stem, 211, 212
    in total hip replacement, 230, 233
        anterior and lateral opening of acetabulum, 232, 236, 242,
                243-244, 245
        for avascular necrosis, 255
        description, 227-228
        infection, 280, 282-283
        intraoperative fracture, 259, 260
        long neck, 253, 257-258, 276, 277
        loosening, 271
        maximum stress areas, 237
        in osteoporatic bone, 264-265
        protrusion of femoral component, 250
        radiolucent methylmethacrylate, 272, 274, 276
        radiopaque methylmethacrylate, 231
        settling, 239
        standard, 252
        straight stem, 249, 252, 253
        untreated dislocation, 248
    variants, 24, 25
Charnley prosthesis, 227, 230, 242
Charnley's modification, intra-articular fusion, 294
Chiari osteotomy, 7
    cerebral palsy, 85, 86, 87
    description, 71, 74
Childhood, hip surgery in, *see* Hip surgery, childhood
Closing-wedge osteotomy, 4, 5, 6
Colonna capsular arthroplasty: 71, 73
Comminuted acetabular fracture, 13
Comminuted intertrochanteric fracture, 183, 187, 191, 195, 196-197
    prosthetic replacement, 175
Compression screw, 129, 135
    in intertrochanteric fractures, 174, 177
    Richard-type, 31

Computed tomography, 300-302
Congenital displacement of hip:
    arthrography, 62, 63
    displaced femoral head, 59
    treatment:
        0-18 months, 62, 64, 65, 66
        persisting to 18 months to 3 years, 64, 66-70
        age 3 and up, 70-74, 85
        from late childhood into adulthood, 72-77
    see also Neurogenic dysfunction of hip, surgery in
Cortex, penetration of, 249-255
Cruess, R. L., 279
Cups, 7, 22. *See also* Cup mold arthroplasty
Cup mold arthroplasty, 4, 7, 8, 15, 22, 258
    Austin-Moore prosthesis in, 169, 170
    bilateral, 218, 219
    complications:
        fracture, 225
        infection, 225-226
        secondary degenerative arthrosis, 221-223, 224
        subluxation and dislocation, 221
    failure, 260
    heteroptic bone formation, 225
    Pyrex cup mold, 218, 219
    radiographic appearances, 220
    shaft cup mold arthroplasty, 219, 220

Debridement, 280, 293-294
Degenerative arthritis, 156, 160, 224
    secondary, 141, 143
Degenerative arthrosis, 20, 160, 161, 258, 259
    Girdlestone arthroplasty, 291
    secondary, 221, 291
    see also Intertrochanteric osteotomies, degenerative arthrosis
Degenerative cysts, 211, 213, 221
    acetabular, 141, 143, 159, 163, 221
Delayed union and nonunion, 137-138, 140, 143
    in degenerative arthrosis, 215
    in intra-articular fusion, 294
Deyerle apparatus, 129, 134, 183, 185, 188
Dislocation, 221, 232
    complications of hip surgery, 46, 51
    in femoral head prosthesis, 156
    neonatal disease, 59
    recognition, 242, 245-249
    total hip replacement, 240-242, 244-245
    see also Congenital displacement of hip; Neurogenic dysfunction
            in hip, surgery in; *and* Subluxation
Displacement of hip, congenital, *see* Congenital displacement of hip
Distal fragment, appliance fixation, 177-178, 187
    medial displacement, 187-189, 192, 193
Dunn, H. K., 262

Ectopic bone, 271
    in Charnley prosthesis, 230

in femoral neck fracture, 131
   as manifestation of infection, 54, 55, 56
   secondary degenerative arthrosis, 221
   see also Heteroptic bone
Enders nail, 175, 177, 179
Epiphysis:
   location, 60-61
   resorption in Legg-Perthes disease, 89, 90-91, 92, 93, 97, 98, 99
   see also Slipped capital femoral epiphysis
Eternal rotation forces, 191, 198-199, 200
Extra-articular fusion, 4. *See also* Hip fusion

Femoral component, drill hole near, 236-237
   total hip replacement, 233, 236
Femoral head replacements, 33
   acetabular protrusion, 152, 157
   appliance, 6, 21
   arthroplasty, 4, 9, 15
   cartilage necrosis, 156, 160, 166
   degenerative arthritis, 156, 160
   dislocation, 156
   fractures, 153-154, 159
   heteroptic bone formation, 167-168
   increased bone density, 151-152, 154
   infection, 166-167
   Judet prosthesis, 145, 146, 148, 149
   limp, 155-156
   loosening, 156-157, 159, 161, 162, 163-164, 165-166
   periostitis, 150-151
   prosthesis sinking into femoral shaft, 152
   radiolucency zone around prosthesis, 152, 156
   resorption of medial femoral neck, 152
   Thompson prosthesis, 150, 152
      in methylmethacrylate, 147
         replaced, 153
         settling, 162
   see also Austin-Moore prosthesis; Femoral neck fractures
Femoral neck fractures, 12, 17, 18
   appliances, 129, 132, 134, 135, 136
      placement, 132, 138, 139
   avascular necrosis, 125, 126-127, 128, 133, 135, 137, 140, 141
   in delayed union and nonunion, 125, 128, 137-138, 140, 141, 143
   in fixation methods, 129
      penetration into acetabulum, 138
   in proper reduction, 123-125
   in varus malreduction, 139
Femoral neck resorption, 51, 53, 237, 238
Fibroblasts, 238
Fixation methods, *see* Femoral neck fractures
Fracture:
   intraoperative and stress, 255, 258-261
   treatment, 3
   see also Femoral head replacement; Femoral neck fractures; Intertrochanterif fractures; *and* Metastases, fracture through
Frejka pillow, 64, 65

Gage's sign, 93, 96, 97, 98
Gallium citrate Ga 67, 299. *See also* Tracer imaging techniques
Garden, R. S., 123, 125, 128
Girdlestone, F. R., 289
Girdlestone arthroplasty, 74, 76, 262, 265, 281, 283, 289-291
   description, 289-291
   modifications, 291
Glutei muscles, 80, 81
   functioning and stability of hip, 48, 50, 51
   gluteus medius, 261
Granulation tissue, 167, 168, 224
Granulomatous reaction, to total hip replacement, 277, 278-279, 280
Greater trochanter:
   fracture, 155, 159
   total hip replacement, 261-263
      problems, 264-265

Harrington, K., 191
Harris, William, 277
Harris prosthesis, 9, 41, 221, 223, 227-228, 233
Hess, W. E., 262
Heteroptic bone:
   cup mold arthroplasty, 225
   femoral head replacement, 166, 167-168
   see also Ectopic bone
High intertrochanteric fracture, 185, 189
Hip arthrodesis, 201. *See also* Intertrochanteric osteotomies, degenerative arthrosis
Hip fusion, 293-294
   extra-articular fusion, 4, 10, 295-297
   hip appearance, 297
   intra-articular fusion, 293-295
   spinal changes, 297
Hip nails, *see* Nails
Hip replacement, *see* Total hip replacement
Hip surgery, adult, *see* Cup mold arthroplasty; Femoral head replacements; Femoral neck fractures; Girdlestone arthroplasty; Hip fusion; Intertrochanteric fractures; Intertrochanteric osteotomies, degenerative arthrosis; Metastases, fracture through; *and* Total hip replacement
   childhood, 119. *See also* Congenital displacement of hip; Legg-Perthes disease; Neurogenic dysfunction of hip; surgery in; *and* Slipped capital femoral epiphysis
Hip surgery:
   complications, 46-55
   effect on appearance of prior, 36
   periosteal reaction, 44, 45
   see also headings under individual complications
Holt nail, 14, 174, 176, 177-178, 182
Hourglass deformity, 61, 63
Hypertrophy, bone, 240

Iliofemoral fusion, 295, 296
Iliopsoas muscle, 80, 81, 82, 187
   functioning and stability of hip, 48, 50-51

Impacting force, *see* Intertrochanteric fractures
Infection:
   complications of hip surgery, 53-54, 54-56
   cup mold arthroplasty, 225-226
   femoral head replacement, 166-167
   femoral neck fracture, 139-143
   periprosthetic, 623
   total hip replacement, 277, 279-281, 282-285
   see also Ectopic bone
Instability, Barlow's test, 59. *See also* Congenital displacement of
      hip
Interference fit, 7
Intertrochanteric fractures, 153-154
   appliance fixation, 176-181, 187
   appliances, 172
      compression screw, 174, 177
      Enders nail, 175, 177, 179
      failure, 182, 186
      Holt nail, 174, 176, 177-178, 182, 183
      Jewett nail, 174, 175, 182, 183, 187, 188, 190, 199
      prosthetic replacement of comminuted, 175
      Smith-Peterson nail, 174
      Zickel nail, 174-175, 177, 178, 186-189
   comminuted, 191, 193, 195
   external rotation forces, 191, 198-199, 200
      high, 185, 189
      hip nails, 172
      impacted, 173
      impacting forces, 182-185, 189
   medial displacement of distal fragment, 187-189, 192, 193
   shear forces, 181-183, 185, 187
   stability through nonanatomic alignment, 181, 182, 184, 185
   stable reduction, 179, 181
   varus angulation forces, 190-191, 194, 195, 196, 197
Intertrochanteric osteotomies, degenerative arthrosis:
   complications, 213, 215
   conversion to total hip replacement, 215
   description, 209, 212
   McMurray medial displacement osteotomy, 209, 210-211, 213,
      214-215
   positioning of fragments, 212
   radiologic changes, 213
   valgus osteotomy, 212, 215
   see also Total hip replacement
Intertrochanteric osteotomies with medial displacement of distal
      fragment, *see* Medial displacement osteotomy
Intra-articular fusion, 4, 10. *See also* Hip fusion
Intramedullary bone, 29, 33
Intramedullary femoral head prosthesis, 7, 21
Ischemia, *see* Legg-Perthes disease
Ischiofemoral fusion, 295, 296

Jarry, L., 138
Jewett nail, 11, 19, 38
   description, 174, 175

   in intertrochanteric fractures, 182, 183, 187, 188, 190, 191, 199
      replaced by Austin-Moore prosthesis, 168, 169
Joint alignment, complication of hip surgery: 46-48
Joint replacements, 7, 24-26
Judet prosthesis, in femoral head replacement, 145, 146, 148-149
   variant of, 21, 33

Ken nail, description, 129, 133, 142-143
   in fractures of femoral neck, 125, 126-127, 128, 139-140
Knowles pins:
   in fractures of femoral neck, 129, 132
   serrated, 12
   in slipped capital femoral epiphysis, 110, 111, 112-113, 114-115, 117
K wires, 136, 137

Lag bolts, 5, 15
Lag screws, 5, 15
Lamellar periosteal reaction, 281, 284-285
Lateral opening of acetabular component, 232, 236
Laurenson, R. D., 62
Legg-Perthes disease, 30, 272
   bilateral, 102-103, 105, 107
   Catterall's groups, 93, 98
   containing femoral head within acetabulum, 102-105, 108
   decreasing force applied to femoral head, 100, 103
   deformed femoral head treatment, 106, 108
   follow-up period, 98-101
   nature of deformity, 92-93, 94, 95, 104
   prevention, of deformity, 100
   recognition of deformity, 93, 96, 106
   stages, 89, 90-92
   tracer imaging techniques in, 299-300
Limp, from femoral head replacements, 155-156
Loosening:
   complications of hip surgery, 48-53
   septic and aseptic, 280
   see also Femoral head replacements
Loosening in total hip replacement:
   confirming presence of, 271-272, 275-277
   granulomatous reaction, 277, 278-279, 280
   methylmethacrylate in, 263, 267-269, 271, 272-277
   settling of prosthesis, 238, 265, 267-271
   stress films, 272, 273, 275-277
Lytic metastasis, 191, 201

McElfresh, E. C., 258
McKee-Farrar prosthesis, 24, 26, 45
   description, 227, 229
   in total hip replacement, 241
McMurray osteotomy, *see* Medial displacement osteotomy
McMurray, T. P., 213
Massie nails, 129, 133
Massie, W. K., 123, 139
Medial displacement, 196, 197
   impaction, 181, 185, 190

Medial displacement osteotomy, 44, 191
  description, 4, 7, 20
  McMurray osteotomy, 214-215, 249, 251, 252, 253, 255
    description, 213
  see also Chiari osteotomy
Meningomyelocele patients, see Myelomeningocele patients
Metabolic disturbances, in slipped capital femoral epiphysis, 113
Metastases, fracture through, 201-202
  lytic, 191, 201
  methylmethacrylate in, 203, 205
  prosthetic replacement of diseased bone, 204, 205
  subtrochanteric fractures, 202-203, 205
  Zickel nail, 202-203, 205
Methacrylate, see Methylmethacrylate
Methylmethacrylate:
  in Austin-Moore prosthesis, 145, 150
  change in bone elasticity, 34-35, 42
  in Charnley-Muller total hip prosthesis, 28
  description, 7-9, 233-234
  to replace diseased bone, 203, 205
  in Thompson prosthesis, 147
  in total hip replacement, 277
    abnormal location, 281-282, 286
    appearance of normal reaction of bone to, 229, 230, 231, 233,
      234-236, 240, 241
    in loosening, 263, 265, 268-269
    position, 234, 237, 238, 239, 281-282, 286
  see also Appliance, response of bone to; Radiolucent
    methylmethacrylate; and Radiopaque methylmethacrylate
Milch osteotomy, 76, 291
Moore prosthesis, 154
  long stem, 154, 159
  see also Austin-Moore prosthesis
Mose sphericity gauge, 98, 99
Muller prosthesis, 21, 153
Multicomponent prosthesis, 228, 235
Murray, 272
Mustard procedures, 81-82
Mustard, W. T., 81
Myelodysplastic child, 81
Myelomeningocele patients, 79-85. See also Neurogenic dysfunction
  of hip, surgery in
Myositis ossificans bone, see Ectopic bone; Heteroptic bone

Nails, 6, 16
  hip, 172
  Smith-Petersen, 17
  see also Jewett nail; Ken nail; and Side plates
Neurogenic dysfunction of hip, surgery in:
  cerebral palsy:
    Chiari pelvic osteotomy, 85, 86, 87
    Salter procedure, 83, 85, 86, 87
    varus osteotomy, 86
  Mustard procedures, 81-82
  myelomeningocele patients:

    L1-L2 level, 79-81
    L3-L4 level, 81-83, 84, 85
    L5 level, 83
    T-12 level, 79
    poliomyelitis, 83, 85
      shelf procedures, 85
    Sharrard procedures, 81-83, 84, 85
  See also Congenital displacement of hip
Nolan, D. R., 282
Nonanatomic alignment, 188. See also Intertrochanteric fractures
Nonunion, 125, 129, 130, 131, 137, 261

O'Hara, J. P., 98
Olsson, S. S., 213
Opening wedge osteotomy, 4, 8. See also Salter innominate bone
  osteotomy
Open reduction, 110, 111
Orofino, C., 110
Orthopedic procedures, 3-4. See also entries under individual
  procedures
Ortolani test, 59
  hip click, 64, 67
Osteoarthritis, 191
Osteophytes, 159, 163, 211, 212, 213, 215-216, 221
Osteoporotic femur, 132, 138
Osteotomies, 3-8
  intertrochanteric, see Intertrochanteric osteotomies, degenerative
    arthrosis
  see also entries under individual osteotomies

Paget's disease, 147, 151, 152, 157, 253
Pain, unexplained, 55-56
  in total hip replacement, 282, 287
Pauwels, 212
Pemberton acetabuloplasty, 71, 72
Periosteal reaction, 245, 254-255
  following second operation, 36, 44-45
  lamellar, 281, 284-285
  periosteal bone, 29
Periostitis, 150-151
Permeative lytic destruction, hip infection, 54, 55
Perthes disease, see Legg-Perthes disease
Pharm band, 235
Pins, 5, 11
  Knowles, 12
  Steinmann, 11, 12
Poliomyelitis, 83
  shelf procedure, 85
Polymethylmethacrylate, see Methylmethacrylate
Posterior femoral neck comminution, 154, 159
Posterior opening of acetabular component, 233
Press-fit total hip prosthesis, 277, 280
Proper reduction, in femoral neck fracture, 32
Prosthesis breakage, 263, 266-267
Proximal femur, fractures of, see Femoral head replacements;

Femoral neck fractures; Intertrochanteric fractures; *and* Metastases, fracture through

Proximal fragment, appliance fixation, 178-179, 180, 181

Pyrex cup mold, 218, 219

Radiolucent methylmethacrylate:
    in Charnley-Muller prosthesis, 272, 274, 276
    description, 31
    loosening, 51, 263, 265
    zone of radiolucency, 236
        around blade, 29-31
        description, 237-238, 241
        loosening, 156-157
        around prosthesis, 9, 28, 152, 156
        around radiopaque methylmethacrylate, 31-32, 41, 42
        between prosthesis and methylmethacrylate, 33-34
    see also Methylmethacrylate

Radiopaque methylmethacrylate, 231, 235
    in Charnley-Muller prosthesis, 27, 28, 43
    description, 31, 263
    see also Methylmethacrylate

Reconstitution, Legg-Perthes disease, 89, 91, 92

Reduction:
    anatomic, 188
    in avascular necrosis, 125, 126-127
    in fractures, 123-125
    in intertrochanteric fractures, 179, 181
    see also Femoral neck fractures

Reossification, Legg-Perthes disease, 89, 91, 92

Resorption:
    femoral neck, 51, 53, 152
    irregular, 54, 56
    osteoclastic, 51
    see also Bone resorption

Resurfacing prosthesis, 228, 235

Richard-type compression screw, 31

Ring, P. A., 263

Ring prosthesis, 227, 228, 263

Rotational osteotomy, 4, 212
    Russin-Silvash prosthesis, 234

Salter innominate bone osteotomy, 8
    cerebral palsy, 83, 85, 86, 87
    congenital subluxation of hip, 68-69
    description, 64, 66, 67, 70
    Legg-Perthes disease, 103, 105, 108
    Steel's modification, 66

Salter, Robert, 92

Salvage procedures, *see* Girdlestone arthroplasty; Hip fusion

Salvati, E., 145

Salvati series, 272

Schanz angulation osteotomy, 75-77

Sclerosis, 29, 140, 152, 155, 221, 277
    acetabular, 141, 151-152, 166, 221
    Legg-Perthes disease, 89-91

Sclerotic bone, 26, 29, 32, 36, 40, 49

Scout film, 53, 54

Screws, 5, 13
    lag, 5, 15
    Richard-type compression, 31

Septic arthritis, use of tracer imaging techniques, 300

Septic loosening, 280

Shaft cup mold arthroplasty, 219, 220

Shantz osteotomy, 291

Sharrard, W. J. W., 79, 81

Sharrard procedures, 81-83, 84, 85

Shear forces, in intertrochanteric fractures, 181-183, 185, 187

Shelf procedure, 72-75
    poliomyelitis, 85

Shenton's line, 60, 61, 65

Side plates, 6, 16, 18
    Jewett, 19
    see also Nails

Simon, G., 61

Simon's line, 60, 61, 65

Sinography, 281

Slipped capital femoral epiphysis:
    complications and surgery, 115, 117, 118
    description and treatment, 110-113, 114, 115, 116, 117
    metabolic disturbances, 113

Smith, F. B., 125

Smith-Petersen, M. N., 128

Smith-Petersen nail:
    femoral neck fracture, 129, 132, 138
    intra-articular fusion, 293, 295
    to side plate, 174

Snyder, C. R., 98, 108

Spica casting, 64, 293

Spinal changes, hip fusion, 297

Splines, 6, 20

SRN prosthesis, 234

Stability, complications of hip surgery:
    joint alignment, 47, 48
    role of muscle length, 48, 50-51

Staples, 6

Steel's modification, 66

Steinmann pins, 11, 12

Stem femoral head prosthesis, 6, 21

Stress films, evaluating loosening in total hip replacement, 272, 273, 275-277

Stress fractures, source of unexplained pain, 282

Subluxation, 9, 80, 81, 146, 221, 228, 232
    complications of hip surgery, 46, 51
    of femoral component, 243
    neonatal disease, 59
    by radiograph, 67, 68
    see also Dislocation; Neurogenic dysfunction of hip, surgery in

Subtrochanteric fracture, 154, 159, 183, 187
    through metastasis, 202-203, 205
        transverse, 187, 190

Subtrochanteric osteotomy, angulation, 75-77
    in fusion, 294, 296, 297
Surgery, *see* Hip surgery
Sustained abduction, 65, 67

Technetium phosphate Te 99m, 339. *See also* Tracer imaging
    techniques
Tenodesis, 82
Thompson prosthesis, replace diseased bone, 204, 205
    settling, 162
    see also Femoral head replacements
Tomogram, 209, 210-211
Total hip replacement:
    acetabular position, 228-229, 232-233, 236
    common types:
        Charnley prosthesis, 227, 230
        McKee-Farrar prosthesis, 227, 229
        nondislocatable, 228, 234
        multicomponent prosthesis, 228, 235
        resurfacing prosthesis, 228, 235
    conversion from intertrochanteric osteotomy, 215, 217
    development, 227
    femoral component position, 233, 236
    metal-on-metal/or plastic, 7, 24, 25
    normal position, 228
    normal radiographic changes, 236-240
    pathologic changes:
        abnormal locations of methylmethacrylate, 281-282, 286
        dislocation and subluxation, 240-242, 245-249
        greater trochanter problems, 261-263, 264-265
        infection, 277, 279-281, 282-285
        intraoperative stress, 255, 258-261
        penetration of acetabular bone, 253, 257-258
        penetration of cortex, 249-255
        prosthesis breakage, 263, 266-267
        unexplained pain, 282, 287
    tracer imaging techniques, 300
    see also Charnley-Muller prosthesis; Loosening in total hip
        replacement
Trabecular bone, 29, 31, 33, 132, 135, 141, 177, 178, 235

amount in contact with appliance, 181, 182
    nonuniform pattern, 181, 185
    see also Delayed union and nonunion
Tracer imaging techniques, 299-301
Transient synovitis of hip, 89
Transverse fracture, 187, 190
Transverse osteotomy, 209, 213
Transverse subtrochanteric fracture, 187, 190
Trochanteric bursitis, 55, 287
Tronzo, R. G., 262
Tronzo prosthesis, 228, 235
Turner-Aufrane prosthesis, 26, 42, 232

Union, delayed, *see* Delayed union and nonunion
Urist cup, 23

Valgus deformity, 79, 80
Valgus osteotomy, 79-81, 113
    angulation arthroplasty, 75-77
    description, 4, 6, 212, 215
    see also Intertrochanteric fractures
Valgus repositioning, in intertrochanteric fracture, 184, 185
Varus angulation, 209-211
    forces at fracture site, 190-191, 194-195
Varus deformity, progressive, 215
Varus derotational osteotomy, 64, 66, 105, 108
Varus malreduction, 139
Varus osteotomy, 79, 80, 81, 253, 255
    in cerebral palsy, 86
    description, 4, 5, 39, 212
    in Legg-Perthes disease, 93, 97, 102-103, 105
Vitallium wires, 218, 258
Von Rosen splint, 64, 65

Waldenstrom-Calve-Legg-Perthes disease, *see* Legg-Perthes disease
Watson-Jones, R., 297
Wiberg's center-edge angle, 71, 99, 100

Zone of radiolucency, *see* Radiolucent methylmethacrylate